Atlas of Intraoperative Frozen Section Diagnosis in Gynecologic Pathology

Pei Hui · Natalia Buza

Atlas of Intraoperative Frozen Section Diagnosis in Gynecologic Pathology

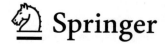 Springer

Pei Hui
Department of Pathology
Yale University School of Medicine
New Haven, CT
USA

Natalia Buza
Department of Pathology
Yale University School of Medicine
New Haven, CT
USA

ISBN 978-3-319-35672-3   ISBN 978-3-319-21807-6 (eBook)
DOI 10.1007/978-3-319-21807-6

Springer Cham Heidelberg New York Dordrecht London
© Springer International Publishing Switzerland 2015
Softcover re-print of the Hardcover 1st edition 2015

Printed on acid-free paper

Springer International Publishing AG Switzerland is part of Springer Science+Business Media (www.springer.com)

To my wife, Ran Wu, with profound gratitude—for her kindness, insight, and support.

Pei Hui

To my wonderful family—Emma, Julia, and Attila—with love.

Natalia Buza

Preface

The conception of this volume originated from the cumulative experience in resolving diagnostic challenges in our daily practice of intraoperative consultation of gynecologic pathology. Gynecologic tumors are among the most frequently encountered frozen section specimens in both academic and community practice settings, yet frozen section evaluation of gynecologic tumors often proves difficult because of the large number of disease entities and their numerous morphological variants. This book reviews the salient clinicopathologic, gross, and microscopic features of gynecologic neoplasms with special focus on indications, limitations, and potential pitfalls of intraoperative frozen section consultation. Strategies to recognize key diagnostic features are emphasized along with discussion of the impact of frozen section diagnosis on the clinical decision-making process at the time of surgery. The book intends to provide detailed practical guidance for intraoperative consultation for pathologists at all career/expertise levels who are involved in frozen section evaluation in their daily clinical practice.

The general classification of lesions in this book follows the 2014 WHO classification of tumors of the female reproductive organs. The format of the book is a concise description of each entity, richly illustrated with high-quality fresh gross and frozen section microscopic images to aid the recognition of morphologic patterns and to serve as a quick reference during the intraoperative consultation. Entities frequently encountered for frozen section evaluation are covered in greater detail and are balanced with less common lesions. It should be emphasized, however, that standard guidelines for the clinical practice of frozen section evaluation are lacking. Trying to provide a uniform approach proves to be difficult, especially since indications for intraoperative frozen section consultation vary significantly among institutions and even among gynecologic oncologists within the same institution.

Without the luxury of ancillary study materials in frozen section diagnosis, we essentially go back to square one as traditional morphologists and rely on the diversity and quality of gross images and frozen section microscopic slides that are available to us. Indeed, this book has taken advantage of the superb collection of gynecologic pathology specimens provided by the outstanding gynecologic oncology service at Yale-New Haven Hospital. We extend our appreciation to Dr. Brian West for his leadership in supporting the Yale Gynecologic Pathology Program. We acknowledge our pathology trainees for their effort in taking high-quality gross images of various gynecologic specimens in the past. Special thanks go to the technical staff in the frozen section diagnostic laboratory at Yale Smilow Cancer Hospital, as the readers will appreciate the quality of microscopic illustrations in this book, all of which were captured from authentic frozen section slides.

New Haven, CT, USA

Pei Hui, MD, PhD
Natalia Buza, MD

Contents

The Purpose of Frozen Section Evaluation in Gynecologic Pathology

The primary function of intraoperative consultation is to provide a tissue evaluation that is as accurate and prompt as possible and to effectively communicate the findings to the operating surgeon to guide subsequent surgical management of the patient [1–4].

To fulfill this function, the intraoperative pathology consultant is expected to provide the following:

- Evaluation of the presence of malignancy
- Assessment of the primary site, histological type, and grade of the tumor
- Assessment of the extent of local tumor invasion and distant metastasis

Less frequently frozen section evaluation is requested to assess tissue sample adequacy to accommodate the following clinical or diagnostic considerations [2]:

- Lesional tissue procurement for drug sensitivity and resistance testing
- Lesional tissue procurement for ancillary diagnostic studies (molecular testing, karyotyping, electron microscopy, etc.)

Considerations to perform frozen section diagnosis may also include:

- Preserving fertility
- Reducing anxiety of the patient and family
- Subsequent risk assessment for disease progression and prognosis
- Financial cost of treatment options

However, there is no standardized practice for surgeons in requesting intraoperative consultation. Indications for frozen section evaluation vary significantly among institutions and even among gynecologic oncologists within the same institution. In principle, a request for intraoperative consultation is acceptable if a tissue sample is submitted with a question for an answer, upon which a real-time clinical decision has to be made for subsequent surgical or medical management of the patient [2, 5]. It is important that the frozen section remains relevant only in the context of broad medical knowledge of the pathologist and judicious utilization by the surgeon, both for the ultimate patient care [6].

Assessment and Sampling of Specimens for Frozen Section Evaluation

Prior to examination of the specimen, careful review of the clinical information and understanding of the clinical expectations for frozen section are crucial for a successful intraoperative consultation. Many specimens are submitted for intraoperative consultation with a specific clinical question, which should guide the initial gross examination to identify the lesion of interest. When the clinical indication is unclear or the orientation of the specimen cannot be determined with certainty, prompt communication with the operating surgeon may be necessary to identify the lesion and to take appropriate tissue sections for frozen section evaluation.

Interpretation of Frozen Section Findings

As a real-time engagement between surgeons and pathologists, frozen section diagnosis frequently offers the most decisive consultation during surgery. Concordance between the frozen and the final histological diagnoses ranges from 96.5 to 98.5 % in the general pathology practice [7–9] with mean and median concordance rates of 96.8 % and 97.4 %, respectively [8]. Common reasons for diagnostic discordance include misinterpretation of the frozen section

P. Hui, N. Buza, *Atlas of Intraoperative Frozen Section Diagnosis in Gynecologic Pathology*,
DOI 10.1007/978-3-319-21807-6_1

(interpretation error), presence of diagnostic tissue only on the permanent section of the frozen tissue block, and diagnostic tissue in the portion of the specimen not sampled by the frozen section (sampling error) [9].

In diagnostic gynecologic pathology, frozen section evaluation is an important tool to assess the local tumor spread and therefore to guide intraoperative decision-making regarding the necessity of lymphadenectomy and/or omentectomy for patients with endometrial cancer. High concordance between the frozen section and final permanent section diagnosis has been consistently reported with concordance rates of 88–89.9 % for tumor grade, 85.4–98.2 % for depth of myometrial invasion, 100 % for cervical involvement, and 92.4 % for lymphovascular invasion [10–12]. In ovarian lesions, the overall accuracy of frozen section diagnosis ranges between 80.7 and 97.1 % for primary [13, 14] and between 78.8 and 90 % for metastatic tumors [15, 16].

Although pathologists should make the best attempt to provide a diagnostic interpretation as precisely and quickly as possible, the frozen section evaluation cannot be thorough in many cases. The inherent limitations of frozen section diagnosis need to be carefully considered and communicated adequately between pathologists and surgeons. Significantly different from routine pathology diagnosis using formalin-fixed paraffin-embedded tissue preparations, frozen section evaluation is limited by suboptimal tissue quality, tissue processing (freezing and cutting) artifacts, often different tissue staining qualities, time restraints, and lack of ancillary study tools. Other significant factors affecting intraoperative consultation include the pathologist's experience, the need of consulting additional pathologist(s)/subspecialty pathologist, involvement of pathology trainees, availability of preoperative diagnostic materials, concurrent multiple frozen sections, and technical issues (e.g., instruments, technical skills of the staff) [17].

Strategies for Successful Intraoperative Consultation

- Understanding the clinical history, reasons for frozen section diagnosis, and surgical management algorithm.
- Requesting and reviewing relevant prior specimens of the patient before the surgery.
- Thorough examination of the gross specimen and appropriate sampling for frozen section evaluation.
- Providing concise frozen section diagnosis followed by effective communication to the surgeon.
- When in doubt, seeking the opinion of experienced colleagues.
- Prompt discussion with the surgeon during frozen section helps resolving a difficult diagnostic interpretation and

unusual or unexpected findings, and requesting additional clinical information when needed.

- The frozen section pathologist should not feel intimidated by an anxious surgeon or pressured by the turn-around time.
- Understanding that the frozen section diagnosis is not intended to replace a comprehensive specimen evaluation. Attaining adequate frozen section diagnosis takes priority over spending more effort in reaching an "ideal" diagnosis by taking additional frozen sections.
- When dealing with small tissue samples, effort should be taken—without compromising the frozen section diagnosis—to preserve diagnostic tissue for permanent, formalin-fixed tissue sections.
- Participation in a frozen section-permanent diagnosis quality assurance program has been associated with sustained improvement in performance by pathologists [18].
- Building a long-term, mutually respectful working relationship between pathologists and surgeons.

References

1. Stout AP. Frozen section diagnosis in surgery. Surg Clin North Am. 1956;335–44.
2. Kindschi GW. Frozen sections. Their use and abuse. JAMA. 1984;251:2559–60.
3. Lechago J. The frozen section: pathology in the trenches. Arch Pathol Lab Med. 2005;129:1529–31.
4. Gal AA, Cagle PT. The 100-year anniversary of the description of the frozen section procedure. JAMA. 2005;294:3135–7.
5. Ackerman LV, Ramirez GA. The indications for and limitations of frozen section diagnosis; a review of 1269 consecutive frozen section diagnoses. Br J Surg. 1959;46:336–50.
6. Taxy JB. Frozen section and the surgical pathologist: a point of view. Arch Pathol Lab Med. 2009;133:1135–8.
7. Novis DA, Gephardt GN, Zarbo RJ. Interinstitutional comparison of frozen section consultation in small hospitals: a College of American Pathologists Q-Probes study of 18,532 frozen section consultation diagnoses in 233 small hospitals. Arch Pathol Lab Med. 1996;120:1087–93.
8. Howanitz PJ, Hoffman GG, Zarbo RJ. The accuracy of frozen-section diagnoses in 34 hospitals. Arch Pathol Lab Med. 1990;114:355–9.
9. Gephardt GN, Zarbo RJ. Interinstitutional comparison of frozen section consultations. A college of American Pathologists Q-Probes study of 90,538 cases in 461 institutions. Arch Pathol Lab Med. 1996;120:804–9.
10. Stephan JM, Hansen J, Samuelson M, McDonald M, Chin Y, Bender D, et al. Intra-operative frozen section results reliably predict final pathology in endometrial cancer. Gynecol Oncol. 2014;133:499–505.
11. Karabagli P, Ugras S, Yilmaz BS, Celik C. The evaluation of reliability and contribution of frozen section pathology to staging endometrioid adenocarcinomas. Arch Gynecol Obstet. 2015;292(2): 391–7.
12. Turan T, Oguz E, Unlubilgin E, Tulunay G, Boran N, Demir OF, Kose MF. Accuracy of frozen-section examination for myometrial invasion and grade in endometrial cancer. Eur J Obstet Gynecol Reprod Biol. 2013;167:90–5.

13. Bige O, Demir A, Saygili U, Gode F, Uslu T, Koyuncuoglu M. Frozen section diagnoses of 578 ovarian tumors made by pathologists with and without expertise on gynecologic pathology. Gynecol Oncol. 2011;123:43–6.

14. Malipatil R, Crasta JA. How accurate is intraoperative frozen section in the diagnosis of ovarian tumors? J Obstet Gynaecol Res. 2013;39:710–3.

15. Stewart CJ, Brennan BA, Hammond IG, Leung YC, McCartney AJ. Accuracy of frozen section in distinguishing primary ovarian neoplasia from tumors metastatic to the ovary. Int J Gynecol Pathol. 2005;24:356–62.

16. Aslam MF, Ghayoori R, Khulpateea N. Adnexal masses: relative accuracy of sonography and frozen section in predicting final pathology. Int J Gynecol Pathol. 2010;30:187–9.

17. Novis DA, Zarbo RJ. Interinstitutional comparison of frozen section turnaround time. A College of American Pathologists Q-Probes study of 32868 frozen sections in 700 hospitals. Arch Pathol Lab Med. 1997;121:559–67.

18. Raab SS, Tworek JA, Souers R, Zarbo RJ. The value of monitoring frozen section-permanent section correlation data over time. Arch Pathol Lab Med. 2006;130:337–42.

Vulva and Vagina

Introduction

Tumors of the vulva and vagina share overall histological classifications of neoplastic lesions into squamous, glandular, melanocytic, and mesenchymal tumors. Squamous carcinoma is by far the most common primary malignancy involving both organs and is related to human papillomavirus infection in the majority of cases. Squamous intraepithelial lesion is the most common preinvasive condition of squamous cell carcinoma. Conventional Mullerian adenocarcinomas are rare malignancies of the vulva and vagina. Extramammary Paget disease represents a special form of intraepithelial glandular malignancy and is only rarely associated with an invasive component. Primary clear cell carcinoma of the vagina has been famous for its association with intrauterine diethylstilbestrol (DES) exposure in the past but is very rare nowadays. Melanoma accounts for 5 % of vulvar cancers and is capable of widespread metastases. A variety of benign and malignant mesenchymal tumors also occur in the vulvar and vaginal regions with benign angiomyofibroblastoma and deep aggressive angiomyxoma primarily involving these areas.

Since both organs are easily accessible for biopsy diagnosis, requests for frozen section diagnosis are relatively uncommon for clinical management of vulvar and vaginal neoplasms. The single most common intraoperative consultation is frozen section evaluation of tumor resection margins for squamous cell carcinoma or adenocarcinoma [1]. Other frozen section indications include presence of multifocal synchronous tumors and assessment of lymph nodes for metastatic disease. Frozen section diagnosis is rarely initiated to rule out malignancy of unexpected vulvar or vaginal mass lesions.

© Springer International Publishing Switzerland 2015
P. Hui, N. Buza, *Atlas of Intraoperative Frozen Section Diagnosis in Gynecologic Pathology*,
DOI 10.1007/978-3-319-21807-6_2

Squamous Lesions

Benign Squamous Lesions

- *Squamous hyperplasia*
  - Benign hyperplastic condition, often associated with lichen sclerosus
  - Presence of acanthosis, hyperkeratosis, and parakeratosis
  - Lack of human papillomavirus cytopathic changes, inflammation, or stromal fibrosis
- *Squamous papilloma*
  - Papillomatous proliferation of bland squamous cells with appropriate maturation and without evidence of human papillomavirus cytopathic changes or dysplasia
- *Condyloma acuminatum*
  - Papillomatous squamous proliferation with fibrous stroma.
  - Marked acanthosis, parakeratosis, and hyperkeratosis are common.
  - Presence of koilocytes.
    - Nuclear enlargement, multinucleation, hyperchromasia, irregular or raisinoid nuclear membranes, and perinuclear halo.
    - Koilocytosis may be focal and involves clusters of superficial squamous cells.
  - Prominent granular cell layer with keratohyalin granules is also characteristic.
- *Seborrheic keratosis*
  - Elevated proliferation of basaloid squamous cells with a smooth, flat base.

- Multiple keratin (horn) cyst formation.
- Hyperkeratosis, acanthosis, and papillomatosis are common.
- Frequently increased melanin pigment in the basal and parabasal layers.
- No cytological atypia or significant mitotic activity.
- May be complicated by human papillomavirus infection (condyloma with features of seborrheic keratosis).
- *Lichen sclerosus (LS)* (Fig. 2.1)
  - Common squamous lesion—a preneoplastic condition to squamous carcinoma that is not associated with human papillomavirus infection.
  - Grossly shiny, flat to wrinkled vulvar lesion and may be associated with scarring.
  - Loss of rete pegs leading to flattened epithelial-stromal junction.
  - Presence of subepithelial homogenization of the stroma and chronic inflammation.
  - May be associated with hyperkeratosis.
  - Retained epithelial maturation and polarity without significant cytological atypia.
  - Differential diagnosis includes lichen planus and stromal fibrosis induced by radiation therapy.
  - The lesion may be associated with differentiated vulvar intraepithelial neoplasia (dVIN).
    - Distinction between LS and dVIN may be difficult on frozen section and is typically not critical for intraoperative management.

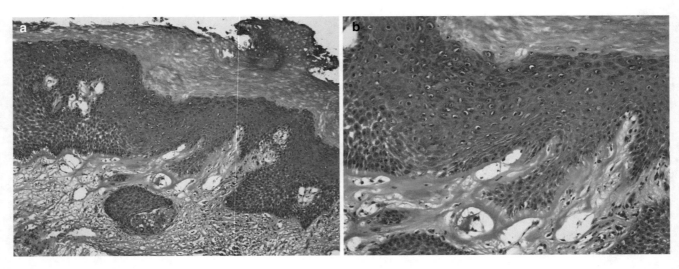

Fig. 2.1 Lichen sclerosus. Hyperkeratotic squamous epithelium with loss of rete pegs at the dermoepidermal junction (**a**) and presence of eosinophilic homogenization of the subepithelial stroma (**b**)

Squamous Intraepithelial Lesion (SIL)/Vulvar and Vaginal Intraepithelial Neoplasia (VIN and VAIN)

- Dysplastic squamous epithelium classified into low and high grade dysplasia.
- *High-grade SIL* consists of dysplastic squamous cells involving two-thirds to entire thickness of squamous mucosa (Fig. 2.2).
  - Marked nuclear atypia, loss of polarity, and mitotic activity in the mid and upper third of epithelium—including abnormal mitotic figures.
  - Absence of stromal invasion.
- Usual squamous intraepithelial lesion includes two histological subtypes: warty and basaloid types.
- *Pagetoid VIN* is characterized by singles or clusters of dysplastic squamous cells embedded within non-dysplastic squamous epithelial cells with normal maturation.
- *Differentiated VIN (dVIN)* is commonly seen in postmenopausal patients and may be associated with lichen sclerosus but is unrelated to human papillomavirus infection [2, 3].
  - Thickened hyperkeratotic squamous epithelium
  - Elongated and branching rete pegs
  - Abnormal maturation of individual or groups of squamous cells with eosinophilic cytoplasm, prominent desmosomes, and macronucleoli in the mid third of epithelium
  - Basal and parabasal dysplastic cells with marked cytological atypia
- Differential diagnosis
  - Paget disease
  - Melanoma
  - Invasive squamous cell carcinoma
- Diagnostic pitfalls/key issues of frozen section diagnosis
  - Suboptimal orientation and tangential sectioning may mimic invasion.
  - In case of dVIN, a high index of suspicion is needed to rule out adjacent invasive well-differentiated squamous cell carcinoma at the time of frozen section diagnosis, as it is not uncommonly associated with invasion.

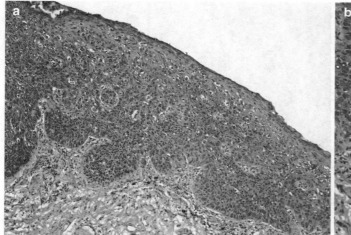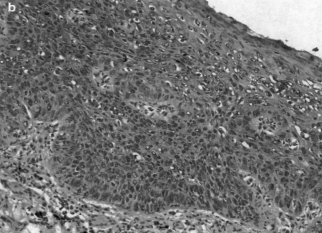

Fig. 2.2 High-grade squamous intraepithelial lesion/vulvar intraepithelial neoplasia 3 (VIN3). Markedly atypical squamous cells involving approximately 2/3 of the squamous epithelium (**a**) low magnification (**b**) high magnification

Squamous Cell Carcinoma (SCC) [4–7]

- Clinical features
  - Most often present in postmenopausal patients
  - Bleeding, dyspareunia, pruritus, and pain
- Gross pathology (Fig. 2.3)
  - Most SCCs are located in the posterior and upper third of the vagina and vulvar lesions are often multifocal.
  - Hyperkeratotic, white, or erythematous plaques to exophytic mass lesions, frequently associated with ulceration.
- Microscopic features
  - Most vaginal squamous cell carcinomas are moderately differentiated and nonkeratinizing, arising in a background of high-grade squamous intraepithelial lesion.
  - Most vulvar squamous cell carcinomas are well differentiated and keratinizing, arising in a background of high-grade squamous intraepithelial lesion, while a smaller proportion of cases are linked to dermatoses or lichen sclerosus.
  - Sheets, nests, or cords of atypical squamous cells invading stroma with desmoplasia.
  - Subtypes of squamous cell carcinoma include keratinizing, basaloid, and warty (Fig. 2.4).
  - Other histological variants include:
    - Verrucous carcinoma
      - Pushing border
      - No significant cytological atypia
      - No obvious stromal invasion
    - Spindle cell/sarcomatoid SCC (Fig. 2.5)
      - Spindle cell proliferation
      - Presence of in situ squamous lesion with focal transition to the spindle component
      - Must be separated from malignant mixed Mullerian tumor

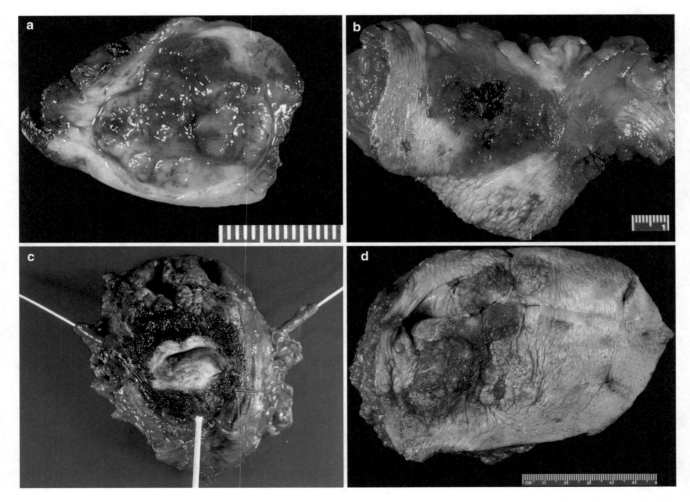

Fig. 2.3 Invasive squamous cell carcinoma. Exophytic masses or plaques with ulcer and hemorrhage involving the vulva (**a**, **b**) and vagina (**c**). Verrucous carcinoma involving the vulva (**d**)

- Papillary squamous cell carcinoma (Fig. 2.6)
  - Surface papillary squamous cell proliferation with stromal cores
  - High-grade dysplastic squamous cells
  - May harbor underlying invasive squamous cell carcinoma
- Differential diagnosis
  - HSIL/VIN3.
  - Vulvar basal cell carcinoma.
  - Sebaceous carcinoma.
  - Vulvar granular cell tumor may induce marked pseudoepitheliomatous squamous hyperplasia mimicking squamous cell carcinoma.
  - Leiomyosarcoma, soft tissue spindle cell sarcomas, and spindle cell melanoma.
- Diagnostic pitfalls/key intraoperative consultation issues
  - Frozen section evaluation to rule out inguinal lymph node metastasis is common (Fig. 2.7).

- Accurate specimen orientation is crucial for frozen section assessment of surgical margins.
- Well-oriented frozen sections help avoiding misinterpretation of tangential sectioning of normal skin structures, squamous hyperplasia, or HSIL/ VIN3/ VAIN3 as invasive squamous carcinoma (Fig. 2.8).
- Large sections to include sufficient tumor border are required to appreciate the overall pushing invasive border to separate verrucous carcinoma from condyloma, squamous papilloma, and pseudoepitheliomatous hyperplasia [8], particularly in association with underlying granular cell tumor.
- Careful search for the presence of definite squamous differentiation and absence of junctional in situ melanoma component to confirm spindle cell squamous cell carcinoma as opposed to spindle cell melanoma or spindle cell sarcomas.

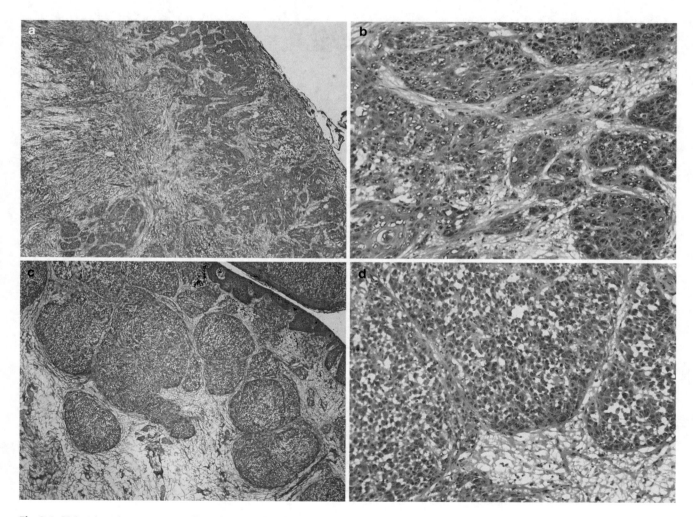

Fig. 2.4 Vulvar invasive squamous cell carcinoma of keratinizing (**a**, **b**) and basaloid type (**c**, **d**)

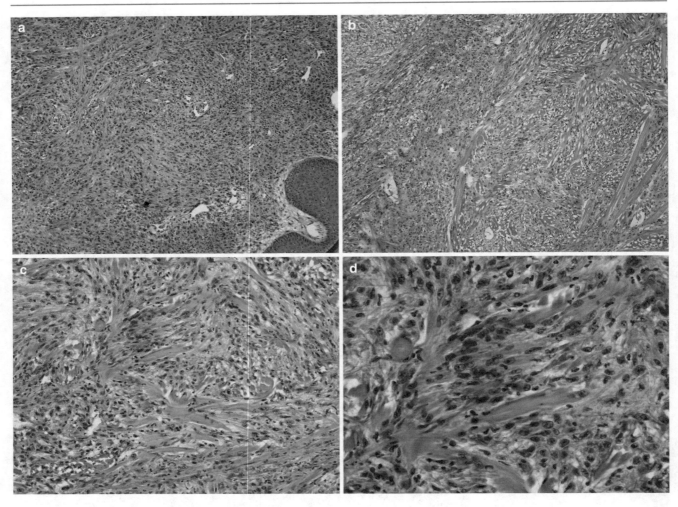

Fig. 2.5 Vulvar spindle cell squamous cell carcinoma. Spindled squamous cell proliferation simulating mesenchymal sarcoma at various magnifications (**a–d**)

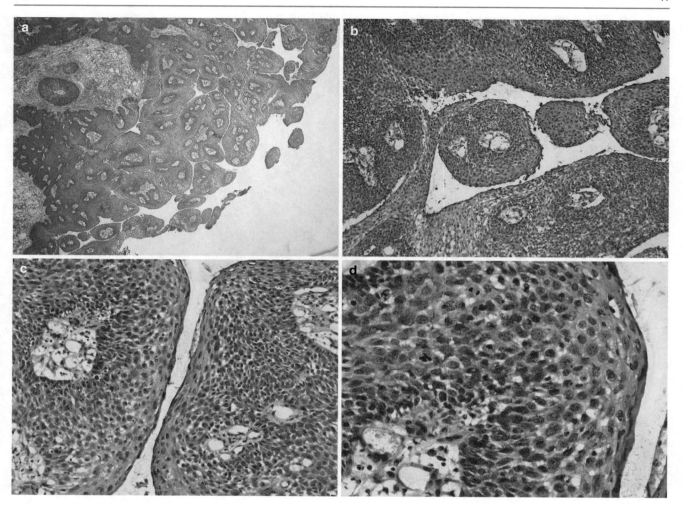

Fig. 2.6 Vulvar papillary squamous cell carcinoma. Papillary proliferation with stromal cores (**a, b**) composed of high-grade dysplastic squamous cells (**c, d**)

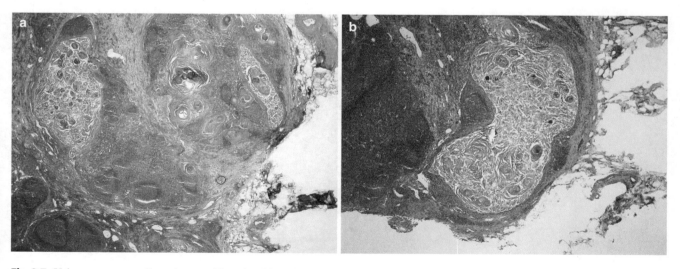

Fig. 2.7 Vulvar squamous cell carcinoma with regional lymph node metastasis. Note the marked maturation of metastatic squamous cell carcinoma with cystic appearance (**a, b**)

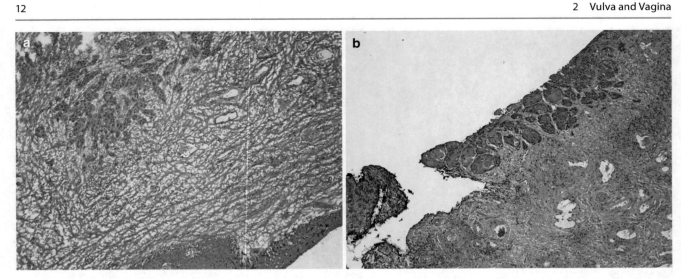

Fig. 2.8 Vulvar squamous cell carcinoma involving surgical margin. Note the microscopic focus of squamous carcinoma involving the stroma of an "en face" section of surgical margin (**a**) and peripheral mucosal margin (**b**)

Superficially Invasive Squamous Cell Carcinoma

- Early stromal invasion, less than 1 mm in depth.
- Singles or irregular clusters of dysplastic epithelial cells extruding from the base of an in situ lesion.
- Isolated tumor nests with paradoxical maturation and haphazard arrangements of tumor cells are highly suggestive of early invasion (Fig. 2.9).

- Stromal response is almost always present, including desmoplasia, edema, and/or lymphoplasmacytic infiltration.
- Differential diagnosis includes high-grade squamous intraepithelial lesion (HSIL) with pseudoinvasion or tangential sectioning.

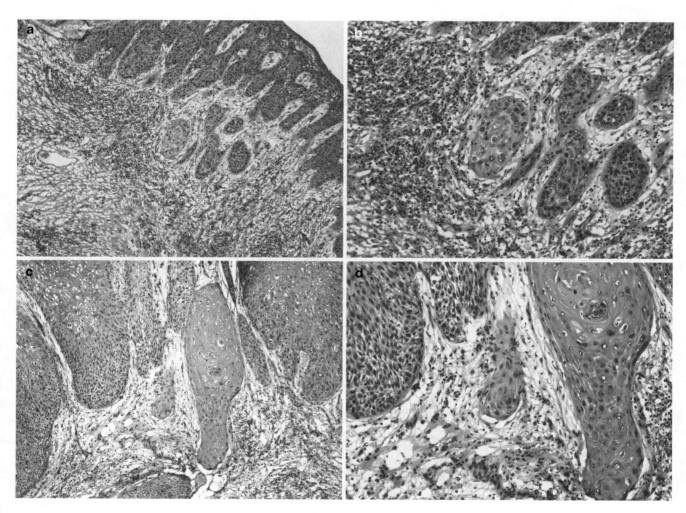

Fig. 2.9 Superficially invasive squamous cell carcinoma. Note detached small atypical squamous nests with characteristic paradoxical maturation and loss of peripheral epithelial palisading beneath the high-grade squamous intraepithelial lesion indicating early stromal invasion (**a–d**)

Basal Cell Carcinoma [9]

- Accounts for 3 % of vulvar cancers.
- Most often occurs in elderly patients.
- Nodular or plaque lesions (Fig. 2.10), which may be pigmented.
- Nests or sheets of uniform basal cell proliferation with peripheral palisading in solid or adenoid glandular patterns (Fig. 2.11).
- Squamous component (metatypical basal carcinoma or basosquamous carcinoma) may be present.

- Differential diagnosis includes basaloid squamous cell carcinoma and other skin adnexal tumors.
- Intraoperative diagnostic separation from basaloid squamous cell carcinoma is important due to a more aggressive behavior of the latter that may require regional lymph node dissection as part of surgical management.
- Basal cell carcinoma should be separated from tangentially sectioned normal hair follicles, particularly at the surgical margin.

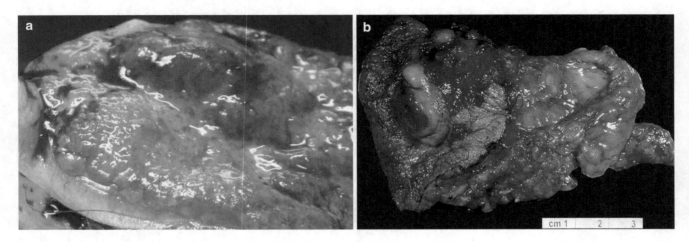

Fig. 2.10 Vulvar basal cell carcinoma. Note the plaque-like (**a**) and nodular lesions (**b**)

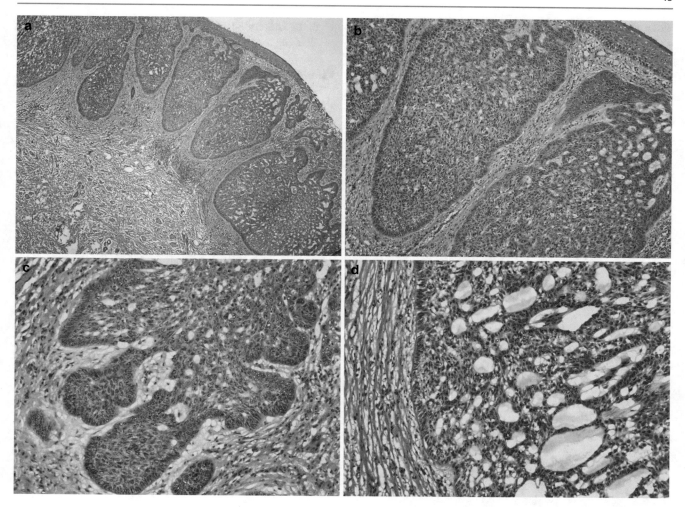

Fig. 2.11 Vulvar basal cell carcinoma (adenoid histological subtype). Note the infiltrating nests or sheets of atypical basal cell proliferation (**a**) with peripheral palisading (**b**, **c**) and adenoid glandular pattern (**c**, **d**)

Glandular Lesions

Benign Glandular Lesions

Tumorlike Lesions

- Bartholin gland hyperplasia: nodular or lobular proliferation of mucinous glands around existing Bartholin duct, frequently associated with cyst formation (Fig. 2.12). Metaplastic changes may occur including squamous metaplasia.
- Vulvar ectopic breast tissue with associated benign conditions (adenosis and papilloma).
- Vaginal adenoma (villous and tubulovillous) and vaginal adenosis
- Prolapsed fallopian tube occasionally occurs after vaginal hysterectomy and may present as a polypoid lesion at the vaginal vault. Disrupted fallopian tube mucosa, frequently with inflammation, fibrosis, and reactive epithelial changes may simulate infiltrating adenocarcinoma [10].

Vulvar Hidradenoma Papilliferum [11]

- Most common benign glandular tumor of the vulva.
- Asymptomatic and small (less than 2 cm), frequently involving the labia majora.
- Histologically well-circumscribed nodular proliferation of compact glandular or tubular epithelial growth with papillary formations and frequently hyalinized stroma.
- The epithelium is, at least focally, double layered with inner tall columnar glandular cells and outer myoepithelial cells.
- May have focal sebaceous and/or squamous differentiation.
- The absence of infiltrative border and minimal cytological atypia attest to its benignancy in its separation from various adenocarcinomas. Presence of mitoses, even frequent, does not necessarily indicate malignancy.

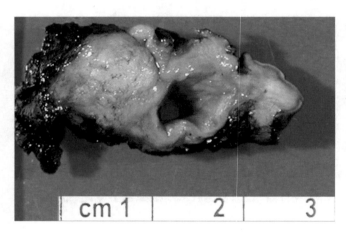

Fig. 2.12 Vulvar Bartholin duct cyst

Vulvar Paget Disease [12–15]

- Clinical features
  - In situ/intraepidermal adenocarcinoma
  - Represents 5 % of vulvar malignancy
  - Almost exclusively seen in Caucasian women, often postmenopausal
- Gross pathology (Fig. 2.13)
  - Red eczematous plaques involving both labia majora and minora
- Microscopic features (Fig. 2.14)
  - Scattered singles or clusters of large, round mucin-containing cells involving the lower half to entire epithelium with frequent tracking into hair follicles or other skin adnexal structures.
  - Focal gland formation may be present within the tumor nests.
  - The tumor cells have abundant pale cytoplasm and central, round nuclei with prominent centrally located nucleoli. Mitoses may be frequent.
  - The disease is often multifocal.
  - An underlying invasive adenocarcinoma can occur, although rarely.
- Differential diagnosis
  - In situ melanoma
  - Colonization of the vulvar epithelium by urothelial or anal carcinomas [16] (secondary Paget disease)
  - VIN with mucinous differentiation and Pagetoid VIN
- Diagnostic pitfalls/key intraoperative consultation issues
  - Presence of glandular structures within the tumor nests is highly suggestive of Paget disease as opposed to melanoma.
  - Frozen section evaluation of surgical margin involvement by vulvar Paget disease may be requested; however, the tumor is often multifocal and the clinical and gross presentation of the disease can be deceptive. Seemingly uninvolved surgical margins may turn out to be positive for microscopic disease.
  - Therefore, generous sampling of the resection margins at the time of frozen section is essential to prevent recurrence.

Bartholin Gland Carcinomas [17]

- Middle-aged to elderly patients.
- Histological transition between normal Bartholin glands and carcinoma components.
- No primary tumor elsewhere.
- Histological variants include squamous cell carcinoma (40 %), adenocarcinoma (25 %), adenoid cystic carcinoma (12 %), and rarely transitional cell carcinoma and various mucinous adenocarcinomas.
- Diagnosis requires the presence of the following: the tumor arises at the location of Bartholin gland and is histologically associated with residual Bartholin gland structures and absence of a known primary carcinoma at other sites.

Adenocarcinoma of the Mammary Type [18]

- Very rare and likely arises from vulvar ectopic breast tissue.
- Histologically the tumor resembles conventional breast ductal and lobular carcinomas.
- At the time of frozen section diagnosis, metastasis from a breast primary must be ruled out before such diagnosis is made.

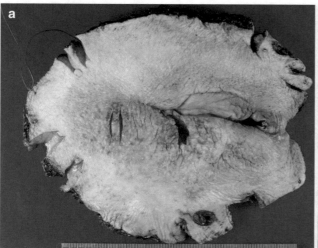 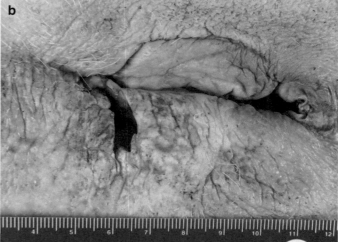

Fig. 2.13 Vulvar Paget disease. Note the red eczematous plaques involving labia majora and minora (multiple sections have been taken for frozen section evaluation of margin involvement) (**a**, **b**)

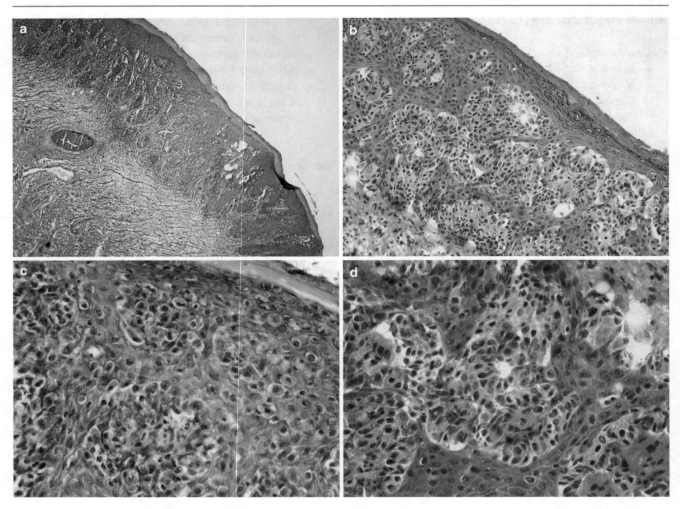

Fig. 2.14 Vulvar Paget disease. Note singles and clusters of large round mucin-containing cells involving the lower half and focally the entire squamous epithelium (**a–c**) with subtle glandular structure formation (**d**)

Mesenchymal Tumors

Although rare, a variety of benign and malignant soft tissue tumors may occur in the vulva and vagina. Relatively common soft tissue tumors and tumorlike lesions are discussed here.

Aggressive Angiomyxoma [19]

- Clinical features
  - Patients in their reproductive age.
  - Frequently presents as painless vulvar or vaginal "cyst" or deep soft tissue mass.
  - Rapid enlargement during pregnancy may occur.
- Gross pathology (Fig. 2.15)
  - Deep-seated soft tissue mass involving mainly pelvico-perineal soft tissue
  - Often more than 10 cm in size with poorly circumscribed borders and irregular extension into adjacent normal structures
  - Gelatinous or rubbery cut surface
- Microscopic features (Fig. 2.16)
  - Hypocellular lesion with abundant edematous to myxoid matrix
  - Uniformly bland, oval to short spindle cells with round nuclei, inconspicuous cytoplasm, and stellate cytoplasmic processes
  - Clusters of various caliber vessels, including medium to large arteries, some of which show characteristic cuffing by prominent eosinophilic collagen
  - Infiltrative tumor border with frequent entrapment of normal adipose tissue or skeletal muscle

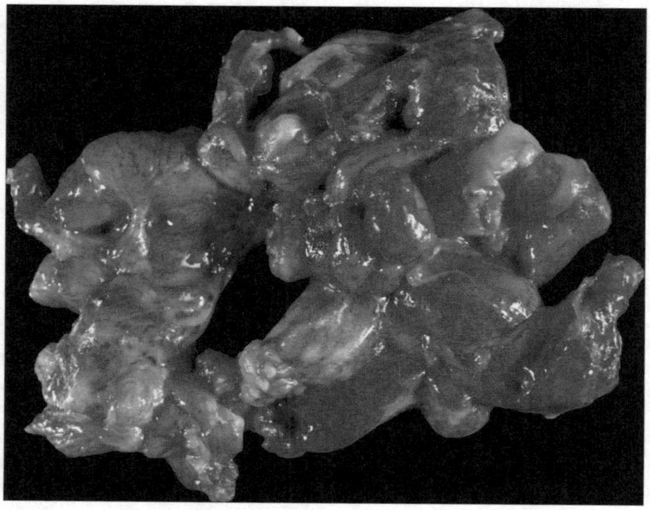

- Differential diagnosis
  - Superficial angiomyxoma
  - Cellular angiofibroma
  - Angiomyofibroblastoma
  - Fibroepithelial stromal polyp
- Diagnostic pitfalls/key intraoperative consultation issues
  - The deep location, infiltrative margin and typical vascular clustering with collagen cuffing separate the tumor from its benign mimics
  - Adequate surgical margin sampling at the time of frozen section is essential to reduce the recurrence rate

Fibroepithelial Stromal Polyp [20, 21]

- Common polypoid lesion in young women.
- Histologically the polypoid lesion is covered by simple, mature squamous epithelium.
- Variable stromal cellularity with bland, spindled, non-atypical cells.
  - Stromal cells may be frequently multinucleated and bizarre raising concern for malignancy.
- Rare cellular pseudosarcomatous variant may show hypercellular stromal cells with marked pleomorphism, nuclear hyperchromasia, mitotic activity of more than 10 mitoses/10 HPF, and even atypical mitoses. This variant is almost invariably seen in a pregnant patient [21].
- Features against a diagnosis of true sarcoma include surface growth only and individually scattered multinucleated stromal cells.

Fig. 2.15 Aggressive angiomyxoma. Note the irregular nodular mass lesions with a gelatinous appearance and tan to pink color

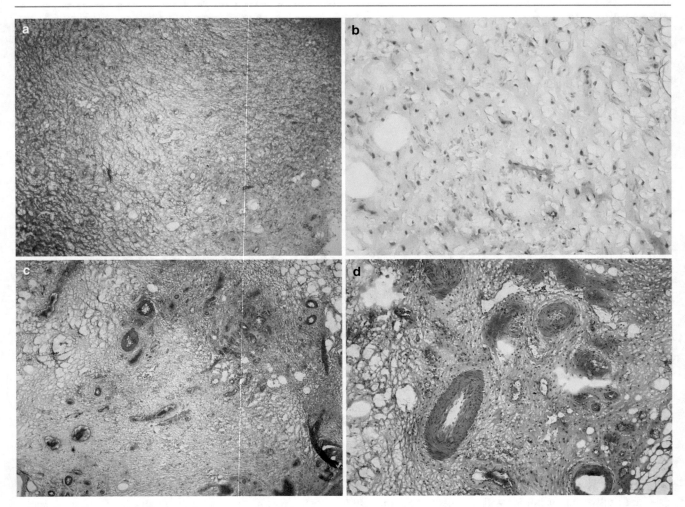

Fig. 2.16 Aggressive angiomyxoma. Hypocellular lesion with myxoid appearance (**a**), short bland spindle cell proliferation (**b**) and characteristic clusters of various caliber vasculature (**c, d**)

Granulation Tissue

- Common polypoid lesion of the vagina or vulva.
- Often involves the upper vagina/vaginal cuff post hysterectomy.
- Soft red, edematous to mucoid polypoid lesion.
- Loose edematous fibrous tissue with delicate capillaries (Fig. 2.17).
- Enriched with acute and chronic inflammatory cells.
- Surface growth, frequently lacking surface epithelium, acute inflammatory infiltrate, and bland cytological features, attests to the nonneoplastic nature of the lesion.

Postoperative Spindle Cell Nodule [22]

- Adult patients around 40 years of age.
- Develops a few months after surgery, commonly hysterectomy.
- Polypoid or nodular lesion of up to several centimeters at the prior surgery site (vaginal vault or cervix).
- The lesion consists of fascicles of spindled myofibroblasts in a background of edema, delicate capillaries, and inflammatory cells.
- Mitoses are numerous but atypical mitoses and cytological atypia are absent.
- Differential diagnosis includes various soft tissue spindle cell sarcomas.

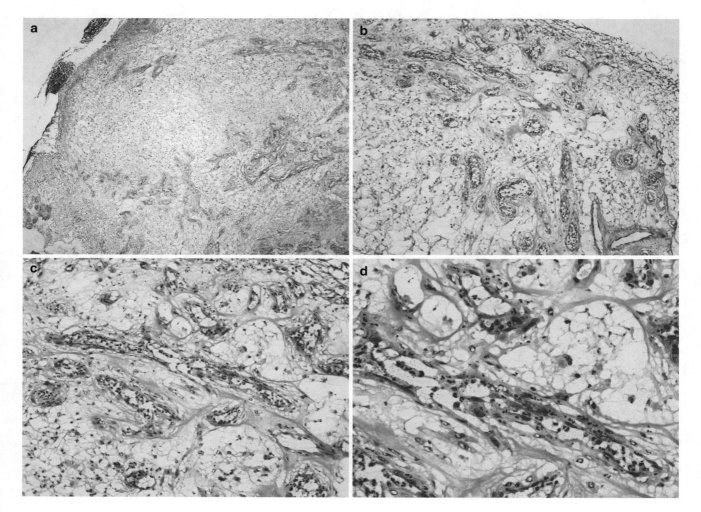

Fig. 2.17 Granulation tissue. Loose edematous fibrous tissue with delicate capillaries (**a, b**) and prominent acute and chronic inflammatory cells (**c, d**)

Angiomyofibroblastoma [23]

- Exclusively arises in vulvovaginal soft tissue of adult women.
- Less than 5 cm in size with sharply defined margins.
- Histologically alternating cellular and hypocellular proliferations of small round epithelioid and spindle cells

with eosinophilic cytoplasm, embedded in an edematous to collagenous matrix (Fig. 2.18).

- Epithelioid tumor cells are typically clustered around capillaries.
- Cytological atypia and mitoses are absent.
- Differential diagnostic separation of this benign lesion from aggressive angiomyxoma is important.

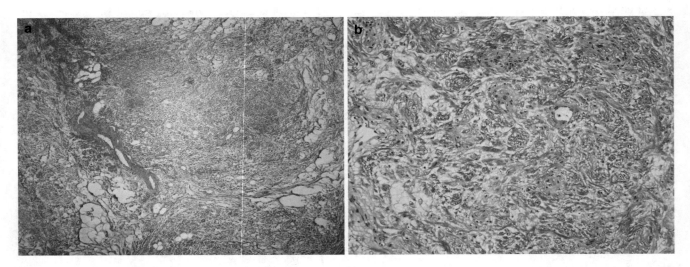

Fig. 2.18 Angiomyofibroblastoma. Note the alternating cellular to hypocellular proliferation of small, round to spindle cells with eosinophilic cytoplasm embedded in a collagenous matrix (**a, b**)

Leiomyoma and Leiomyosarcoma

- Rare vulvar and vaginal tumors.
- Leiomyomas are much more common that leiomyosarcomas.
- Most leiomyomas are conventional mature smooth muscle tumors (Fig. 2.19).
- Epithelioid and myxoid leiomyomas can also occur.
- Diagnostic criteria of malignancy are similar to those of soft tissue leiomyosarcoma (Fig. 2.20), including presence of two of the following: more than 5 cm in size, more than 5 mitotic figures per 10 high-power fields, and moderate or severe cytological atypia. Lesions that fulfill some, but not all, of the above criteria may be interpreted as smooth muscle tumor of uncertain malignant potential (STUMP) at the time of frozen section (Fig. 2.21).

Botryoid Rhabdomyosarcoma (Sarcoma Botryoides) [24, 25]

- Patients under 5 years of age with history of rapid tumor growth.
- Soft, polypoid, or lobulated vaginal lesion.
- Myxoid to edematous stroma containing primitive round to spindle, mitotically active cells.
- Presence of cambium layer—condensation of small tumor cells underneath the mucosal surface—with recognizable rhabdomyoblasts.
- The differential diagnosis includes fibroepithelial stromal polyp with atypical stromal cells.
- The tumor can be deceptively bland.
  - Careful search for small, mitotically active atypical cells or rhabdomyoblasts with cross striations in the cambium layer is important for intraoperative frozen section diagnosis.

Proximal Epithelioid Sarcoma [26, 27]

- Primarily occurs in the genital area.
- More aggressive behavior than that of the distal counterpart.
- Multinodular growth with large eosinophilic epithelioid cells.
- The differential diagnosis includes poorly differentiated carcinoma and melanoma. Presence of an in situ melanocytic lesion favors malignant melanoma.

Granular Cell Tumor [28, 29]

- Middle-aged adult patients.
- Asymptomatic solitary mass involving labia majora.
- Grossly well-circumscribed firm mass of less than 4 cm with a tan, solid cut surface.
- Nests or cords of round to polygonal cells with abundant granular cytoplasm and small but distinct centrally located nuclei.
- Mitoses and cytological atypia are absent.
- Not uncommonly infiltrative tumor border.
- At the time of frozen diagnosis, striking pseudoepitheliomatous hyperplasia of the overlying squamous epithelium may lead to erroneous impression of invasive squamous cell carcinoma if the underlying granular cell tumor is not appreciated.
- Malignant granular cell tumor has been reported; however, reliable histological parameters have not been defined to predict malignancy.
- Complete tumor excision with surgical margin evaluation is necessary to avoid local recurrence.

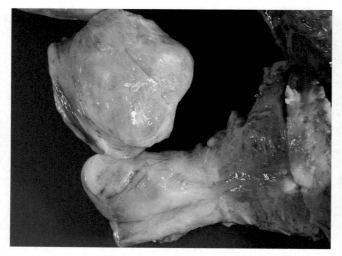

Fig. 2.19 Vaginal leiomyoma. Well-circumscribed nodular lesion with a rubbery, tan-white cut surface

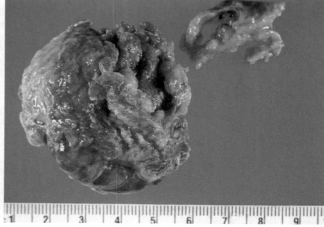

Fig. 2.20 Vaginal leiomyosarcoma. Note the fleshy soft tissue mass and ill-defined tumor borders

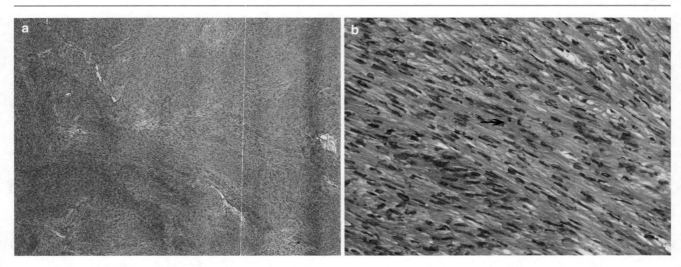

Fig. 2.21 Vaginal smooth muscle tumor of uncertain malignant potential (STUMP). Note the cellular proliferation of smooth muscle cells (**a**) with mitotic activity (*arrow*) but lack of significant cytological atypia and coagulative tumor cell necrosis (**b**)

Miscellaneous Tumors

Malignant Melanoma [30]

- Clinical features
  - 5–10 % of vulvar or vaginal cancers (second most common vulvar cancer)
  - Elderly Caucasian patients with atypical pigmented lesion that may be associated with preexisting melanocytic nevi
  - May present with pruritus, bleeding, and mass lesion
- Gross pathology (Fig. 2.22)
  - Unevenly pigmented asymmetric plaques or nodules with irregular border.
  - Amelanotic melanoma occurs in 25 % of the cases.
  - Satellite tumor nodules may be seen.
- Microscopic features
  - Three histological subtypes: acral/mucosal lentiginous (60 %), nodular, and superficial spreading.
  - Large, round epithelioid tumor cells with eosinophilic cytoplasm, large central nuclei, and prominent nucleoli in most cases.
  - Spindle cell variant of melanoma seen in one-third of cases.
  - Intracytoplasmic melanin pigment may be seen.
  - Vertical growth phase melanoma shows frequent prominent perineural involvement and desmoplasia.
- Differential diagnosis
  - Dysplastic melanocytic nevi
  - Vulvar Paget disease
  - Squamous intraepithelial lesions
  - Poorly differentiated carcinomas, particularly spindle cell variant of squamous cell carcinoma
  - Lymphomas

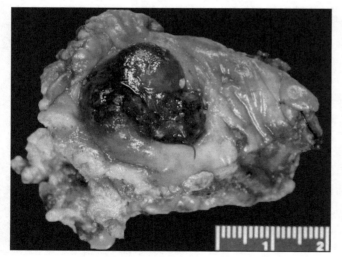

Fig. 2.22 Vulvar melanoma. Pigmented asymmetric nodule with irregular borders

- Diagnostic pitfalls/key intraoperative consultation issues
  - Frozen section evaluation of melanoma is not encouraged [1].
  - Lesions of uncertain diagnosis at any level should be deferred to permanent section diagnosis.

Lymphomas [31, 32]

- Primary vaginal and vulvar lymphomas account for roughly 1/3 of cases; the remaining 2/3 of cases are due to secondary involvement.
- Diffuse large B-cell lymphoma is the most common type of both primary and secondary vulvar and vaginal lymphomas.
- Vulvar and vaginal lymphomas may be misdiagnosed on frozen section as poorly differentiated carcinoma.
- High index of suspicion at the time of frozen section diagnosis is important for preserving fresh lesional tissue for further hematopathology workup.
- Frozen section interpretation as suspicious for lymphoproliferative disorder is sufficient.

Primary Yolk Sac Tumor [33, 34]

- Occurs in children less than 4 years old.
- Vaginal polypoid lesion with bleeding and elevated serum AFP.
- The histological features are similar to its ovarian counterpart with common reticular growth pattern, presence of Schiller-Duval bodies, and eosinophilic hyalin globules [see Chap. 9].
- Common differential diagnosis includes clear cell carcinoma.

Clear Cell Carcinoma [35, 36]

- Vaginal clear cell carcinoma related to diethylstilbestrol (DES) exposure in patients of less than 20 years of age is rarely encountered nowadays. Sporadic clear cell carcinoma is seen in perimenopausal and postmenopausal populations.
- Vaginal bleeding or discharge is typical clinical presentation.
- Most tumors are superficially invasive at presentation.
- Histological patterns include tubulocystic, papillary, and solid, with tubulocystic pattern being the most common.
- Vaginal adenosis, cervical ectropion, transverse septum, and cervical ridges are commonly associated with clear cell carcinoma of the vagina.
- Marked cytological atypia with hobnailing and frequent mitoses are present in most tumors.

References

1. Smith-Zagone MJ, Schwartz MR. Frozen section of skin specimens. Arch Pathol Lab Med. 2005;129:1536–43.
2. Yang B, Hart WR. Vulvar intraepithelial neoplasia of the simplex (differentiated) type: a clinicopathologic study including analysis of HPV and p53 expression. Am J Surg Pathol. 2000;24:429–41.
3. van de Nieuwenhof HP, Bulten J, Hollema H, Dommerholt RG, Massuger LF, van der Zee AG, et al. Differentiated vulvar intraepithelial neoplasia is often found in lesions, previously diagnosed as lichen sclerosus, which have progressed to vulvar squamous cell carcinoma. Mod Pathol. 2011;24:297–305.
4. Steeper TA, Piscioli F, Rosai J. Squamous cell carcinoma with sarcoma-like stroma of the female genital tract. Clinicopathologic study of four cases. Cancer. 1983;52:890–8.
5. Carlson JA, Ambros R, Malfetano J, Ross J, Grabowski R, Lamb P, et al. Vulvar lichen sclerosus and squamous cell carcinoma: a cohort, case control, and investigational study with historical perspective; implications for chronic inflammation and sclerosis in the development of neoplasia. Hum Pathol. 1998;29:932–48.
6. Otton GR, Nicklin JL, Dickie GJ, Niedetzky P, Tripcony L, Perrin LC, Crandon AJ. Early-stage vaginal carcinoma—an analysis of 70 patients. Int J Gynecol Cancer. 2004;14:304–10.
7. Grayson W, Cooper K. A reappraisal of "basaloid carcinoma" of the cervix, and the differential diagnosis of basaloid cervical neoplasms. Adv Anat Pathol. 2002;9:290–300.
8. Gualco M, Bonin S, Foglia G, Fulcheri E, Odicino F, Prefumo F, et al. Morphologic and biologic studies on ten cases of verrucous carcinoma of the vulva supporting the theory of a discrete clinicopathologic entity. Int J Gynecol Cancer. 2003;13:317–24.
9. Mulvany NJ, Rayoo M, Allen DG. Basal cell carcinoma of the vulva: a case series. Pathology. 2012;44:528–33.
10. Varnholt H, Otis CN, Nucci MR, Johari VP. Fallopian tube prolapse mimicking aggressive angiomyxoma. Int J Gynecol Pathol. 2005;24:292–4.
11. Scurry J, van der Putte SC, Pyman J, Chetty N, Szabo R. Mammary-like gland adenoma of the vulva: review of 46 cases. Pathology. 2009;41:372–8.
12. Fanning J, Lambert HC, Hale TM, Morris PC, Schuerch C. Paget's disease of the vulva: prevalence of associated vulvar adenocarcinoma, invasive Paget's disease, and recurrence after surgical excision. Am J Obstet Gynecol. 1999;180(1 Pt 1):24–7.
13. Goldblum JR, Hart WR. Vulvar Paget's disease: a clinicopathologic and immunohistochemical study of 19 cases. Am J Surg Pathol. 1997;21:1178–87.
14. Willman JH, Golitz LE, Fitzpatrick JE. Vulvar clear cells of Toker: precursors of extramammary Paget's disease. Am J Dermatopathol. 2005;27:185–8.
15. Shaco-Levy R, Bean SM, Vollmer RT, Papalas JA, Bentley RC, Selim MA, Robboy SJ. Paget disease of the vulva: a histologic study of 56 cases correlating pathologic features and disease course. Int J Gynecol Pathol. 2010;29:69–78.
16. Wilkinson EJ, Brown HM. Vulvar Paget disease of urothelial origin: a report of three cases and a proposed classification of vulvar Paget disease. Hum Pathol. 2002;33:549–54.
17. Cardosi RJ, Speights A, Fiorica JV, Grendys Jr EC, Hakam A, Hoffman MS. Bartholin's gland carcinoma: a 15-year experience. Gynecol Oncol. 2001;82:247–51.
18. Kazakov DV, Spagnolo DV, Kacerovska D, Michal M. Lesions of anogenital mammary-like glands: an update. Adv Anat Pathol. 2011;18:1–28.
19. Fetsch JF, Laskin WB, Lefkowitz M, Kindblom LG, Meis-Kindblom JM. Aggressive angiomyxoma: a clinicopathologic study of 29 female patients. Cancer. 1996;78:79–90.
20. Ostor AG, Fortune DW, Riley CB. Fibroepithelial polyps with atypical stromal cells (pseudosarcoma botryoides) of vulva and vagina. A report of 13 cases. Int J Gynecol Pathol. 1988;7:351–60.
21. Nucci MR, Young RH, Fletcher CD. Cellular pseudosarcomatous fibroepithelial stromal polyps of the lower female genital tract: an underrecognized lesion often misdiagnosed as sarcoma. Am J Surg Pathol. 2000;24:231–40.
22. Proppe KH, Scully RE, Rosai J. Postoperative spindle cell nodules of genitourinary tract resembling sarcomas. A report of eight cases. Am J Surg Pathol. 1984;8:101–8.
23. Nielsen GP, Rosenberg AE, Young RH, Dickersin GR, Clement PB, Scully RE. Angiomyofibroblastoma of the vulva and vagina. Mod Pathol. 1996;9:284–91.
24. Newton Jr WA, Gehan EA, Webber BL, Marsden HB, van Unnik AJ, Hamoudi AB, et al. Classification of rhabdomyosarcomas and related sarcomas. Pathologic aspects and proposal for a new classification—an Intergroup Rhabdomyosarcoma Study. Cancer. 1995;76:1073–85.
25. Daya DA, Scully RE. Sarcoma botryoides of the uterine cervix in young women: a clinicopathological study of 13 cases. Gynecol Oncol. 1988;29:290–304.
26. Guillou L, Wadden C, Coindre JM, Krausz T, Fletcher CD. "Proximal-type" epithelioid sarcoma, a distinctive aggressive neoplasm showing rhabdoid features. Clinicopathologic, immunohistochemical, and ultrastructural study of a series. Am J Surg Pathol. 1997;21:130–46.
27. Hasegawa T, Matsuno Y, Shimoda T, Umeda T, Yokoyama R, Hirohashi S. Proximal-type epithelioid sarcoma: a clinicopathologic study of 20 cases. Mod Pathol. 2001;14:655–63.
28. Lack EE, Worsham GF, Callihan MD, Crawford BE, Klappenbach S, Rowden G, Chun B. Granular cell tumor: a clinicopathologic study of 110 patients. J Surg Oncol. 1980;13:301–16.
29. Wolber RA, Talerman A, Wilkinson EJ, Clement PB. Vulvar granular cell tumors with pseudocarcinomatous hyperplasia: a comparative analysis with well-differentiated squamous carcinoma. Int J Gynecol Pathol. 1991;10:59–66.
30. Ragnarsson-Olding BK, Nilsson BR, Kanter-Lewensohn LR, Lagerlof B, Ringborg UK. Malignant melanoma of the vulva in a nationwide, 25-year study of 219 Swedish females: predictors of survival. Cancer. 1999;86:1285–93.
31. Vang R, Medeiros LJ, Silva EG, Gershenson DM, Deavers M. Non-Hodgkin's lymphoma involving the vagina: a clinicopathologic analysis of 14 patients. Am J Surg Pathol. 2000;24:719–25.
32. Kosari F, Daneshbod Y, Parwaresch R, Krams M, Wacker HH. Lymphomas of the female genital tract: a study of 186 cases and review of the literature. Am J Surg Pathol. 2005;29:1512–20.
33. Copeland LJ, Sneige N, Ordonez NG, Hancock KC, Gershenson DM, Saul PB, Kavanagh JJ. Endodermal sinus tumor of the vagina and cervix. Cancer. 1985;55:2558–65.
34. Flanagan CW, Parker JR, Mannel RS, Min KW, Kida M. Primary endodermal sinus tumor of the vulva: a case report and review of the literature. Gynecol Oncol. 1997;66:515–8.
35. Herbst AL, Robboy SJ, Scully RE, Poskanzer DC. Clear-cell adenocarcinoma of the vagina and cervix in girls: analysis of 170 registry cases. Am J Obstet Gynecol. 1974;119:713–24.
36. Waggoner SE, Mittendorf R, Biney N, Anderson D, Herbst AL. Influence of in utero diethylstilbestrol exposure on the prognosis and biologic behavior of vaginal clear-cell adenocarcinoma. Gynecol Oncol. 1994;55:238–44.

Uterine Cervix

3

Introduction

Squamous cell carcinoma is the most common cervical malignancy and is caused by high-risk human papillomavirus (HPV) with viral DNA integration into the host cell genome [1]. Most tumors are conventional squamous cell carcinomas of either keratinizing or nonkeratinizing large cell type. Common histological variants include verrucous, basaloid, papillary, lymphoepitheliomatous, and spindled squamous carcinomas. Invasive adenocarcinoma of the cervix now represents 10–20 % of all cervical cancers. Similar to squamous carcinoma, high-risk HPV, particularly type 18, is the causal agent for most of the cases. The histological spectrum of cervical adenocarcinomas includes usual endocervical adenocarcinoma, endometrioid adenocarcinoma, gastrointestinal-type mucinous carcinoma and its variants including minimal deviation adenocarcinoma (adenoma malignum), villoglandular adenocarcinoma, adenoid basal carcinoma, adenosquamous carcinoma, serous carcinoma, and clear cell carcinoma. Malignant stromal tumors of the cervix are uncommon. Many reactive, metaplastic, and tumorlike conditions may simulate various malignant processes of the cervix.

Common scenarios for intraoperative consultation include evaluation for the presence of malignancy of an unexpected cervical mass and/or assessment of the extent of tumor involvement—depth of tumor invasion and margin status—and lymph node metastasis. Intraoperative pathologic evaluation of pelvic lymph nodes may be requested before hysterectomy to rule out advanced disease. More recently frozen section evaluation of sentinel lymph nodes has also been introduced to the surgical management of cervical malignancy. In young patients, the most common reason for performing frozen section evaluation of a cervical cone excision, trachelectomy, or biopsy is to maximize the chance of preserving fertility by doing limited surgery for an early cervical cancer.

© Springer International Publishing Switzerland 2015
P. Hui, N. Buza, *Atlas of Intraoperative Frozen Section Diagnosis in Gynecologic Pathology*,
DOI 10.1007/978-3-319-21807-6_3

Tumorlike Conditions of the Cervix

Endocervical Polyp

- Usually single and less than 1 cm in size (Fig. 3.1).
- Histologically, the polyp consists of varying proportions of squamous and endocervical glandular epithelium and stromal components.
- The overall appearance can be adenomatous, cystic, fibrous, or inflammatory (Fig. 3.2).
- Differential diagnosis
  - Mullerian adenosarcoma
- Diagnostic pitfalls/key intraoperative consultation issues
  - Unlike adenosarcoma, benign endocervical polyps are characterized by absence of periglandular stromal cell condensation and papillary intraglandular protrusions and lack of epithelial atypia and stromal mitotic activity.

Tunnel Clusters

- Localized proliferation of endocervical glands, commonly seen in multigravida women.
- Type A tunnel cluster is noncystic, consisting of crowded endocervical glands with round borders. Irregular glands with mild atypia may be seen, but mitotic activity is generally absent.
- Type B tunnel cluster consists of round clusters of packed glands with cystic dilatation that are covered by flattened epithelial cells.
- Both types may involve deeper cervical stroma.
- Differential diagnosis
  - Minimal deviation adenocarcinoma (MDA)
- Diagnostic pitfalls/key intraoperative consultation issues
  - Tunnel clusters can be diagnostically separated from MDA primarily by absence of significant cytological atypia, absence of desmoplastic stromal response, and their overall lobular growth pattern and sharp lesional border.

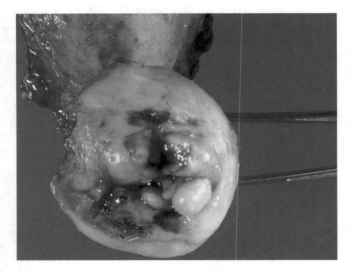

Fig. 3.1 Endocervical polyp. White-tan polypoid lesions of several millimeters with adjacent mucosal erosion and hemorrhage in this example

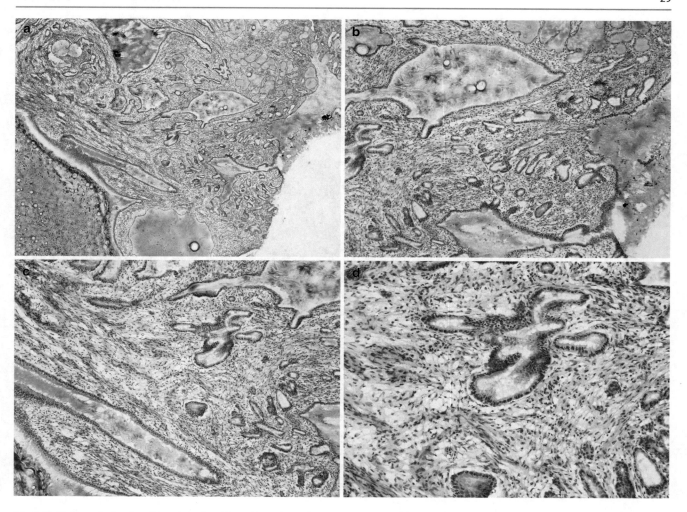

Fig. 3.2 Endocervical polyp. Note the polypoid configuration, edematous stroma (**a**, **b**) and variable number of benign endocervical glands (**c**, **d**)

Deep Nabothian Cyst

- Deeply seated, cystically dilated, mucin-filled endocervical glands (Fig. 3.3).
- Extravasated mucin pools may be present.
- Cysts are lined by bland columnar or flattened endocervical glandular epithelium.

- Differential diagnosis
  - Minimal deviation adenocarcinoma (MDA)
- Diagnostic pitfalls/key intraoperative consultation issues
  - Lack of a mass lesion, and absence of infiltrative glands and significant cytological atypia separates nabothian cysts from minimal deviation adenocarcinoma.

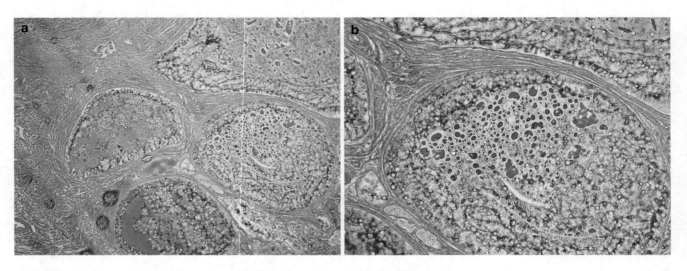

Fig. 3.3   Deep nabothian cyst. Deeply seated, cystically dilated endocervical glands filled with mucin (**a**, **b**)

Lobular and Diffuse Laminar Endocervical Glandular Hyperplasia [2, 3]

- Benign mucinous glandular proliferations, in a lobular or diffuse laminar pattern.
- May be deeply seated lobular mass lesions involving cervical stroma, exceeding 1 cm in size (Fig. 3.4).
- Both types show crowded hyperplastic glands lined by mucin-producing endocervical glandular epithelial cells.
- Both may have mild cytological atypia and low mitotic activity (2 per 10 high-power fields.
- In diffuse laminar hyperplasia, the lesion shows a band-like distribution below the endocervical mucosal surface.

Although confluent in growth pattern, the demarcation from the stroma is sharp and smooth (Fig. 3.5).

- Differential diagnosis
  - Mucinous endocervical adenocarcinomas, including minimal deviation adenocarcinoma, intestinal-type mucinous adenocarcinoma, and mucinous adenocarcinoma NOS
- Diagnostic pitfalls/key intraoperative consultation issues
  - Endocervical glandular hyperplasia may be separated from endocervical adenocarcinomas by its superficial location, non-infiltrative border, and absence of significant cytological atypia and desmoplastic stromal response.

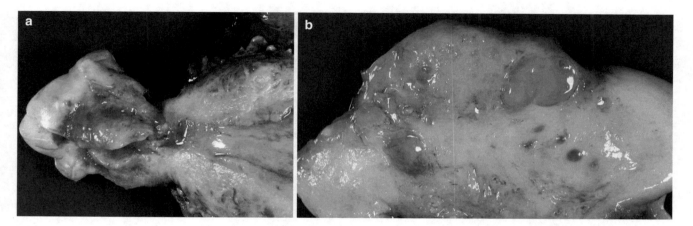

Fig. 3.4 Diffuse laminar endocervical glandular hyperplasia. Note the ill-defined, mucoid mass lesion involving the endocervix (**a, b**)

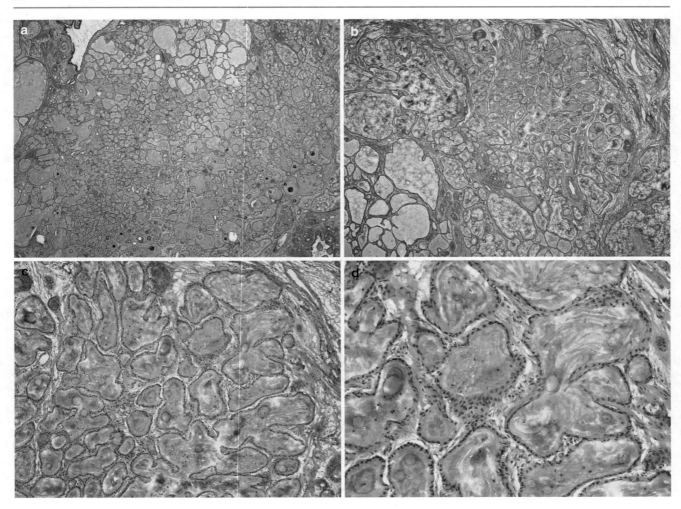

Fig. 3.5 Diffuse laminar endocervical glandular hyperplasia. Note diffuse hyperplastic proliferation of endocervical glands (**a**) well-demarcated from the adjacent endocervical stroma (**b, c**) and absence of cytological atypia or mitotic activity (**d**)

Microglandular Hyperplasia (MGH) [4–6]

- Incidental microscopic finding or may be a grossly polypoid lesion.
- Polypoid, reticular, cribriform, and rarely solid proliferation of closely packed small- to medium-sized endocervical glands with conspicuously neutrophil-rich stroma (Fig. 3.6).
- Relatively uniform endocervical glandular cells with subnuclear vacuoles, associated squamous metaplasia, often with reserve cell hyperplasia imparting on a double-layered epithelial appearance.
- Mild nuclear atypia may be present.
- Mitoses are usually rare but occasional cases may show higher mitotic activity (rarely up to 11 mitoses/10 HPF).

- Differential diagnosis
  - Clear cell carcinoma
  - Endometrioid adenocarcinoma—endometrial or endocervical primary
  - Mucinous adenocarcinoma—endometrial or endocervical primary
- Diagnostic pitfalls/key intraoperative consultation issues
  - Absence of infiltrative growth and lack of significant cytological atypia separate florid microglandular hyperplasia from adenocarcinoma.
  - Endometrial microglandular adenocarcinoma, unlike MGH, is characterized by absence of a reserve cell layer, often presence of significant cytological atypia and continuity with endometrial rather than endocervical tissue

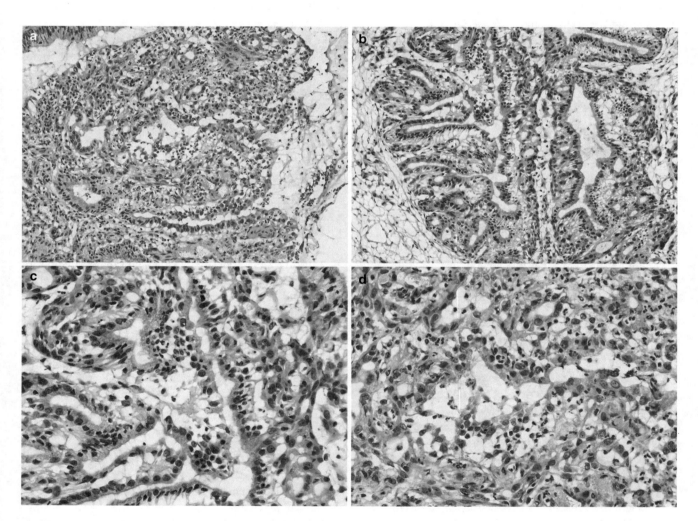

Fig. 3.6 Microglandular hyperplasia. Note the closely packed small- to medium-sized endocervical glands (**a**, **b**), uniform endocervical cells with noticeable reserve cell layer in some glands (**c**) and the presence of neutrophils in the stroma (**d**)

Chronic Endocervicitis

- Intense lymphoid hyperplasia with marked squamous metaplasia and secondary lymphoid follicle formation.
- Surface papillary epithelial proliferation with associated lymphoid follicles (papillary cervicitis) may be seen.
- Rarely, a lymphoid germinal center may be confused with high-grade squamous intraepithelial lesion involving endocervical glands, due to its pleomorphic lymphoid cell population and frequent mitotic activity.

Lymphoma-Like Lesions [7, 8]

- Adult patients.
- May present with vaginal bleeding or discharge.
- Thickened or erythematous, friable mucosa.
- Band-like subepithelial mixed lymphoid infiltrate consisting of reactive large centroblasts or immunoblasts and mature plasma cells.
- Lack of a mass lesion and deep involvement separates it from true lymphoma.

Arias-Stella Reaction [9]

- Generally focal, may appear papillary on gross examination.
- Enlarged glandular cells with abundant clear cytoplasm and apically located hyperchromatic nuclei (hobnail cells).
- The lesion may closely resemble clear cell carcinoma. The overall normal glandular distribution, degenerative nature of nuclei, absence of mitoses, and concurrent pregnancy or hormone use are typical features of Arias-Stella reaction.

Mesonephric Hyperplasia [10–12]

- Typically located at the lateral aspect of cervix.
- Glandular proliferation in a lobular or irregular distribution around a centrally located duct.
- Glands are lined by cuboidal or low columnar epithelial cells.
- No significant nuclear atypia or mitotic activity.
- Characteristic intraluminal dense eosinophilic secretion is present.
- Pseudostratification, papillary tufting, and bridging are compatible with benign mesonephric hyperplasia.
- Differential diagnosis
  - Mesonephric adenocarcinoma
- Diagnostic pitfalls/key intraoperative consultation issues
  - Diffuse mesonephric hyperplasia may pose a significant diagnostic challenge on frozen section.
  - Significant cytological atypia, desmoplastic stromal response, presence of luminal necrotic debris, perineu-

ral invasion, lymphovascular invasion, and haphazard infiltrative growth are features of mesonephric carcinoma.

Endocervicosis [13]

- Patients may have a history of uterine surgery (e.g., caesarean section).
- Nodular to cystic mass lesion consisting of variably sized and shaped glands infiltrating the outer cervical stroma.
- Columnar to flattened endocervical glandular cells without significant cytological atypia and absence of mitotic activity.
- Stromal response to extravasated mucin may be present.
- Differential diagnosis
  - Minimal deviation adenocarcinoma
  - Metastatic well-differentiated adenocarcinoma, particularly when the lesion also involves adjacent organs including bladder, cul-de-sac, and vaginal apex
- Diagnostic pitfalls/key intraoperative consultation issues
  - Separation of endocervicosis from an adenocarcinoma is based on lack of cytological atypia, mitosis, and stromal response.

Endometriosis

- Frequent lesion of the cervix.
- Deep cervical endometriosis is usually associated with pelvic endometriosis.
- Typical endometrial stroma with hemorrhage or hemosiderin pigment around proliferative-type endometrial glands.
- Differential diagnosis
  - Cervical adenocarcinoma in situ
- Diagnostic pitfalls/key intraoperative consultation issues
  - In contrast to cervical adenocarcinoma in situ, endometriosis lacks significant cytological atypia, nuclear stratification, apically located mitotic figures, and numerous apoptotic bodies.

Tubo-endometrial Metaplasia [14]

- Common lesion of the cervix and may be related to a prior cervical procedure (e.g., loop excision).
- Glands with tubal and/or endometrioid differentiation.
- Oxyphilic changes with increased eosinophilic cytoplasm and enlarged nuclei may be present.
- Absence of significant cytological atypia and mitotic activity and presence of tubal-type ciliated cells are helpful features separating tubo-endometrioid metaplasia from cervical adenocarcinoma in situ

Squamous Metaplasia

- Very common condition involving the cervical transformation zone or an endocervical polyp.
- Squamous metaplasia may be extensive, frequently involving endocervical glands, simulating squamous intraepithelial lesion or even invasive squamous cell carcinoma (Fig. 3.7).
- Papillary immature squamous metaplasia may simulate papillary squamous cell carcinoma.
- Frequently associated with marked inflammation.
- Absence of cytological atypia and stromal invasion confirm the diagnosis.

Transitional Metaplasia

- Typically occurs in peri- and postmenopausal women
- Transitional-type epithelial cells with small, oval nuclei replacing the full thickness of squamous epithelium
- Streaming of nuclei with frequent nuclear grooves
- Absence of significant cytological atypia and mitotic activity
- Differential diagnosis
  - High-grade squamous intraepithelial lesion (cervical intraepithelial neoplasia 3; CIN3)
- Diagnostic pitfalls/key intraoperative consultation issues
  - Unlike transitional metaplasia, high-grade dysplasia is characterized by loss of epithelial polarity, marked cytological atypia with increased nuclear to cytoplasmic ratio, and mitotic activity, often with atypical mitoses.

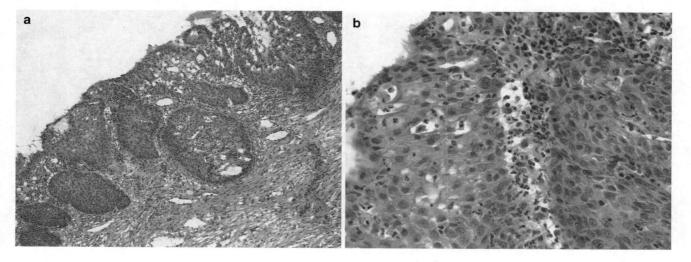

Fig. 3.7 Squamous metaplasia at the cervical transformation zone. Metaplastic squamous epithelium frequently extends into the endocervical glands (**a**). Note the absence of significant cytological atypia and lack of true stromal invasion (**b**)

Squamous Cell Carcinoma

Squamous Intraepithelial Lesion

- The most common precursor lesion of cervical squamous carcinoma.
- Almost always associated with human papillomavirus (HPV) infection, particularly high-risk HPV in high-grade intraepithelial lesion (HSIL).
- HSIL mostly occurs in patients in their mid twenties to mid thirties.
- Dysplastic squamous cells occupy at least 2/3 of the epithelium with loss of polarity in HSIL. Low grade intraepithelial lesion (LSIL) has dysplastic cells limited to the lower third of the epithelium.

- Histological features include nuclear enlargement, high nuclear/cytoplasmic ratio, coarse chromatin, thickened nuclear membrane, and easily identifiable mitoses and atypical mitoses in HSIL (Fig. 3.8).
- Differential diagnosis
  - Immature squamous metaplasia
  - Papillary squamous metaplasia
  - Transitional metaplasia
  - Reactive epithelial changes

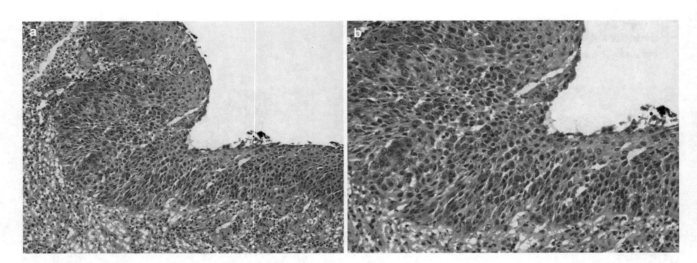

Fig. 3.8 High-grade squamous intraepithelial lesion (*HSIL*). Dysplastic squamous cells occupy approximately two-thirds of the epithelium (**a**, **b**)

Invasive Squamous Cell Carcinoma (SCC)

- Clinical features
  - Most common cervical cancer.
  - Associated with high-risk HPV infection and preceded by high-grade squamous intraepithelial lesion (HSIL).
  - Mean patient age is 55 years, but a third of cases occur in women less than 35 years of age.
  - Most common clinical symptoms are vaginal bleeding, discharge, and/or pelvic pain.
- Gross pathology (Fig. 3.9)
  - Pink, friable, commonly exophytic polypoid or papillary growth, or ulcerative surface lesion.
  - Almost always located at the cervical transformation zone.
  - Advanced tumors may show gross infiltration to various adjacent organs, e.g., parametrium, vagina, or uterine corpus.
- Microscopic features [15] (Fig. 3.10)
  - Proliferation of tumor cells in sheets and nests with anastomosing bands or single infiltrating cells.
  - Desmoplastic stromal response is common.
  - Tumor cells with variable amount of cytoplasm, large nuclei, and conspicuous nucleoli.
  - Keratinizing-type SCC
    - Shows obvious squamous maturation including keratin pearl formation
  - Nonkeratinizing-type SCC
    - Composed of medium-sized, atypical squamous cells without obvious keratin pearl formation, but individual tumor cell keratinization is often present
  - Superficially invasive SCC
    - Associated with HSIL and histologically similar to vulvar superficially invasive SCC (see Chap. 2)
    - Small irregular nests of highly atypical dysplastic epithelial cells, frequently with abrupt keratinization (paradoxical maturation)
    - Presence of stromal response, including stromal edema, desmoplasia, or prominent inflammatory changes
- Variants of squamous carcinoma [16–23]
  - Verrucous carcinoma
    - Highly differentiated variant with undulating surface simulating condyloma or squamous papilloma.
    - Hyperkeratosis is common.
    - Minimal cytological atypia and low mitotic activity.
    - Multiple tumor blocks may be required for frozen section evaluation to reveal its pushing and bulbous invasive border.
  - Warty SCC
    - Well-differentiated variant with a warty surface and architecture similar to condyloma

- Basaloid SCC
  - Aggressive tumor with characteristic peripheral palisading of primitive high-grade tumor cells.
  - Brisk mitotic activity and geographic necrosis.
  - Absence of stromal response.
  - Individual keratinization may be present, but keratin pearls are typically absent.
- Papillary squamous/squamotransitional carcinoma
  - Resembles urothelial carcinoma with high-grade cells arranged in papillary fronds with stromal cores.
  - Adequate sampling for frozen section is important to include the tumor base to rule out possible coexistence of an invasive component.
- Lymphoepitheliomatous variant
  - Syncytial growth of large tumor cells with vesicular nuclei, prominent nucleoli and surrounding marked inflammatory infiltrate
- Spindle cell or sarcomatoid SCC
  - Rare variant of SCC with more aggressive clinical behavior.
  - Histologically sarcomatoid spindle cell proliferation that may merge with conventional SCC.
  - It should be separated from malignant mixed Mullerian tumor (MMMT).
    - In contrast to spindle cell SCC, MMMT has distinct squamous carcinomatous and sarcomatous components without merging between the two.
- Differential diagnosis
  - HSIL extensively involving endocervical glands
  - Gestational trophoblastic lesions: epithelioid trophoblastic tumor, placental site nodule, and ectopic decidua
  - Clear cell carcinoma, solid variant vs. SCC with large amount of cytoplasmic glycogen
  - Neuroendocrine carcinoma, particularly small cell carcinoma vs. poorly differentiated SCC
  - Sarcomas vs. spindle cell/sarcomatoid SCC
  - Melanoma
  - Reactive and tumorlike conditions including exuberant squamous metaplasia, extensive inflammation, and pseudoinvasion of squamous epithelium induced by prior surgical procedure
- Diagnostic pitfalls/key intraoperative consultation issues
  - Trachelectomy procedure may be used for management of early cervical cancer in young patients [24].
    - At least 5 mm proximal surgical margin clearance is recommended and the margin status should be reported on frozen section evaluation [25].
  - Frozen section evaluation of a cervical cone excision is labor intensive and time consuming and may compromise precise characterization of the tumor. If

possible, discussion with submitting physician to defer for permanent sections should be attempted [26].

– Presence of HSIL with focal transition to spindled invasive component is a helpful hint for the diagnosis of spindle cell SCC.

  • Absence of sharply demarcated carcinomatous and sarcomatous components separates spindle cell SCC from malignant mixed Mullerian tumor.

– Microinvasive/superficially invasive SCC vs. HSIL involving endocervical glands.

  • Loss of peripheral palisading with markedly atypical cells, stromal response, and abrupt tumor cell keratinization (abnormal or paradoxical maturation) are features of invasion.

  • When in doubt, a frozen diagnosis of "high-grade squamous intraepithelial lesion, cannot rule out invasion" may be communicated to the surgeon.

– Sentinel lymph node evaluation for cervical cancer [27, 28]

  • Sentinel lymph node evaluation may be performed at the time of hysterectomy for cervical cancer.

• In the absence of uniform guidelines, grossly identifiable lymph nodes should be serially sectioned and submitted for frozen section evaluation followed by careful microscopic examination, particularly at the subcapsular sinus region to identify microscopic metastases (Fig. 3.11).

– Most common differential diagnosis of metastatic cervical carcinoma in a lymph node includes endosalpingiosis and endometriosis.

  • Both lesions lack malignant cytological atypia.

  • In contrast to subscapular sinus location of metastatic carcinoma, endosalpingiosis is found within the fibrous capsule of the lymph node [see Chap. 8] or nodal medullary sinuses.

  • Endometriosis may be found inside subscapular sinuses, and it is also associated with endometrial stroma around the glandular epithelium.

  • Other rare mimics include transported mesothelial cells within the nodal capsule and ectopic decidua in pregnant patients and should not be over-interpreted as metastatic disease.

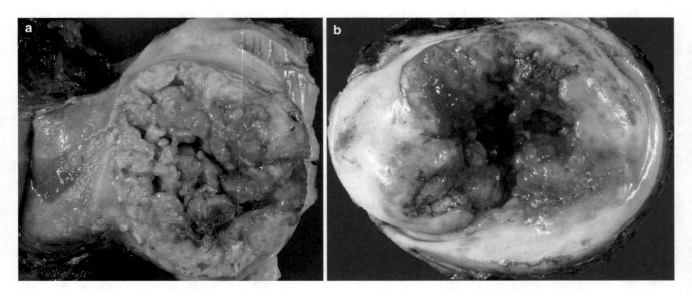

Fig. 3.9 Cervical invasive squamous cell carcinoma. Note the friable, exophytic mass lesions with hemorrhage and necrosis (**a, b**)

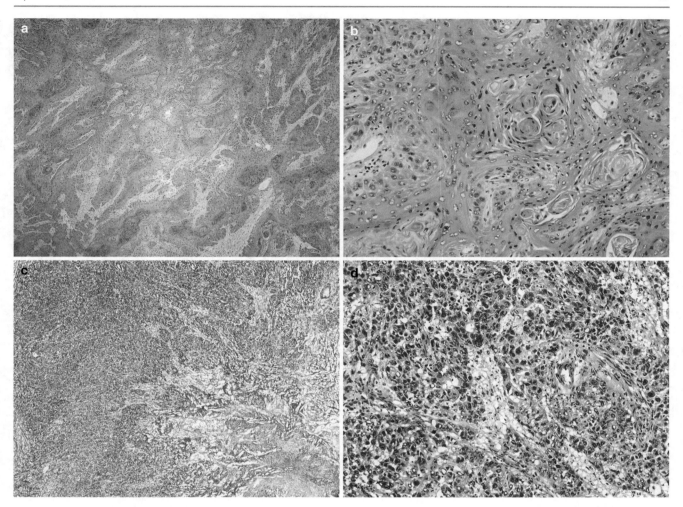

Fig. 3.10 Cervical invasive squamous cell carcinoma. Keratinizing well-differentiated (**a**, **b**) and poorly differentiated histological subtypes (**c**, **d**)

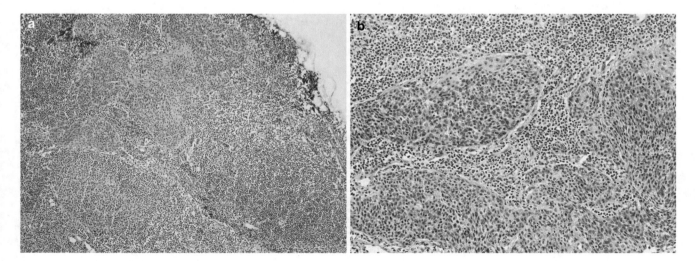

Fig. 3.11 Cervical squamous cell carcinoma metastasis in a regional lymph node (**a**, **b**)

Adenocarcinoma of the Cervix

Endocervical Adenocarcinoma In Situ (AIS) [24]

- Mostly seen in patients in their thirties and forties.
- History of abnormal glandular cells on Pap smear is often present.
- Most cases are associated with high-risk human papillomavirus (HPV) infection, mainly HPV 18.
- Primarily affects the transformation zone, frequently as multifocal and discontinuous "skip" lesions.
- Diagnosis of adenocarcinoma in situ should be made based on the presence of the following histological findings:
  - Cellular crowding with nuclear stratification.
  - Moderate to severe nuclear atypia including hyperchromasia and nucleomegaly.
  - Readily identifiable mitotic figures: often located in the apical portion of cells—"jumping mitoses"—and apoptotic bodies.
  - Additional features include intraglandular epithelial branching, budding or cribriforming.
- Three subtypes of AIS can be seen:
  - *Typical/usual AIS* with uniform zone of apical cytoplasmic mucin of the endocervical cells.
  - *Intestinal variant* with goblet cells and argentaffin and Paneth cells.
  - *Endometrioid variant* with lack of mucin production.
  - AIS may coexist with squamous intraepithelial lesion or invasive squamous cell carcinoma.
- Differential diagnosis
  - Early invasive endocervical adenocarcinoma
  - Endometrial adenocarcinoma extending to/involving endocervical mucosa
  - Reactive cytological atypia including radiation-induced cytological changes
  - Lower uterine segment endometrium (especially on trachelectomy margin evaluation)
  - Atypical oxyphilic change (metaplasia)
- Diagnostic pitfalls/key intraoperative consultation issues
  - Separation of AIS from early invasive adenocarcinoma can be difficult at the time of frozen section diagnosis (see below).
    - Frozen section diagnosis of "at least in situ adenocarcinoma, defer to permanent sections to rule out invasion" may suffice for intraoperative management.
  - Reactive cytological atypia may show nuclear enlargement and multinucleation without crowding and increased mitotic activity.

Invasive Endocervical Adenocarcinoma (Usual Type) [29]

- Clinical features
  - Represents 10–15 % of all cervical cancer.
  - Patients present with abnormal bleeding and mass lesion in 80 % of the cases.
- Gross pathology (Fig. 3.12)
  - Exophytic mass lesion is seen in around 50 % of the cases.
  - Ulcerative or infiltrative lesions leading to barrel-shaped cervix are not uncommon.
- Microscopic features
  - Endocervical adenocarcinoma (conventional or usual type) (Fig. 3.13) represents 80–90 % of all cervical adenocarcinomas.
  - Complex proliferation of medium-sized glands with angulated, papillary branching to cribriforming configurations.
  - Pseudostratified epithelial cells with eosinophilic to amphophilic cytoplasm and minimal mucin production.
  - Obvious nuclear atypia with conspicuous nucleoli, brisk mitotic activity with "jumping" mitotic figures in the apical zone of the epithelium and frequent apoptotic bodies are characteristic.
  - Common architectural variations include cribriforming, microcystic, microglandular, papillary villous, and solid growth patterns [30, 31].
- Differential diagnosis
  - Endocervical adenocarcinoma in situ
  - Endometrioid adenocarcinoma of the cervix
  - Villoglandular adenocarcinoma of the cervix
  - Endometrial carcinoma with cervical involvement
  - Metastatic adenocarcinoma
  - Various nonneoplastic glandular lesions including lobular or diffuse endocervical glandular hyperplasia, tunnel clusters, and microglandular hyperplasia.
- Diagnostic pitfalls/key intraoperative consultation issues
  - Separation of early invasive adenocarcinoma from extensive in situ adenocarcinoma is based on the neoplastic glands showing growth configurations incompatible with the normal endocervical glandular distribution, including:
    - Continuous or band-like growth of dysplastic glands involving large areas of cervical mucosa.
    - Glandular complexity including closely packed glands, marked variations of gland size and shape, and extensive cribriforming are highly suspicious for invasion.

- Deeply seated glands or glands in close proximity to larger vasculature.
- In some early invasive lesions, budding of single cells or clusters of dysplastic cells from an in situ adenocarcinoma along with stromal response is diagnostic of early invasion.
- Separation of AIS from early invasive adenocarcinoma can be difficult at the time of frozen section diagnosis (see below). Frozen section interpretation of "at least in situ adenocarcinoma, defer for permanent sections to rule out invasion" may suffice for clinical management.
– For trachelectomy procedures in early cervical adenocarcinoma of young patients (Fig. 3.14), at least 5 mm proximal surgical margin clearance is recommended [25].

– Separation of usual endocervical adenocarcinoma from endometrioid or villoglandular adenocarcinoma of the cervix is based on their distinct histological features (see below).
  - Precise separation of histological subtypes of invasive cervical adenocarcinoma is not critical for intraoperative surgical management.
– Superficial mucosal location, well-circumscribed border, and lack of the following: infiltrative growth, significant cytological atypia, mitotic activity, and stromal response, are features of nonneoplastic glandular lesions.

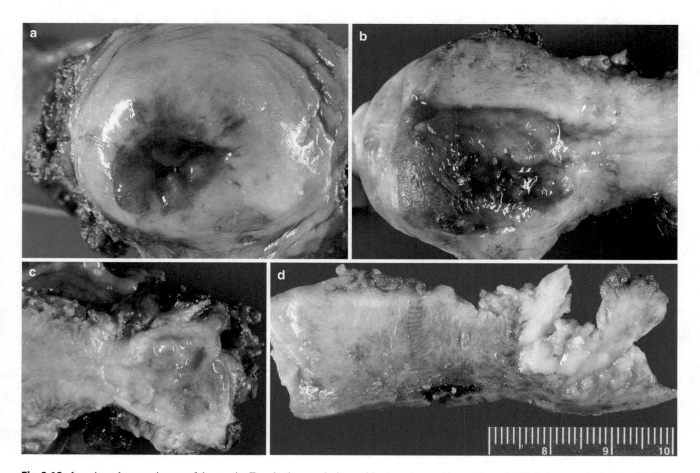

Fig. 3.12 Invasive adenocarcinoma of the cervix. Exophytic mass lesions with ulceration and hemorrhage (**a**, **b**) or deep cervical stromal infiltration (**c**, **d**)

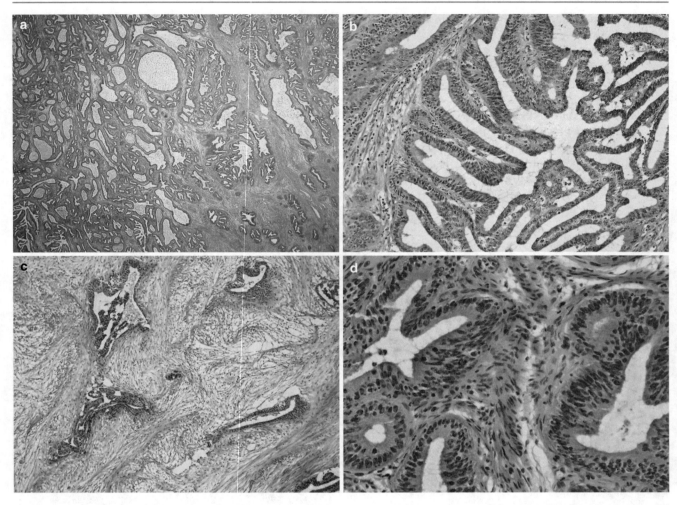

Fig. 3.13 Cervical adenocarcinoma, usual type. Note the complex glandular proliferation with angulated, papillary configuration (**a**, **b**) and infiltrative growth with desmoplastic stromal response (**c**). Pseudostratified mucin-poor epithelial cells have eosinophilic to amphophilic cytoplasm and many mitotic figures in the apical zone of the epithelium—"jumping mitotic figures" (**d**)

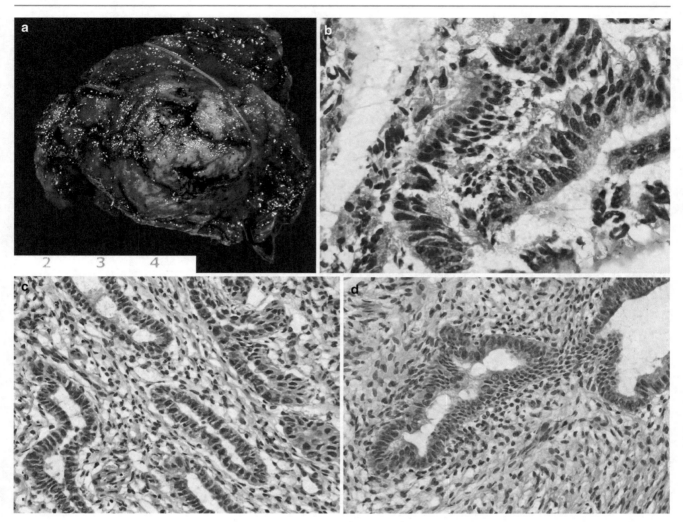

Fig. 3.14 Trachelectomy for endocervical adenocarcinoma. Appropriate specimen orientation is important for assessing the surgical (endocervical) margin involvement, e.g., inking the endocervical margin, (**a**). Endocervical adenocarcinoma shows hyperchromatic, enlarged nuclei, increased nuclear to cytoplasmic ratio, and loss of polarity (**b**). Benign glandular mimics include lower uterine segment endometrial glands (especially at the trachelectomy margin) (**c**) or tubal metaplastic epithelium (**d**)

Microscopic Variants of Cervical Adenocarcinoma

Villoglandular Adenocarcinoma [32]

- Commonly occurs in young women in their forties.
- Exophytic tumor without deep stromal invasion in most cases (Fig. 3.15).
- Histologically characterized by long and slender papillae, surfaced by flat tumor cells without tufting.
- Mild to moderately atypical cells of endocervical origin or endometrioid type in rare cases.

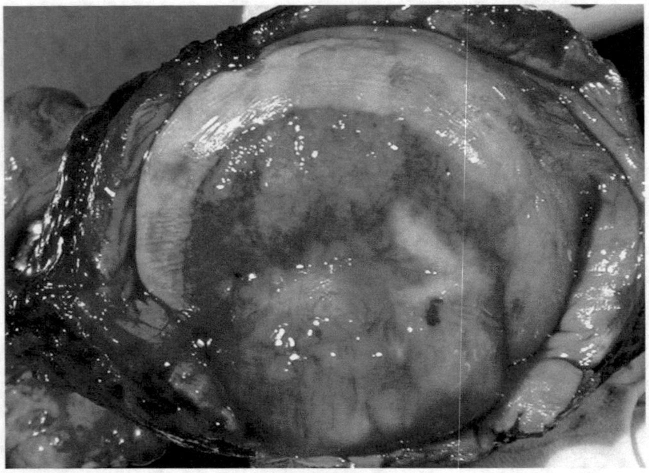

- Differential diagnosis includes serous and other types of adenocarcinoma.
- At the time of intraoperative frozen consultation, the presence of low nuclear grade, apical cytoplasmic clearing, and smooth luminal surface without tufting separate villoglandular adenocarcinoma from serous carcinoma.
  - Precise separation of histological subtypes of invasive cervical adenocarcinoma is not critical for intraoperative surgical management.

Fig. 3.15 Villoglandular adenocarcinoma of the cervix. Note the exophytic lesion with mucoid secretion involving the cervical os

Endometrioid Adenocarcinoma [29, 33]

- Rare histological subtype, which may be associated with cervical endometriosis.
- Endometrioid histology with various growth patterns and grades.
- Presence of ciliated tumor cells, squamous differentiation, and round to oval glands separates it from usual-type endocervical carcinoma.

- Diagnostic separation from an endometrial endometrioid carcinoma largely depends on the location of the tumor, absence of endometrial hyperplasia, and presence of associated cervical in situ carcinoma or foci of usual-type endocervical adenocarcinoma.
- Synchronous endocervical and endometrial adenocarcinomas can also occur. Careful morphologic assessment may identify the histological evidence of two distinctly different, independent primary tumors (Fig. 3.16a–d).

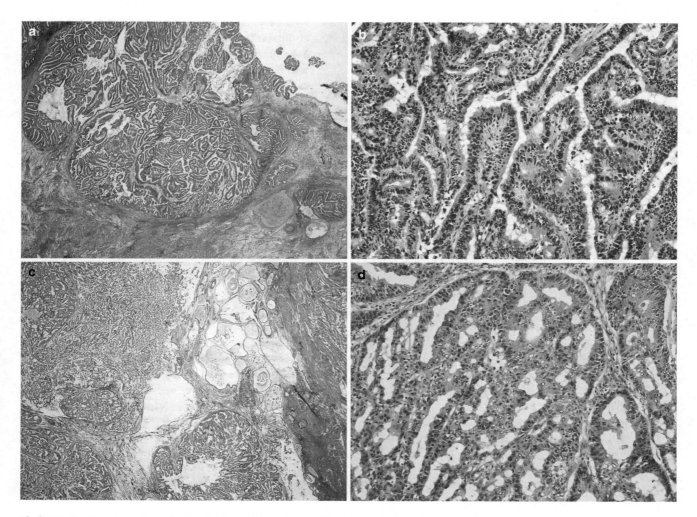

Fig. 3.16 Synchronous endocervical and endometrial carcinomas. Note the two independent tumors involving the cervix (usual-type endocervical adenocarcinoma) (**a, b**) and the endometrium (well-differentiated endometrioid carcinoma) (**c, d**)

Mucinous Carcinomas

- *Mucinous carcinomas* are recognized by their cytoplasmic mucin content in contrast to the minimal mucin production of usual-type endocervical adenocarcinomas [2].
  - *Intestinal-type mucinous adenocarcinoma* resembles colorectal adenocarcinoma and is histologically characterized by the presence of goblet cells and Paneth cells.
  - *Gastric-type mucinous adenocarcinoma* is featured by simple, but irregular to cystic glands of variable sizes. Cribriform to focal solid patterns may also be seen. The tumor cells have distinct cell borders and contain abundant clear to eosinophilic apical cytoplasm and basally located nuclei with obvious nuclear atypia.
  - *Mucinous carcinoma of signet-ring type consists* of focal or diffuse signet-ring cells [34].
  - *Minimal deviation adenocarcinoma (adenoma malignum or well-differentiated mucinous carcinoma of gastric type).*
    - Rare mucinous carcinoma with deceptively benign-looking glands.
    - Firm indurated mass leading to barrel-shaped cervix.
    - Deep invasion of haphazardly distributed open glands of highly variable sizes and unusual shapes is characteristic (Fig. 3.17).
    - Tumor cells contain abundant mucin with basally located nuclei.
    - Unequivocal dysplastic glands and/or single or clusters of infiltrating tumor cells with stromal response (Fig. 3.18).
    - Close juxtaposition of glands to large caliber vessels, involvement of lower uterine segment myometrium or parametrium, and presence of lymphovascular or perineural invasion.
- Differential diagnosis
  - Endocervical glandular hyperplasia of either lobular or diffuse type
  - Endocervicosis
  - Tunnel clusters
  - Mesonephric hyperplasia
  - Mesonephric adenocarcinoma
  - Cervical involvement by mucinous endometrial adenocarcinoma
- Diagnostic pitfalls/key intraoperative consultation issues
  - Separation from various nonneoplastic conditions is based on their superficial mucosal location, well-circumscribed border, and lack of infiltrative growth, significant cytological atypia, mitotic activity, and stromal response.
  - Separation from mesonephric and mucinous carcinomas is based on their distinct histological features (see each subheading), although such distinction is not crucial at the time of intraoperative consultation.

Glassy Cell Carcinoma [35]

- Occurs in young patients less than 35 years of age
- Sheets of large, poorly differentiated tumor cells with abundant homogenous eosinophilic or amphophilic cytoplasm with distinct cell borders
- Large round to oval nuclei with prominent macronucleoli, brisk mitotic activity, and presence of dense inflammatory infiltrate (eosinophils, lymphocytes, and plasma cells)
- Differential diagnosis
  - Squamous cell carcinoma of large cell nonkeratinizing type
  - Undifferentiated carcinoma
  - Lymphoepithelioma-like carcinoma
- Diagnostic pitfalls/key intraoperative consultation issues
  - Diagnostic separation from carcinomas of other histological subtypes is based on their distinct histology features (see each subheading), although such distinction is not crucial at the time of intraoperative consultation.

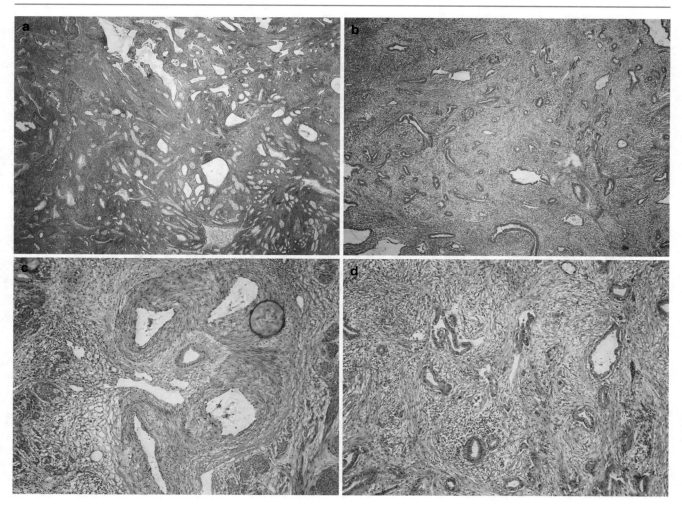

Fig. 3.17 Minimal deviation adenocarcinoma, gastric type. Note the deceptively benign-looking glands deeply invading the cervical stroma in a haphazard fashion (**a**, **b**) with focal close juxtaposition to large caliber vessels (**c**) and stromal response (**d**)

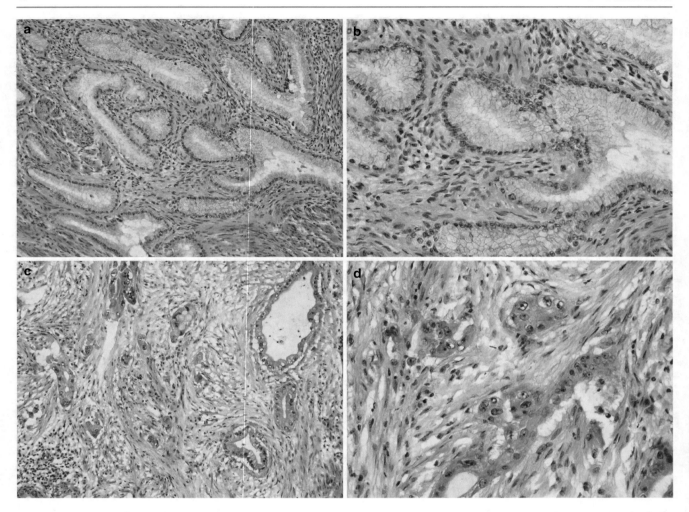

Fig. 3.18 Minimal deviation adenocarcinoma, gastric type. Note the abnormally shaped glands (**a**), abundant cytoplasmic mucin and basally located nuclei (**b**), and foci of infiltrating, markedly atypical cells in singles or clusters with stromal response (**c**, **d**)

Adenosquamous Carcinoma [36]

- Variant of cervical carcinoma with both squamous and glandular differentiation and a more aggressive clinical behavior.
- Unequivocal gland formation must be present for the diagnosis (Fig. 3.19).
- May coexist with high-grade squamous intraepithelial lesion and adenocarcinoma in situ.
- Differential diagnosis
  - Squamous cell carcinoma with cytoplasmic mucin
  - Usual-type adenocarcinoma with focal squamous differentiation (metaplasia)
  - Squamous cell carcinoma with clear cell change
- Diagnostic pitfalls/key intraoperative consultation issues
  - Diagnostic separation from carcinomas of other histological subtypes is based on their distinct histological features (see each subheading), although such distinction is not crucial at the time of intraoperative consultation.

Adenoid Basal Carcinoma [37, 38]

- Mostly occurs in postmenopausal patients.
- The tumor usually does not reach the mucosal surface.
- Lobules of widely spaced round to oval nests of small uniform cells with peripheral palisading, resembling basal cell carcinoma.
- Central cyst formation with squamous or glandular differentiation.
- Frequently associated with surface high-grade squamous intraepithelial lesion (HSIL).
- Differential diagnosis
  - Adenoid cystic carcinoma
  - Benign adenoid basal hyperplasia
- Diagnostic pitfalls/key intraoperative consultation issues
  - Absence of pseudocysts and intraluminal hyalin material are helpful features for separation from adenoid cystic carcinoma.
  - Adenoid basal hyperplasia is a benign lesion simulating adenoid basal carcinoma, but is limited to within 0.5 mm of the overlying mucosal surface with direct surface extension.

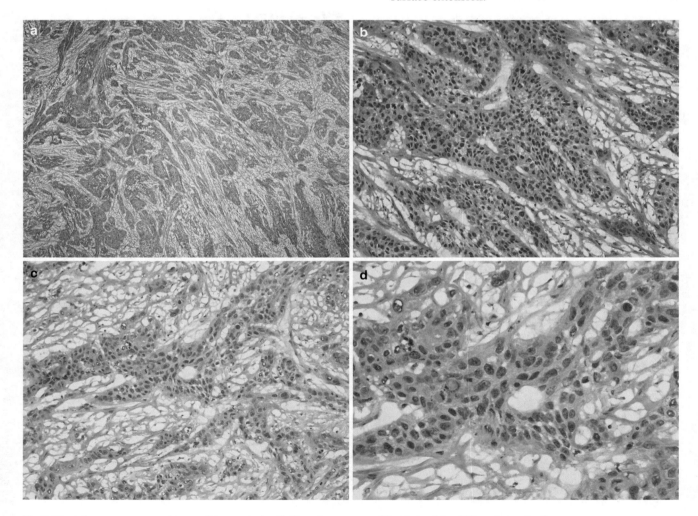

Fig. 3.19 Adenosquamous carcinoma of the cervix (**a–d**). Note the presence of focal glandular differentiation (**c**, **d**)

Adenoid Cystic Carcinoma [37]

- Round to oval tumor nests with characteristic cribriform-ing due to the presence of bluish pseudocysts/cylindrical hyaline basement membrane material.
- Palisading of tumor cells along the basement membrane is often found.
- Small basaloid cells of varying sizes with angulated nuclei and high nuclear to cytoplasmic ratio.
- Lymphovascular invasion is common.
- Differential diagnosis
  - Adenoid basal carcinoma (see above)
  - Basaloid squamous cell carcinoma with adenoid cystic carcinoma-like growth pattern
- Diagnostic pitfalls/key intraoperative consultation issues
  - Diagnostic separation from the above entities is based on their distinct histological features (see each subheading), although such distinction is not crucial at the time of intraoperative consultation.

Mesonephric Adenocarcinoma [10]

- Typically presents with vaginal bleeding in patients in their fifties.
- Exophytic or infiltrative mass lesion with frequent deep invasion into the lateral cervical wall (Fig. 3.20).
- Generally ductal growth pattern with tubular glands of varying sizes.
- Intraluminal eosinophilic secretion is characteristic.
- Papillary, endometrioid, retiform, sex-cord-like, or spindled solid patterns may be seen focally or diffusely in some cases (Fig. 3.21)
- The neoplastic glands are lined by a single layer of non-mucinous cuboidal cells.
- Cytological atypia may be minimal, but careful search usually helps identifying individual or clustered tumor cells with overt atypia in most cases, particularly in association with desmoplastic stromal response.
- Differential diagnosis
  - Benign mesonephric hyperplasia
  - Usual-type endocervical adenocarcinoma
  - Clear cell carcinoma
  - Endometrioid carcinoma
  - Minimal deviation adenocarcinoma

- Diagnostic pitfalls/key intraoperative consultation issues
  - Presence of deep and haphazard infiltration involving the outer third of the cervical wall, areas of desmoplastic stromal response with associated individual or clusters of overtly malignant cells, intraluminal necrotic debris, easily identifiable mitotic figures, and perineural and vascular wall invasion are in favor of mesonephric carcinoma over hyperplasia.
  - Tubulocystic growth pattern and clear cells with hobnailed nuclei are not features of mesonephric adenocarcinoma, rather are commonly seen in clear cell carcinoma.
  - The presence of adjacent mesonephric hyperplasia or remnants may help separating mesonephric adenocarcinoma from endometrioid adenocarcinoma of the cervix.
  - Diagnostic separation from other types of cervical carcinomas is not crucial at the time of intraoperative consultation.

Serous Carcinoma [39]

- The incidence of primary cervical serous carcinoma has two peaks: reproductive age of <40 years and postmenopausal population over 65 years of age.
- Vaginal bleeding and abnormal Pap smear are the most common clinical findings.
- Gross and microscopic features are similar to those of endometrial serous carcinoma.
- Differential diagnosis
  - Usual endocervical adenocarcinoma
  - Secondary involvement by primary endometrial serous carcinoma
- Diagnostic pitfalls/key intraoperative consultation issues
  - In contrast to serous carcinoma, usual endocervical adenocarcinoma has relatively uniform tumor cells and lesser degree of nuclear atypia.
  - Frozen section diagnostic separation from primary endometrial serous carcinoma relies on the absence—or minimal extent—of uterine corpus lesion.
  - While cervical serous carcinoma can occur in patients younger than 40 years old, primary endometrial serous carcinoma in this age group is exceedingly rare.

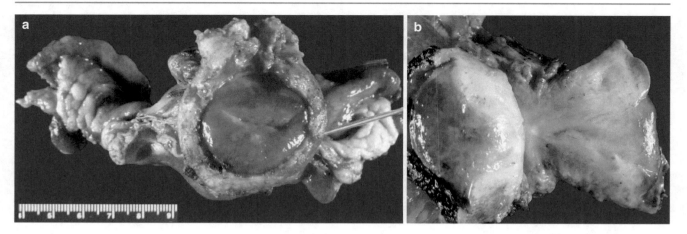

Fig. 3.20 Mesonephric adenocarcinoma of the cervix. Note the diffuse enlargement of the cervical wall by tumor infiltration in this example (**a**, **b**)

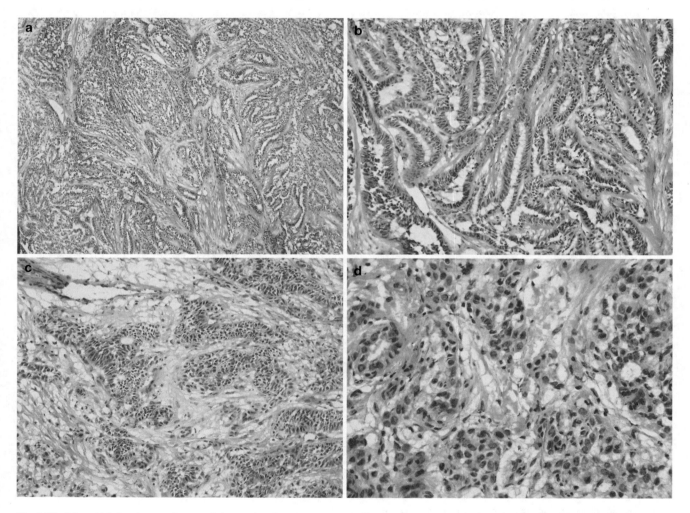

Fig. 3.21 Mesonephric adenocarcinoma of the cervix. Note the tubular glands of varying sizes lined by uniform epithelial tumor cells with mild cytological atypia (**a–d**)

Clear Cell Carcinoma [40]

- High-grade adenocarcinoma, that is histologically identical to that of the endometrium.
- Cervical clear cell carcinoma related to DES exposure is seen in patients of less than 20 years of age and is rare nowadays. Sporadic clear cell carcinoma occurs in peri- and postmenopausal populations.
- Most common growth pattern is tubulocystic.
- Differential diagnosis
  - Microglandular hyperplasia
  - Arias-Stella reaction
  - Serous carcinoma
  - Mesonephric adenocarcinoma
- Diagnostic pitfalls/key intraoperative consultation issues
  - Separation from nonneoplastic conditions is based on the presence of a mass lesion, infiltrative growth, significant cytological atypia, mitotic activity, and stromal response
  - Diagnostic separation from mesonephric or serous carcinomas is not crucial at the time of intraoperative consultation.

Neuroendocrine Carcinomas [41–43]

- Very rare cervical malignancies (<4 % of all cervical cancers).
- Low-grade neuroendocrine tumor (typical and atypical carcinoid tumors or grade 1 and 2 neuroendocrine tumors) is very rare and is histologically identical to those seen in the gastrointestinal tract.
  - Grade 1 neuroendocrine tumor is characterized by its organoid, insular, nested, or trabecular growth of small uniform cells with abundant cytoplasm, granular chromatin, and visible nucleoli. Moderate nuclear atypia and mitotic activity define a grade 2 neuroendocrine tumor.
- High-grade neuroendocrine carcinomas include small cell and large cell neuroendocrine carcinomas (Fig. 3.22).
  - They occur at a wide range of age from 20s to 80s.
  - *High-grade neuroendocrine carcinoma of the small cell type* is similar to small cell carcinoma of the lung, consisting of nests to sheets of monotonous proliferation of small cells with minimal cytoplasm, dense chromatin, inconspicuous nucleoli, and nuclear molding. Mitoses and apoptotic bodies are numerous. Single to extensive tumor cell necrosis with frequent crushing artifact is common, so is lymphovascular invasion.
  - *High-grade neuroendocrine carcinoma of the large cell type* is characterized by medium to large, highly atypical cells with abundant cytoplasm and numerous mitoses. Geographic necrosis, peripheral nuclear palisading, and cytoplasmic granules are common findings. Focal glandular formation may be present.
- Differential diagnosis
  - Serous carcinoma
  - Poorly differentiated adenocarcinoma
  - Basaloid squamous cell carcinoma
- Diagnostic pitfalls/key intraoperative consultation issues
  - Frozen diagnostic separation of the two types of high-grade neuroendocrine carcinoma or distinction from other cervical cancers is not crucial for intraoperative surgical management.

Metastatic Carcinomas

- Various malignant tumors may metastasize to the cervix.
- The most common primary sites include endometrium, breast, and gastrointestinal tract.
- Cervical involvement by endometrial carcinoma is primarily a result of direct extension, but mucosal colonization by detached fragments of endometrial carcinoma may also occur, leading to skip tumor involvement ("drop metastasis").
  - When endometrial endometrioid adenocarcinoma extends to the cervical stroma, the tumor may assume a deceptively mature appearance simulating a benign process (see Chap. 4).
- Cervical involvement by metastatic breast carcinoma generally presents as diffuse tumor spread that may also involve multiple other gynecologic organs (see Chap. 4).
- Cervical involvement by primary colonic adenocarcinoma usually results from direct extension.
- Diagnostic pitfalls/key intraoperative consultation issues
  - In patients with a history of malignancy at other sites, morphologic comparison with the prior specimen(s)—if available at the time of frozen section—should be pursued.

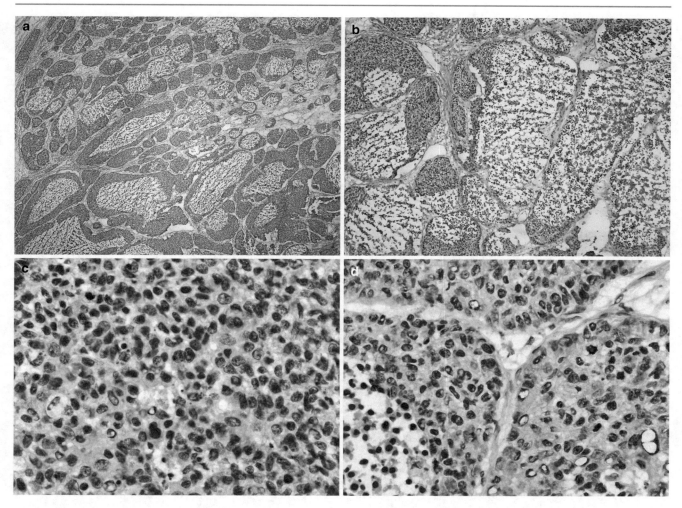

Fig. 3.22 Large cell neuroendocrine carcinoma of the cervix. Large sheets (**a**) of highly atypical cells with nuclear molding, brisk mitotic activity, geographic necrosis, and peripheral nuclear palisading (**b–d**)

Mesenchymal Tumors and Mixed Epithelial and Mesenchymal Tumors

Smooth Muscle Tumors

- Leiomyoma occasionally occurs in the cervix (Fig. 3.23).
- Primary cervical leiomyosarcoma is exceedingly rare.
- The diagnostic criteria essentially follow those of uterine smooth muscle tumors (Fig. 3.24).

Mullerian Adenosarcoma

- Patients present with vaginal bleeding and may have history of recurrent cervical polyps.
- Grossly polypoid endocervical mass.
- Histologically biphasic tumor consisting of cystic glands surrounded by low-grade cellular stromal condensation (cuffing) with frequent papillary intraglandular infoldings.
- Mitotic figures are present (generally >2/10 HPF) and are best identified within the hypercellular periglandular areas.

- Mullerian-type glandular epithelium (endocervical, proliferative endometrial, or tubal epithelium) with mild to moderate cytological atypia.
- Areas of hypocellular stroma and marked hyalinization may be seen.
- Sarcomatous overgrowth is diagnosed when the pure sarcomatous element comprises at least 25 % of the tumor, often showing high-grade morphology [44].
- Differential diagnosis
  - Malignant mixed Mullerian tumor (carcinosarcoma)
  - Adenofibroma
  - Endocervical polyp
- Diagnostic pitfalls/key intraoperative consultation issues
  - Absence of a sharply demarcated malignant epithelial component separates adenosarcoma from malignant mixed Mullerian tumor.
  - Unlike adenosarcoma, benign endocervical polyp and adenofibroma are characterized by absence of periglandular stromal cell condensation and lack of epithelial atypia and stromal mitotic activity.

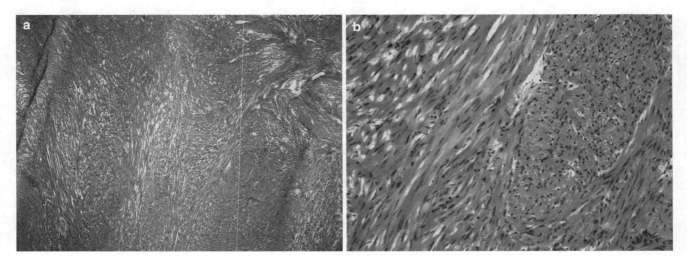

Fig. 3.23 Cervical leiomyoma (**a**, **b**). Typical proliferation of mature smooth muscle cells of benign leiomyoma

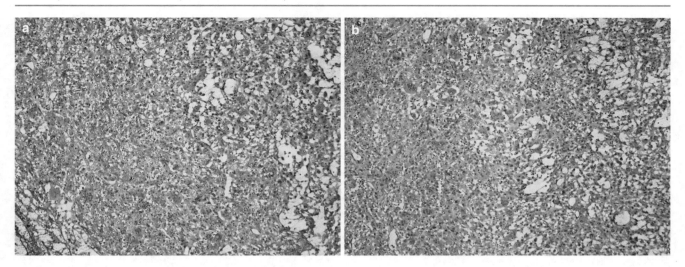

Fig. 3.24 Cervical primary high-grade epithelioid leiomyosarcoma (**a**, **b**). Note the highly pleomorphic proliferation of large epithelioid cells with striking nuclear atypia, multinucleation, and tumor cell necrosis

Malignant Mixed Mullerian Tumor (Carcinosarcoma)

- Most often occurs in postmenopausal patients, presenting with vaginal bleeding.
- Large polypoid mass protruding from the cervical os.
- Histologically sharply demarcated carcinoma and sarcoma components.

- Carcinomatous component is generally of endocervical type (usual cervical adenocarcinoma, squamous cell carcinoma or adenoid basal carcinoma) (Fig. 3.25).
- Sarcomatous component is often of homologous type, including fibrosarcoma or endometrial stromal sarcoma.
- Differential diagnosis includes Mullerian adenosarcoma (see above).

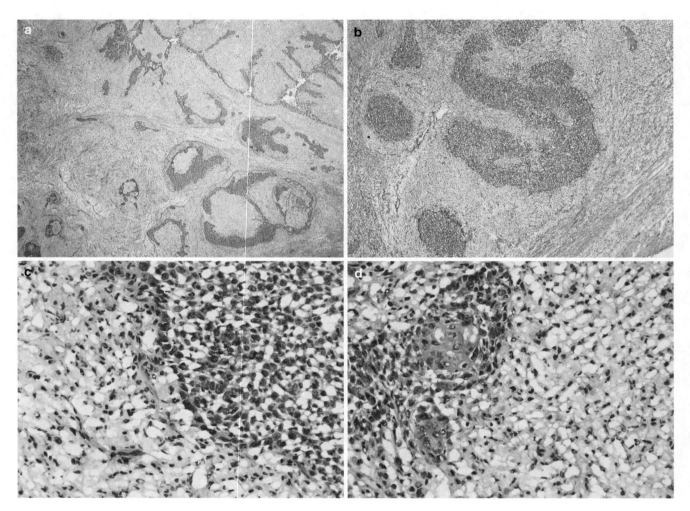

Fig. 3.25 Cervical malignant mixed Mullerian tumor (MMMT). Note the poorly differentiated squamous carcinoma as the epithelial component and homologous sarcoma as the mesenchymal component in this example (**a–d**)

Lymphomas

- Diffuse large B-cell lymphoma is the most common lymphoma involving the cervix [45].
- Clinically presents with constitutional symptoms (low-grade fever, night sweats, and weight loss) and elevated serum LDH.
- Diffuse or nodular enlargement of the cervix with white-tan, soft, fleshy cut surface (Fig. 3.26).
- Histologically the tumor consists of diffuse proliferation of medium to large atypical lymphoid cells (Fig. 3.27a–c).
- Touch cytology preparation may help identifying atypical lymphoid cells (Fig. 3.27d).
- Differential diagnosis
  - Poorly differentiated carcinoma
  - Lymphoepitheliomatous SCC
  - Reactive lymphoid hyperplasia
- Diagnostic pitfalls/key intraoperative consultation issues
  - High index of suspicion at the time of frozen section diagnosis is important to avoid misinterpretation as poorly differentiated carcinoma and unnecessary surgical staging.
  - Unlike diffuse large B-cell lymphoma, poorly differentiated carcinoma has nested growth pattern and lacks cytological features of atypical lymphoid cells.
  - In contrast to large B-cell lymphoma, lymphepitheliomatous SCC has a syncytial growth of large epithelial cells with significant amount of cytoplasm and lack of cytological features of atypical lymphoid cells.
  - Reactive lymphoid hyperplasia does not form a mass lesion and shows well-defined reactive germinal centers and a background of mixed small lymphocytes and plasma cells.
  - When the diagnosis of lymphoma is suspected, fresh tissue sample should be triaged for additional hematopathology diagnostic workup at the time of intraoperative consultation.

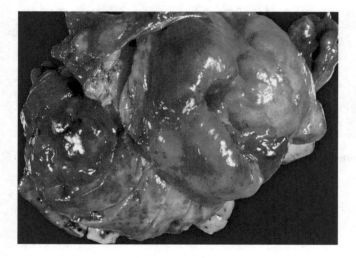

Fig. 3.26 Diffuse large B-cell lymphoma (*DLBCL*). Note the diffuse gross involvement of the cervix

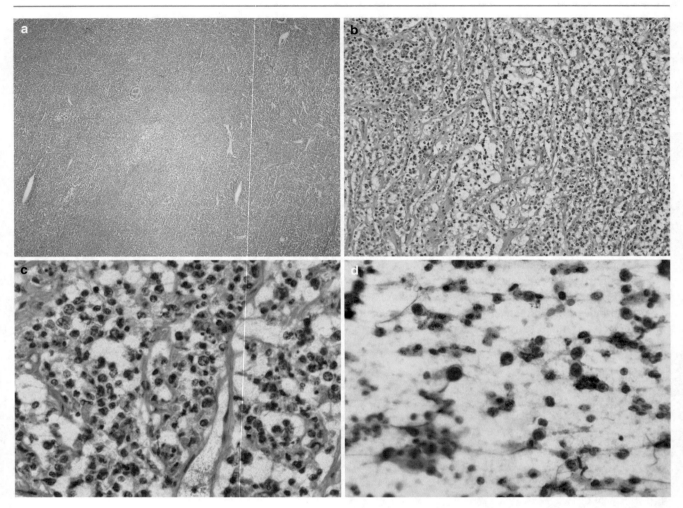

Fig. 3.27 Diffuse large B-cell lymphoma (*DLBCL*). Note the diffuse proliferation of atypical lymphoid cells of various sizes (**a–c**) and the presence of atypical lymphoblasts in the touch cytological preparation (**d**)

References

1. Arbyn M, Castellsagué X, de Sanjosé S, Bruni L, Saraiya M, Bray F, Ferlay J. Worldwide burden of cervical cancer in 2008. Ann Oncol. 2011;22:2675–86.
2. Mikami Y, McCluggage WG. Endocervical glandular lesions exhibiting gastric differentiation: an emerging spectrum of benign, premalignant, and malignant lesions. Adv Anat Pathol. 2013;20:227–37.
3. Jones MA, Young RH, Scully RE. Diffuse laminar endocervical glandular hyperplasia. A benign lesion often confused with adenoma malignum (minimal deviation adenocarcinoma). Am J Surg Pathol. 1991;15:1123–9.
4. Young RH, Clement PB. Pseudoneoplastic glandular lesions of the uterine cervix. Semin Diagn Pathol. 1991;8:234–49.
5. Abi-Raad R, Alomari A, Hui P, Buza N. Mitotically active microglandular hyperplasia of the cervix: a case series with implications for the differential diagnosis. Int J Gynecol Pathol. 2014;33:524–30.
6. Young RH, Scully RE. Atypical forms of microglandular hyperplasia of the cervix simulating carcinoma. A report of five cases and review of the literature. Am J Surg Pathol. 1989;13:50–6.
7. Ma J, Shi QL, Zhou XJ. Lymphoma-like lesion of the uterine cervix: report of 12 cases of a rare entity. Int J Gynecol Pathol. 2007;26(2):194–8.
8. Geyer JT, Ferry JA, Harris NL, Young RH, Longtine JA, Zukerberg LR. Florid reactive lymphoid hyperplasia of the lower female genital tract (lymphoma-like lesion): a benign condition that frequently harbors clonal immunoglobulin heavy chain gene rearrangements. Am J Surg Pathol. 2010;34:161–8.
9. Nucci MR, Young RH. Arias-Stella reaction of the endocervix: a report of 18 cases with emphasis on its varied histology and differential diagnosis. Am J Surg Pathol. 2004;28:608–12.
10. Silver SA, Devouassoux-Shisheboran M, Mezzetti TP, Tavassoli FA. Mesonephric adenocarcinomas of the uterine cervix: a study of 11 cases with immunohistochemical findings. Am J Surg Pathol. 2001;25:379–87.
11. Ferry JA, Scully RE. Mesonephric remnants, hyperplasia, and neoplasia in the uterine cervix. A study of 49 cases. Am J Surg Pathol. 1990;14:1100–11.
12. Seidman JD, Tavassoli FA. Mesonephric hyperplasia of the uterine cervix: a clinicopathologic study of 51 cases. Int J Gynecol Pathol. 1995;14:293–9.
13. Young RH, Clement PB. Endocervicosis involving the uterine cervix: a report of four cases of a benign process that may be confused with deeply invasive endocervical adenocarcinoma. Int J Gynecol Pathol. 2000;19:322–8.
14. Oliva E, Clement PB, Young RH. Tubal and tubo-endometrioid metaplasia of the uterine cervix. Unemphasized features that may cause problems in differential diagnosis: a report of 25 cases. Am J Clin Pathol. 1995;103:618–23.
15. Kurman RJ, Carcanglu ML, Herrington CS, Young RH. WHO classification of tumours of female reproductive organs. 4th ed. Lyon: International Agency for Research on Cancer (IARC); 2014.
16. Degefu S, O'Quinn AG, Lacey CG, Merkel M, Barnard DE. Verrucous carcinoma of the cervix: a report of two cases and literature review. Gynecol Oncol. 1986;25:37–47.
17. Grayson W, Cooper K. A reappraisal of "basaloid carcinoma" of the cervix, and the differential diagnosis of basaloid cervical neoplasms. Adv Anat Pathol. 2002;9:290–300.
18. Mirhashemi R, Ganjei-Azar P, Nadji M, Lambrou N, Atamdede F, Averette HE. Papillary squamous cell carcinoma of the uterine cervix: an immunophenotypic appraisal of 12 cases. Gynecol Oncol. 2003;90:657–61.
19. Martorell MA, Julian JM, Calabuig C, Garcia-Garcia JA, Perez-Valles A. Lymphoepithelioma-like carcinoma of the uterine cervix. Arch Pathol Lab Med. 2002;126:1501–5.
20. Steeper TA, Piscioli F, Rosai J. Squamous cell carcinoma with sarcoma-like stroma of the female genital tract. Clinicopathologic study of four cases. Cancer. 1983;52:890–8.
21. Young RH, Oliva E. Transitional cell carcinomas of the urinary bladder that may be underdiagnosed. A report of four invasive cases exemplifying the homology between neoplastic and non-neoplastic transitional cell lesions. Am J Surg Pathol. 1996;20:1448–54.
22. Willett GD, Kurman RJ, Reid R, Greenberg M, Jensen AB, Lorincz AT. Correlation of the histologic appearance of intraepithelial neoplasia of the cervix with human papillomavirus types. Emphasis on low grade lesions including so-called flat condyloma. Int J Gynecol Pathol. 1989;8:18–25.
23. Brinck U, Jakob C, Bau O, Fuzesi L. Papillary squamous cell carcinoma of the uterine cervix: report of three cases and a review of its classification. Int J Gynecol Pathol. 2000;19:231–5.
24. Martinelli F, Schmeler KM, Johnson C, Brown J, Euscher ED, Ramirez PT, Frumovitz M. Utility of conization with frozen section for intraoperative triage prior to definitive hysterectomy. Gynecol Oncol. 2012;127:307–11.
25. Ismiil N, Ghorab Z, Covens A, Nofech-Mozes S, Saad R, Dubé V, Khalifa MA. Intraoperative margin assessment of the radical trachelectomy specimen. Gynecol Oncol. 2009;113:42–6.
26. Gu M, Lin F. Efficacy of cone biopsy of the uterine cervix during frozen section for the evaluation of cervical intraepithelial neoplasia grade 3. Am J Clin Pathol. 2004;122:383–8.
27. Jewell EL, Huang JJ, Abu-Rustum NR, Gardner GJ, Brown CL, Sonoda Y, et al. Detection of sentinel lymph nodes in minimally invasive surgery using indocyanine green and near-infrared fluorescence imaging for uterine and cervical malignancies. Gynecol Oncol. 2014;133:274–7.
28. Kadkhodayan S, Hasanzadeh M, Treglia G, Azad A, Yousefi Z, Zarifmahmoudi L, Sadeghi R. Sentinel node biopsy for lymph nodal staging of uterine cervix cancer: a systematic review and meta-analysis of the pertinent literature. Eur J Surg Oncol. 2015;41:1–20.
29. Young RH, Clement PB. Endocervical adenocarcinoma and its variants: their morphology and differential diagnosis. Histopathology. 2002;41:185–207.
30. Young RH, Scully RE. Uterine carcinomas simulating microglandular hyperplasia. A report of six cases. Am J Surg Pathol. 1992;16:1092–7.
31. Tambouret R, Bell DA, Young RH. Microcystic endocervical adenocarcinomas: a report of eight cases. Am J Surg Pathol. 2000;24:369–74.
32. Young RH, Scully RE. Villoglandular papillary adenocarcinoma of the uterine cervix. A clinicopathologic analysis of 13 cases. Cancer. 1989;63:1773–9.
33. Jiang L, Malpica A, Deavers MT, Guo M, Villa LL, Nuovo G, et al. Endometrial endometrioid adenocarcinoma of the uterine corpus involving the cervix: some cases probably represent independent primaries. Int J Gynecol Pathol. 2010;29:146–56.
34. Balci S, Saglam A, Usubutun A. Primary signet-ring cell carcinoma of the cervix: case report and review of the literature. Int J Gynecol Pathol. 2010;29:181–4.
35. Kato N, Katayama Y, Kaimori M, Motoyama T. Glassy cell carcinoma of the uterine cervix: histochemical, immunohistochemical, and molecular genetic observations. Int J Gynecol Pathol. 2002;21:134–40.
36. Samlal RA, Ten Kate FJ, Hart AA, Lammes FB. Do mucin-secreting squamous cell carcinomas of the uterine cervix metastasize more frequently to pelvic lymph nodes? A case-control study? Int J Gynecol Pathol. 1998;17:201–4.

37. Parwani AV, Smith Sehdev AE, Kurman RJ, Ronnett BM. Cervical adenoid basal tumors comprised of adenoid basal epithelioma associated with various types of invasive carcinoma: clinicopathologic features, human papillomavirus DNA detection, and P16 expression. Hum Pathol. 2005;36:82–90.

38. Ferry JA. Adenoid basal carcinoma of the uterine cervix: evolution of a distinctive clinicopathologic entity. Int J Gynecol Pathol. 1997;16:299–300.

39. Zhou C, Gilks CB, Hayes M, Clement PB. Papillary serous carcinoma of the uterine cervix: a clinicopathologic study of 17 cases. Am J Surg Pathol. 1998;22:113–20.

40. Thomas MB, Wright JD, Leiser AL, Chi DS, Mutch DG, Podratz KC, Dowdy SC. Clear cell carcinoma of the cervix: a multi-institutional review in the post-DES era. Gynecol Oncol. 2008;109:335–9.

41. McCluggage WG, Kennedy K, Busam KJ. An immunohistochemical study of cervical neuroendocrine carcinomas: neoplasms that are commonly TTF1 positive and which may express CK20 and P63. Am J Surg Pathol. 2010;34:525–32.

42. Gilks CB, Young RH, Gersell DJ, Clement PB. Large cell neuroendocrine [corrected] carcinoma of the uterine cervix: a clinicopathologic study of 12 cases. Am J Surg Pathol. 1997;21:905–14.

43. Rekhi B, Patil B, Deodhar KK, Maheswari A, Kerkar RA, Gupta S, et al. Spectrum of neuroendocrine carcinomas of the uterine cervix, including histopathologic features, terminology, immunohistochemical profile, and clinical outcomes in a series of 50 cases from a single institution in India. Ann Diagn Pathol. 2013;17:1–9.

44. Gallardo A, Prat J. Mullerian adenosarcoma: a clinicopathologic and immunohistochemical study of 55 cases challenging the existence of adenofibroma. Am J Surg Pathol. 2009;33:278–88.

45. Frey NV, Svoboda J, Andreadis C, Tsai DE, Schulster SJ, Elstrom R, et al. Primary lymphomas of the cervix and uterus: the University of Pennsylvania's experience and a review of the literature. Leuk Lymphoma. 2006;47:1894–901.

Endometrial Epithelial Lesions

4

Introduction

Among endometrial epithelial lesions, common nonneoplastic conditions (metaplasia, hormone-related changes, endometrial polyp, and gestational alterations) can mimic malignant or premalignant lesions of the endometrium. Endometrial carcinoma is the most common cancer of the female genital tract [1]. Long-term estrogen overload due to obesity, hormone replacement, oral contraceptives, and smoking are significantly associated with the most common subtype, endometrioid adenocarcinoma (type 1 endometrial cancer, 70–80 %) [2] and its precursor lesion—atypical endometrial hyperplasia. A smaller subset of endometrial cancers (10–15 %) is represented by serous and clear cell carcinomas (type 2 endometrial cancer) [3] that are high grade by definition and almost always occur in postmenopausal women. Mixed carcinoma is defined by the presence of two histological subtypes of epithelial malignancy, one of which is type 2 (serous or clear cell carcinoma) and the minor component constitutes at least 5 % of the entire tumor [4]. The current (2014) WHO classification of endometrial carcinomas [4] is summarized in Table 4.1. Other histological subtypes of endometrial carcinoma are rare, including neuroendocrine tumors and undifferentiated/dedifferentiated carcinomas.

The primary goal of intraoperative consultation for endometrial malignancy at the time of hysterectomy is to identify patients who are at high risk of pelvic and para-aortic lymph node involvement [5] and to avoid secondary staging surgery or suboptimal extended chemoradiation.

Table 4.1 2014 World Health Organization classification of endometrial carcinomas

Histological type	Subtype	Histological variant	Histological variant
Endometrioid carcinoma	Conventional	With squamous differentiation	With mucinous differentiation
	Secretory		
	Villoglandular		
	Microglandular		
	Sertoliform		
	Ciliated		
Mucinous carcinoma			
Serous carcinoma	Serous endometrial intraepithelial carcinoma (SEIC)		
Clear cell carcinoma			
Neuroendocrine tumors	Low grade	Carcinoid tumor	
	High grade	Small cell neuroendocrine carcinoma (SCNEC)	Large cell neuroendocrine carcinoma (LCNEC)
Undifferentiated carcinoma	Dedifferentiated	With trophoblastic differentiation	
Mixed carcinomas			

Data from Kurman et al. [4]

© Springer International Publishing Switzerland 2015
P. Hui, N. Buza, *Atlas of Intraoperative Frozen Section Diagnosis in Gynecologic Pathology*,
DOI 10.1007/978-3-319-21807-6_4

Indications for Frozen Section Diagnosis

- Unexpected uterine mass
- Clinical suspicion for endometrial malignancy without preoperative biopsy diagnosis
- Confirming the diagnosis of carcinoma suspected on a prior biopsy
- Assessing the overall FIGO grade of tumor
- Determining the depth of myometrial invasion and extent of cervical involvement
- Identifying a high-grade (type 2) carcinoma component (serous, clear cell, or malignant mixed Mullerian tumor)

In general, high-risk histological parameters include presence of type 2 carcinoma component, deep myometrial involvement, cervical stromal invasion, and adnexal metastasis. Although the grade of endometrial cancer is often available as a result of preoperative biopsy or curettage, endometrioid adenocarcinoma is not uncommonly heterogeneous with an admixed type 2 tumor component [6]. Therefore, gynecologic oncologists may request a frozen section even when the preoperative biopsy diagnosis is an endometrioid carcinoma.

Discrepancy between the endometrial biopsy/curettage and the staging hysterectomy is common with regard to tumor grade (31–54 % of cases), and the final grade is equally likely to be higher and lower than that of the prior biopsy [6, 7]. It is important to keep in mind that frozen section evaluation of endometrial cancer is not optimal, with significant disagreement reported between the frozen section and permanent diagnosis in terms of tumor grade, depth of myometrial invasion, cervical involvement, and lymph node metastasis. Such inherent limitation in predicting the final tumor grade and stage must be carefully considered by both the pathologist and gynecologic oncologist [8].

Specimen Processing for Intraoperative Consultation

- Careful gross examination of the anterior and posterior endo-myometrium is important to identify the presence of invasive carcinoma.
- For grossly identifiable lesions, one or two full-thickness sections of uterine wall should be submitted to evaluate the maximum depth of myometrial penetration. Sections of anterior and posterior cervix contiguous to the lower uterine segment should be submitted to assess cervical involvement.
- If there is no grossly identifiable tumor or the preoperative biopsy showed atypical complex hyperplasia, representative anterior and posterior endo-myometrial sections should be submitted for frozen section evaluation.
- Careful gross examination of adnexa is necessary, and frozen section evaluation of any suspicious lesions should be performed if endometrial malignancy is found.

Tumorlike Conditions

Endometrial Polyp [9–11]

- Endometrial polyp is found in about 24 % of women in the general population and is a rather common finding in patients receiving tamoxifen treatment for breast cancer.
- It may be sessile or pedunculated, single or multiple with size ranging from less than 1 cm to filling up the entire endometrial cavity (Fig. 4.1). Tamoxifen-related endometrial polyps tend to be large, multiple, and fibrotic grossly.
- Polypoid configuration, fibrotic stroma, thick-walled vasculature, crowded, and/or irregular endometrial glands that may be proliferative, atrophic, or even secretory (Fig. 4.2).
- Endometrial polyps in postmenopausal patients often have a more prominent fibrotic stoma and less glandular component. Metaplastic changes of the glandular epithelium, particularly endocervical-type mucinous metaplasia are common.
- Endometrial polyps may be involved by preneoplastic conditions including complex mucinous changes, complex papillary proliferation, atypical hyperplasia (>10 % of cases), and early adenocarcinoma (2–3 % of cases).
- Differential diagnosis
  - Polypoid adenomyoma
  - Atypical polypoid adenomyoma
  - Adenosarcoma
- Diagnostic pitfalls/key intraoperative consultation issues
  - Endometrial polyp is separated from polypoid adenomyoma and atypical polypoid adenomyoma by lack of a significant smooth muscle component.
  - Endometrial polyp is separated from adenosarcoma by absence of periglandular stromal cell condensation, cytological atypia, and stromal cell mitotic activity.
  - In postmenopausal patients, careful screening for incidental minute foci of serous endometrial intraepithelial carcinoma (SEIC) within an endometrial polyp is important to ensure appropriate staging surgery at the time of frozen section examination.

Metaplastic and Reactive Changes [12–14]

- Various endometrial metaplastic or reactive changes are frequently associated with or mimic neoplastic lesions of the endometrium.
- Different types of metaplasias often coexist within the same specimen.
- Eosinophilic and papillary syncytial metaplasias are often associated with endometrial breakdown, particularly abnormal bleeding.

- Squamous metaplasia (often forming squamous morules) can be seen in benign endometrium, endometrioid adenocarcinoma, and its precursor—atypical endometrial hyperplasia.
- Tubal or ciliated metaplasia has tubal-type epithelium and is often found in normal proliferative endometrium or in isolated glands of atrophic endometrium.
- Clear cell metaplasia involves endometrial glands and shows clear cytoplasm containing glycogen.
- Secretory changes can be superimposed on either hyperplasia or carcinoma with columnar cells having sub- or supranuclear vacuoles.
- Mucinous changes, including papillary mucinous proliferation, are almost always of the endocervical type and can be seen in benign (endometrial polyp), premalignant, and malignant conditions.
- Diagnostic pitfalls/key intraoperative consultation issues
  - Recognition of metaplastic changes on frozen section at the time of hysterectomy relies on lack of invasion, absence of significant cytological atypia, and minimal mitotic activity.
  - Mucinous changes with or without cytological atypia should prompt additional sampling to rule out a well-differentiated endometrioid carcinoma [15]. Highly complex mucinous proliferation with cribriform and branching villous epithelium and cytological atypia has a high frequency of associated carcinoma. Additional sections of the endometrium may be necessary to rule out invasive carcinoma at the time of intraoperative consultation.

Arias-Stella Reaction [16, 17]

- Seen in patients with concurrent gestation, trophoblastic disease, or high-dose progestin use.
- It may mimic tubulocystic histology of clear cell carcinoma by its glandular irregularity, cellular budding, striking nuclear atypicality, hobnailing, and clear cytoplasm.
- Differential diagnosis
  - Clear cell carcinoma
- Diagnostic pitfalls/key intraoperative consultation issues
  - Aria-Stella reaction is separated from clear cell carcinoma by its overall normal endometrial glandular distribution, absence of mitotic activity, and degenerative nuclear chromatin pattern.
  - Inquiry about concurrent gestational status or history of hormone therapy at the time of intraoperative consultation is helpful to confirm the diagnosis.

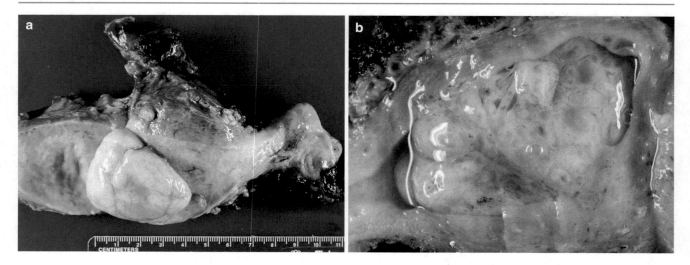

Fig. 4.1 Endometrial polyp. Pedunculated (**a**) or sessile (**b**) polypoid lesions that may fill the entire endometrial cavity

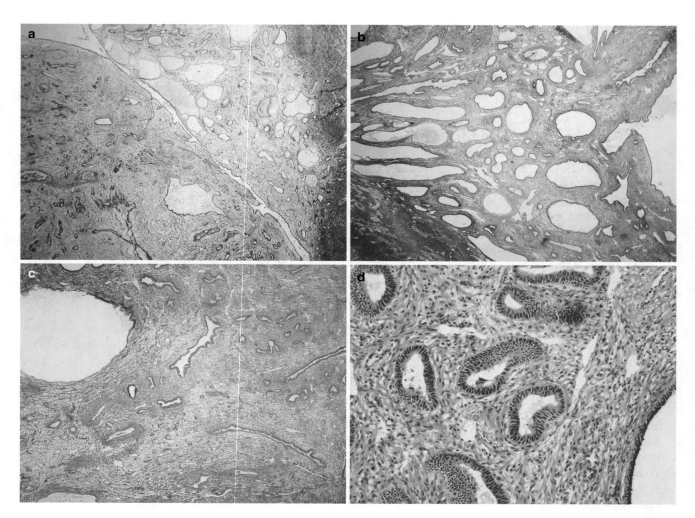

Fig. 4.2 Endometrial polyp. Note the polypoid configuration, fibrotic stroma, thick-walled vasculature, and irregular endometrial glands (**a–c**) and absence of cytological atypia (**d**)

Endometrial Hyperplasia [18–20]

- Clinical features
  - Perimenopausal patients often with obesity, polycystic ovary syndrome, and diabetes.
  - Atypical hyperplasia is generally considered a precursor lesion to endometrioid adenocarcinoma.
- Gross pathology
  - Gross appearance is variable ranging from no obvious lesion to diffuse or polypoid endometrial thickening (Fig. 4.3).
- Microscopic features
  - Hyperplasia without atypia (Fig. 4.4)
    - Diffuse glandular proliferation with abnormal glandular architecture—irregular shapes (cystic, pouching, and branching glands) and variable sizes.
    - Either abundant (simple hyperplasia) or diminished stroma resulting in glandular crowding and back-to-back glandular configurations (complex hyperplasia).
    - Columnar or pseudostratified glandular cells with variable mitotic activity.
    - Lesser degree of proliferative process may be designated as disordered proliferative endometrium, showing isolated glandular abnormalities scattered within otherwise normal proliferative endometrium.
  - Atypical hyperplasia (Fig. 4.5)
    - Hyperplasia with cytological atypia.
- Diagnostic features of cytological atypia include:
  - Cytoplasmic eosinophilia
  - Loss of nuclear polarity
  - Nuclear enlargement, rounding, and variation in size
  - Thickening of the nuclear membrane and chromatin clumping
    - Nuclear atypia should involve a significant number or clusters of glandular cells.
    - Comparison with adjacent background normal, non-metaplastic endometrial glands is helpful to identify nuclear atypia.
    - Metaplastic changes—particularly mucinous metaplasia—frequently involve endometrial hyperplasia (Fig. 4.6).
- Differential diagnosis
  - Grade 1 endometrioid adenocarcinoma (see below)
  - Various endometrial epithelial metaplasias
  - Irregular endometrial glands at the basalis
  - Highly compact secretory endometrium
  - Endometrial polyp
  - Atypical polypoid adenomyoma
- Diagnostic pitfalls/key intraoperative consultation issues
  - The single most important issue at the time of intraoperative consultation is to rule out carcinoma.
  - Grossly the most suspicious areas should be sampled for frozen sections.
  - Separation of atypical from non-atypical hyperplasia may be difficult but is not crucial at the time of frozen section evaluation.
  - Up to 40 % of hysterectomy specimens of patients with a biopsy diagnosis of atypical hyperplasia harbor grade 1 endometrioid carcinoma [21].
  - When atypical hyperplasia is diagnosed on frozen sections without definite evidence of carcinoma (Fig. 4.7), the entire endometrium needs to be submitted later for permanent microscopic examination. The surgeon should be informed of the possibility of endometrial carcinoma on permanent sections.

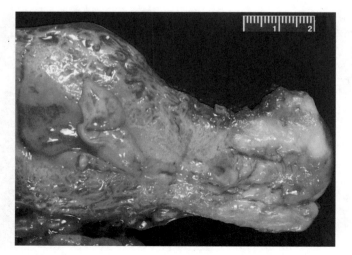

Fig. 4.3 Endometrial hyperplasia. Note the areas of marked endometrial thickening

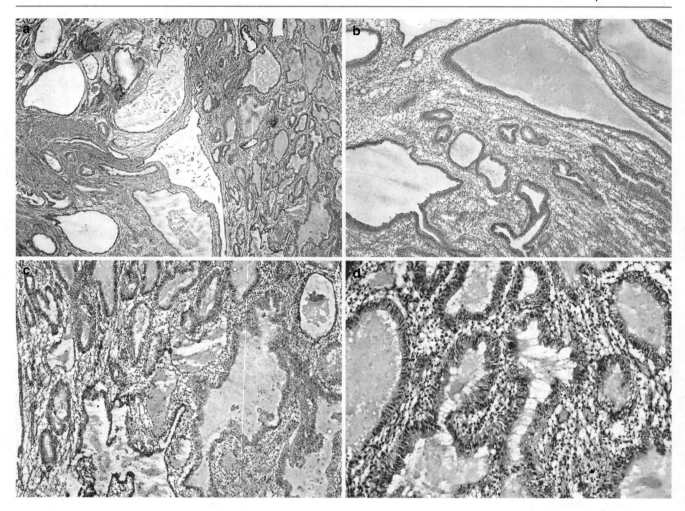

Fig. 4.4 Hyperplasia without atypia (simple hyperplasia without atypia). Diffuse proliferation of both glandular and endometrial stromal components with abnormal glandular architecture including cystic pouching and branching and absence of nuclear atypia (**a–d**)

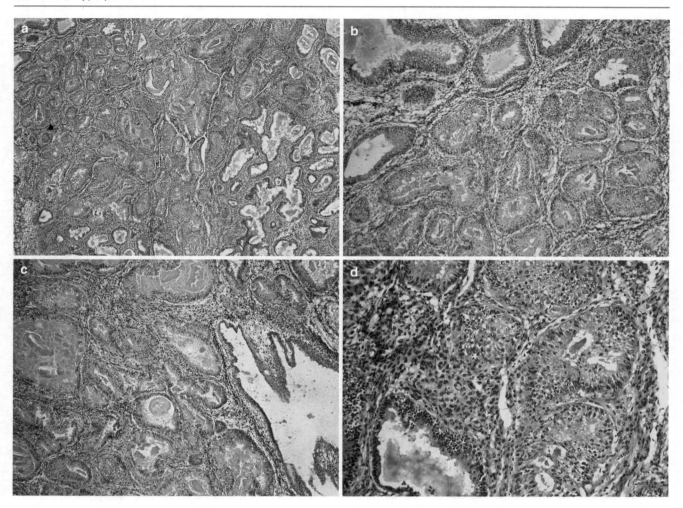

Fig. 4.5 Atypical hyperplasia (complex atypical hyperplasia). Note the glandular crowding (**a**, **b**) and the presence of cytological atypia including cytoplasmic eosinophilia, loss of nuclear polarity, nuclear enlargement, and rounding (**c**, **d**)

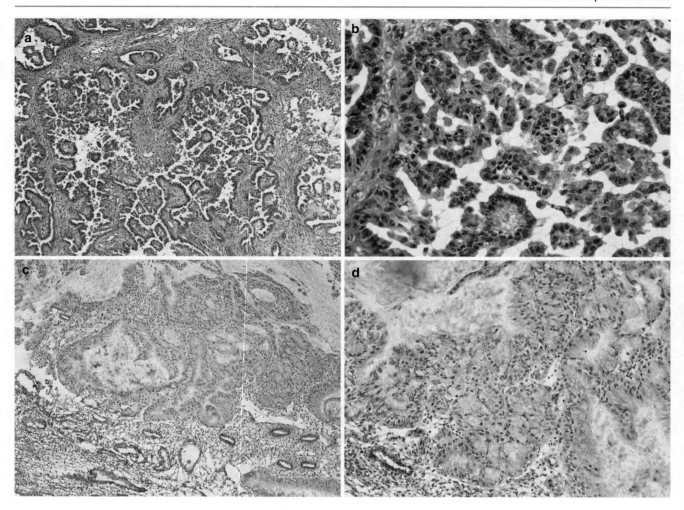

Fig. 4.6 Complex mucinous changes of the endometrium. Note the mucinous epithelium with a complex papillary configuration (**a**, **b**) or complex glandular patterns with mild nuclear atypia (**c**, **d**)

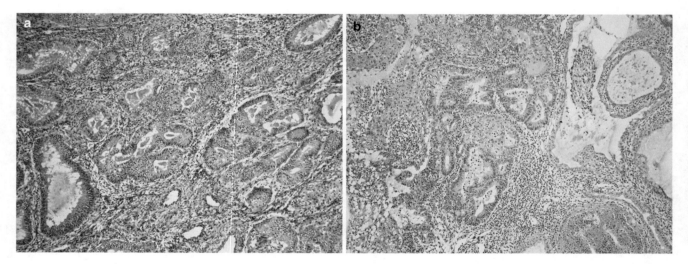

Fig. 4.7 Atypical hyperplasia bordering on well-differentiated endometrioid carcinoma. Note the foci of markedly atypical endometrial glands with intraglandular crowding and cribriform architecture (**a**, **b**)

Endometrioid Adenocarcinoma [4, 22]

- Clinical features
  - In its pure form, the tumor represents 60 % of all uterine cancers and 20 % are mixed with other types of carcinomatous components.
  - Most cases occur in postmenopausal patients and present with vaginal bleeding.
  - Most patients have unopposed estrogen stimulation, due to obesity, chronic anovulation (e.g., polycystic ovary syndrome in a young patient), estrogen-producing ovarian tumors, estrogen replacement therapy, and breast cancer patients receiving tamoxifen treatment.
  - Lynch syndrome is a genetic predisposing factor for endometrial carcinomas, particularly endometrioid type.
  - Often preceded by atypical endometrial hyperplasia.

- Gross pathology (Fig. 4.8)
  - Single to multiple discrete polypoid masses or diffuse, exophytic endometrial growth.
  - Occasional cases may have an endophytic/infiltrative growth pattern with no obvious gross lesion.
  - Necrosis and hemorrhage are common.
- Microscopic features
  - Confluent proliferation with glandular, villoglandular, or cribriform patterns (Fig. 4.9).
  - Stratified glandular epithelium consisting of columnar tumor cells sharing a common apical cytoplasmic border, imparting on a smoothly contoured luminal surface (Fig. 4.10).
  - Tumor cells have variable cytological atypia and mitotic activity.
  - Ciliated tumor cells are common.

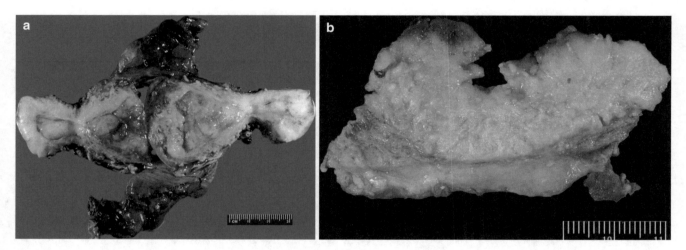

Fig. 4.8 Endometrioid adenocarcinoma. Multiple polypoid mass lesions involving the endometrium (**a**) and myometrium (**b**)

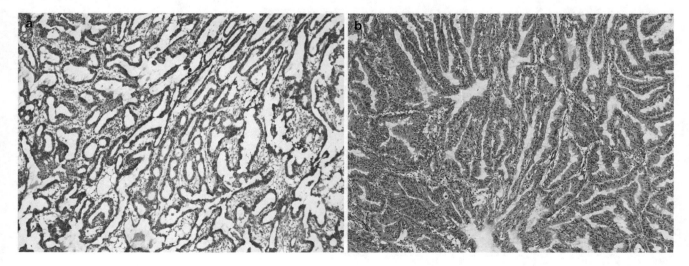

Fig. 4.9 Well-differentiated endometrioid adenocarcinoma. Note the presence of confluent, open glandular proliferation without a solid growth pattern (**a**, **b**)

- Focal mucinous differentiation (<50 % of the entire tumor) is not an infrequent finding.
- Frequent squamous differentiation, including mature (squamous morules, papillary surface squamous differentiation to overt keratinization) and immature types (squamous metaplasia to squamous carcinomatous changes).
- Eosinophilic papillary syncytial metaplasia, luminal necrotic debris, and stromal foamy macrophages are also common.
- Percentage of solid glandular growth determines the histological grade (FIGO grade) [23]: 5 % or less solid glandular component in FIGO grade 1, >5–50 % in grade 2, and >50 % in grade 3 tumors. Low FIGO grade tumor is upgraded by 1 grade when nuclear grade 3 involves more than 50 % of the entire tumor [24] (Figs. 4.11 and 4.12).
- Variants of endometrioid adenocarcinomas [25–32].

- *Secretory carcinoma:* endometrioid adenocarcinoma with a glandular growth pattern and tumor cells containing uniform subnuclear and/or supranuclear vacuolization.
- *Ciliated cell carcinoma:* glandular growth pattern with extensive ciliated epithelial cells involving at least 75 % of the entire lesion.
- *Villoglandular variant:* slender, delicate papillary fronds with thin, minimal stroma (Fig. 4.13).
- *Non-villous papillary endometrioid carcinoma:* non-villous branching and budding papillae simulating serous carcinoma on low magnification, but the tumor cells are columnar with low nuclear grade (Fig. 4.14).
- *Microglandular endometrioid adenocarcinoma* (Fig. 4.15): often mixed with conventional endometrioid adenocarcinoma with mucinous differentiation; areas of the tumor show microglandular growth pattern simulating endocervical microglandular hyperplasia.

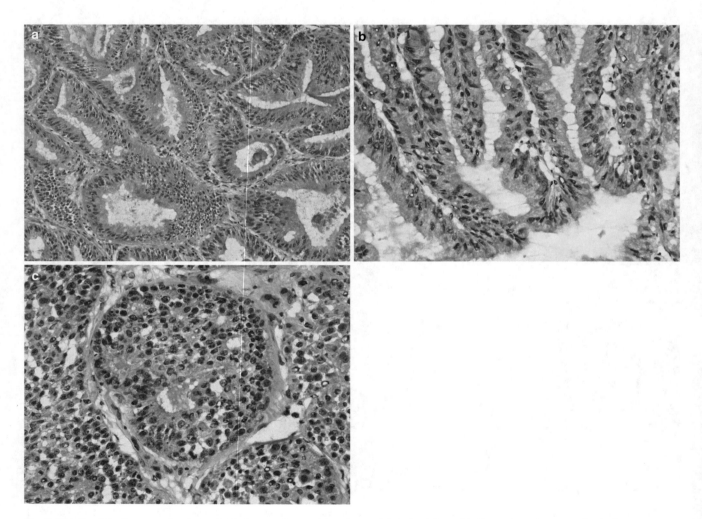

Fig. 4.10 Glandular features of endometrioid adenocarcinoma. Note the stratified glandular epithelium with columnar cells sharing a common apical cytoplasmic border, resulting in a smoothly contoured luminal surface (**a–c**)

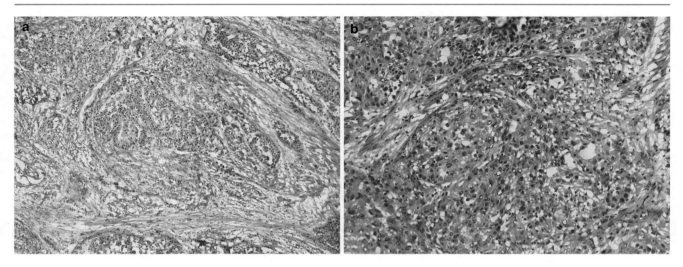

Fig. 4.11 FIGO grade 2 endometrioid adenocarcinoma. Note the presence of focal solid growth pattern (**a**, **b**)

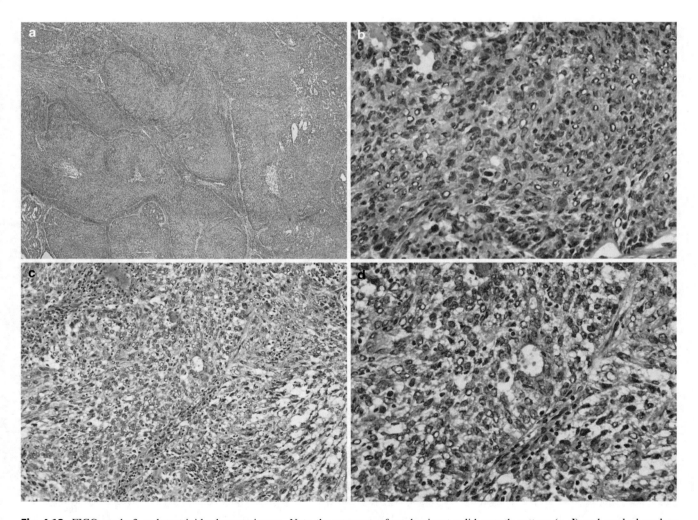

Fig. 4.12 FIGO grade 3 endometrioid adenocarcinoma. Note the presence of predominant solid growth pattern (**a–d**) and marked nuclear atypia (**c**, **d**)

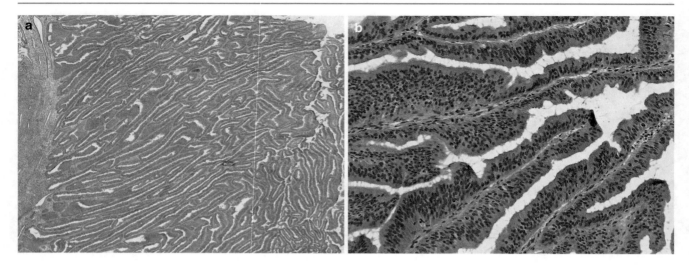

Fig. 4.13 Villoglandular endometrioid adenocarcinoma. Note the slender, delicate papillary fronds with thin or minimal stroma (**a, b**) and mild nuclear atypia (**b**)

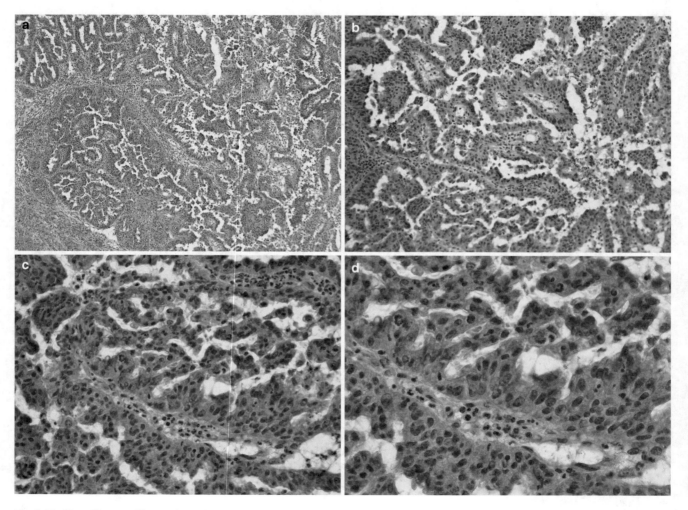

Fig. 4.14 Non-villous papillary endometrioid adenocarcinoma. Note the presence of non-villous papillae with short branching and budding, simulating serous carcinoma at low magnification (**a, b**). However, low nuclear grade with minimal mitotic activity is seen at higher magnification (**c, d**)

- *Sertoliform endometrioid adenocarcinoma:* rare, well-differentiated endometrioid carcinoma showing focal or predominant cords to small, hollow tubular glands simulating Sertoli cell tumor of the ovary. The diagnosis relies on finding areas merging with conventional endometrioid carcinoma. Absence of endometrial stromal tumor component separates this variant from endometrial stromal tumor with sex-cord differentiation and uterine tumor resembling ovarian sex-cord tumor.
- Differential diagnosis
  - Atypical complex hyperplasia
  - Serous carcinoma versus villoglandular, and non-villous papillary endometrioid adenocarcinoma
  - Clear cell carcinoma versus secretory endometrioid adenocarcinoma and endometrioid adenocarcinoma with squamous differentiation/clear cytoplasmic changes
  - Endocervical adenocarcinoma involving endometrium
  - Metastatic carcinomas from other sites (commonly breast and gastrointestinal origins)
- Diagnostic pitfalls/key intraoperative consultation issues
  - Separation of endometrial atypical hyperplasia from invasive carcinoma can be difficult, particularly at the time of frozen section evaluation. Thefollowing findings are indicative of carcinoma [18, 27] (see Fig. 4.7).
    - Desmoplastic stroma with fibroblasts or myofibroblasts rigidly existing between the atypical glands.
    - Stromal space replaced by aggregates of foamy macrophages or eosinophilic collagen.
    - Expansile glands with confluent, cribriforming pattern or extensive papillation.

- When borderline histological findings are present and no gross invasion is found, frozen section interpretation as "markedly atypical hyperplasia, bordering on well-differentiated endometrioid carcinoma" may be communicated.
  - Lymphovascular invasion: true lymphovascular invasion should be carefully separated from mechanically displaced tumor cells, which is increasingly common in hysterectomy specimens obtained by robotic surgery. True lymphovascular invasion in the absence of myoinvasion by a low-grade endometrioid adenocarcinoma is very uncommon.
  - Cervical involvement (Fig. 4.16):
    - Cervical involvement is seen in 20 % of endometrial carcinomas.
    - In rare cases, pseudo-maturation of endometrioid adenocarcinoma when involving the deep cervical stroma may lead to deceptively benign looking glands—small tubular glands with less atypical tumor cells that may contain eosinophilic secretion, therefore simulating mesonephric remnants and hyperplasia. The haphazard infiltrative growth pattern and merging with corpus endometrioid carcinoma confirms true cervical invasion.
    - Mucosal involvement only and free-floating tumor tissue in the cervical canal does not affect clinical stage of the tumor.
  - The presence of grade 3 nuclei in an architecturally FIGO grade 1 tumor suggests serous carcinoma.
  - Separation of dedifferentiated endometrioid carcinoma from an otherwise conventional FIGO grade 1 or 2 adenocarcinoma is important for prognosis due to the more aggressive nature of the former (see later in this chapter).

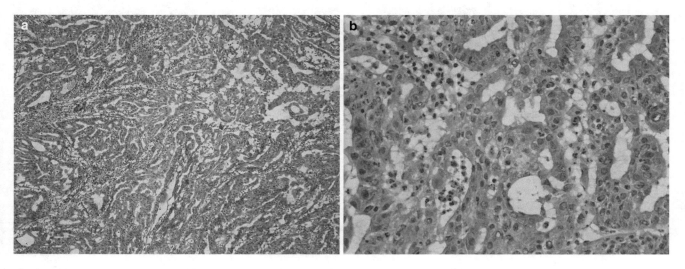

Fig. 4.15 Microglandular endometrioid adenocarcinoma. Note the well-differentiated endometrioid adenocarcinoma with microglandular growth pattern and inflammatory cells, simulating endocervical microglandular hyperplasia (**a**, **b**)

- High index of suspicion is important to avoid misinterpretation of metastatic carcinoma as endometrial primary. In patients with prior history of malignancy, particularly those of breast and gastrointestinal primaries, morphologic comparison with the prior specimen(s)—if available at the time of frozen section—should be made.
- Myometrial invasion pattern [33–35]:
  - Common types of myometrial invasion by endometrioid adenocarcinoma include expansile/pushing invasion, infiltrative invasion, and the microcystic elongated and fragmented (MELF) pattern of invasion (Fig. 4.17).
  - Distinction between superficial myometrial invasion and irregular endo-myometrial junction may not be crucial at the time of frozen section diagnosis.
  - Pseudo-myometrial invasion—adenomyosis involved by carcinoma. The presence of adjacent benign endometrial glands within the same focus, particularly surrounded by a rim of endometrial stroma, and lack of stromal response indicate adenomyosis colonized by carcinoma (see Fig. 4.17c).
- Carcinoma involving the isthmic (intramyometrial) portion of fallopian tube may simulate myoinvasion. Awareness of the anatomic location of the frozen section near the fallopian tube origin and circumferential arrangement of smooth muscle are helpful features to avoid overinterpretation as deep myometrial invasion.
- Myoinvasion by gaping neoplastic glands lined by tufting and stratified epithelium with grade 3 nuclei is a feature of serous carcinoma, not well-differentiated endometrioid carcinoma.
- MELF invasion pattern is associated with high risk of lymph node metastasis. It is recognized by the haphazard infiltration, irregular and frequently broken glands with marked desmoplastic stromal response, and presence of inflammatory cells (see Fig. 4.17d).
- Endometrioid carcinoma may arise from atypical polypoid adenomyoma (Fig. 4.18).

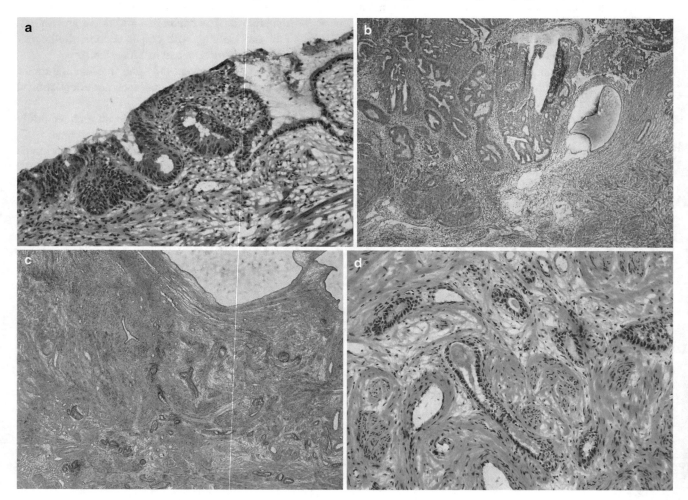

Fig. 4.16 Cervical involvement by endometrioid adenocarcinoma. The tumor may involve the endocervical mucosa (**a**) and stroma (**b**) and may assume deceptively benign-appearing tubular or cystic glandular patterns (**c, d**). Note the deep, haphazard infiltration of cervical stroma (**c**) and proximity to large-caliber vessels (**d**)

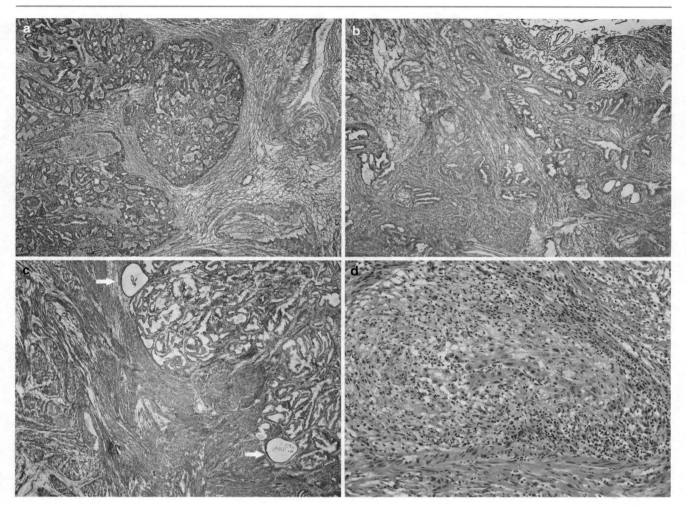

Fig. 4.17 Uterine myometrial invasion and pseudo-myoinvasion. Superficial myometrial invasion may present in either a confluent glandular pattern with a pushing front into the myometrium (**a**) or an infiltrative pattern (**b**). Superficial adenomyosis involved by carcinoma is recognized by the presence of adjacent benign endometrial glands (*arrows*, **c**). The microcystic elongated and fragmented (MELF) pattern of myoinvasion is recognized by its haphazard infiltration by broken neoplastic glands and marked desmoplastic stromal response with inflammation (**d**)

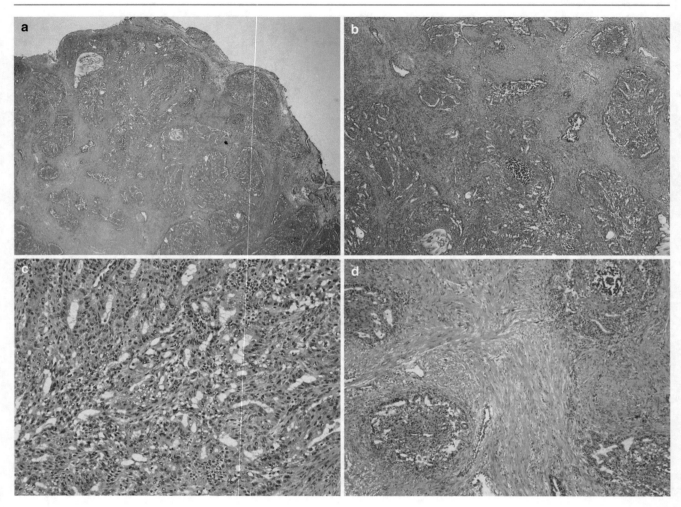

Fig. 4.18 Well-differentiated endometrioid adenocarcinoma arising in an atypical polypoid adenomyoma (APA). Note the well-differentiated endometrioid carcinoma involving areas of glandular component of APA (**a–c**). Focal typical histological features of APA are present (**d**)

Mucinous Carcinoma [15, 36]

- Mucinous carcinoma is defined by at least 50 % of tumor cells showing cytoplasmic mucin production
- Clinical characteristics are similar to those of conventional endometrioid adenocarcinoma.
- Gross lesions may have a soft mucoid appearance.
- Majority of tumors consist of glandular cells with apical pale mucin, arranged in glandular (Fig. 4.19), cribriforming, villoglandular, or microglandular patterns (Fig. 4.20).
- Myoinvasive component frequently shows well-differentiated endometrioid carcinoma with lesser degree of mucinous differentiation.
- Tumor grading is similar to that of the conventional endometrioid carcinoma—most mucinous carcinomas are grade 1 tumors.

- Differential diagnosis
  - Endocervical mucinous adenocarcinoma involving endometrium
  - Complex mucinous changes of the endometrium
  - Microglandular hyperplasia of the cervix (when tumor involves cervix or low uterine segment endometrium)
- Diagnostic pitfalls/key intraoperative consultation issues
  - In contrast to mucinous carcinoma, complex mucinous changes lack stromal invasion (see atypical hyperplasia).
  - Microglandular endometrioid adenocarcinoma involving the cervix is typically contiguous with the endometrial tumor in contrast to the isolated finding of microglandular hyperplasia involving only the endocervix or an endocervical polyp.
  - Separation from endocervical mucinous carcinoma primarily relies on the location of the tumor.

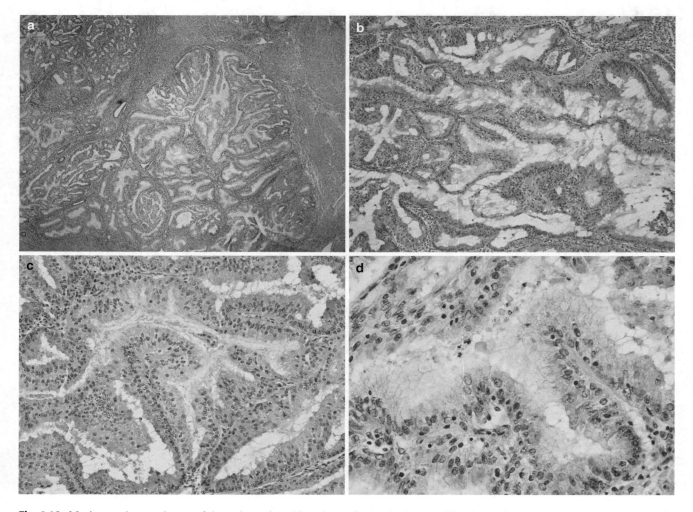

Fig. 4.19 Mucinous adenocarcinoma of the endometrium. Note the confluent glandular proliferation with open lumens (**a, b**), relatively mild nuclear atypia, and presence of intracytoplasmic mucin in the majority of the tumor cells (**c, d**)

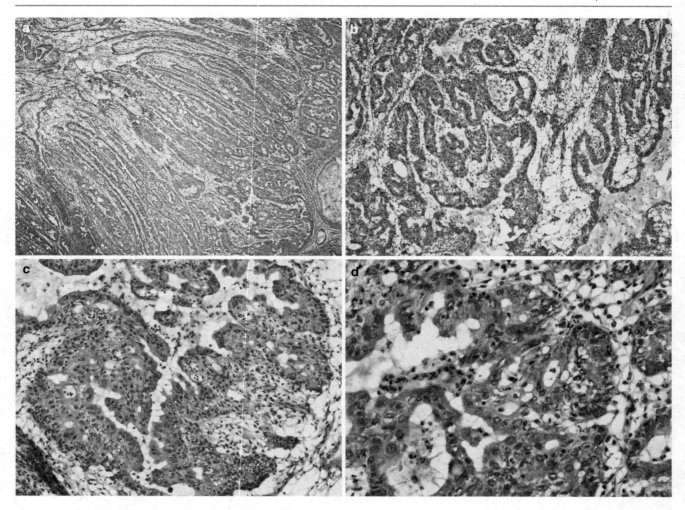

Fig. 4.20 Mucinous endometrial adenocarcinoma with microglandular pattern. Note the presence of cytoplasmic mucin and microglandular growth pattern simulating benign microglandular hyperplasia of the cervix (**a–d**)

Serous Carcinoma

- Clinical features [11, 37–39]:
  - Accounts for 10 % of all endometrial cancers.
  - Almost always occurs in postmenopausal patients and is typically not associated with obesity or estrogen overload.
  - Pelvic irradiation is a risk factor.
  - Postmenopausal bleeding is the most common symptom, although many patients are asymptomatic.
- Gross pathology (Fig. 4.21)
  - Full-blown serous carcinoma is indistinguishable from endometrioid adenocarcinoma macroscopically.
  - Minimal serous carcinoma frequently involves an endometrial polyp in a background of atrophic endometrium.
- Microscopic features
  - Various growth patterns including the following (Fig. 4.22):
    - Complex papillary growth of mostly short blunt cellular papillae with minimal stroma, cellular buds, and detached floating cell clusters.
    - Irregular slit-like glandular spaces or microcysts.
    - Glandular pattern is not uncommon.
    - Solid nest or sheets rarely exist.
  - Gaping irregular glandular pattern when invading the myometrium (Fig. 4.23).
  - Characteristic scalloped/serrated glandular or luminal surfaces as a result of markedly uneven stratification of tumor cells (Fig. 4.24).
  - Frequent lymphovascular invasion.
  - Grade 3 nuclear atypia (Fig. 4.25)
    - Marked nuclear pleomorphism, karyomegaly, and hyperchromasia.
    - Bizarre nuclei, multinucleation, and hobnailing are common.
    - Characteristic macronucleoli, often cherry red in color with a perinucleolar halo.
    - Ubiquitous mitoses with frequent atypical forms.
  - 50 % of serous carcinomas are mixed with an endometrioid or clear cell carcinoma component.
  - Background endometrium is almost always atrophic or shows an endometrial polyp.
- Differential diagnosis
  - Well-differentiated endometrioid carcinoma including villoglandular and non-villous papillary variants
  - Poorly differentiated endometrioid carcinoma with high nuclear grade
  - Clear cell carcinoma
  - Undifferentiated carcinoma
  - Malignant mixed Mullerian tumor
  - Metastatic carcinomas
  - Metaplastic or reactive benign conditions (papillary syncytial metaplasia, radiation changes, Arias Stella reaction) that mimic serous endometrial intraepithelial carcinoma (SEIC), particularly when involving an endometrial polyp
- Diagnostic pitfalls/key intraoperative consultation issues
  - The key intraoperative issue is to identify or confirm the presence of serous carcinoma, either pure or mixed, to ensure appropriate surgical staging (Table 4.2).
    - Complete surgical staging including omentectomy and para-aortic lymph node dissection is commonly performed for serous carcinoma.
    - In constract, the extent of surgical staging may vary for endometrioid carcinoma. Complete surgical staging is recommended for those with deep myometrial invasion and high-grade histology, while less extensive surgical staging may be appropriate for low-grade and non-myoinvasive tumors.
  - Endometrial serous carcinoma almost always occurs in postmenopausal patients. Diagnosis of endometrial serous carcinoma in a premenopausal woman should be avoided, unless it is a secondary involvement from a cervical or ovarian primary.
  - Villoglandular and non-villous papillary endometrioid carcinomas may simulate serous carcinoma at low magnification. Both villoglandular and non-villous papillary endometrial carcinomas have a nonstratified, single layer of low-grade tumor cells (see Figs. 4.13 and 4.14).
  - Microglandular endometrioid carcinoma can be separated from endometrial serous carcinoma by its typical cribriform glands and generally low nuclear grade, rather than slit-like growth pattern and high nuclear grade in endometrial serous carcinoma.
  - Clear cell carcinoma is separated from serous carcinoma mainly by histological and cytological findings (see Table 4.2).
  - Presence of distinct sarcomatous elements is diagnostic of malignant mixed Mullerian tumor (carcinosarcoma).
  - Serous endometrial intraepithelial carcinoma (Fig. 4.26) and minimal invasive serous carcinoma (intramucosal invasive serous carcinoma of < 1 cm) (Fig. 4.27) frequently involve or arise from an endometrial polyp [11, 40].
  - Early serous carcinoma can be an incidental finding—recognition of the lesion at the time of frozen section is clinically relevant to ensure appropriate surgical staging and to avoid a second surgery, as up to 50 % of these cases already have extrauterine spread at the time of hysterectomy.

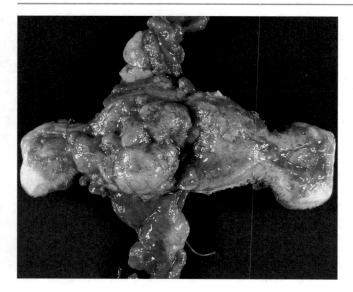

Fig. 4.21 Endometrial serous carcinoma. Note the presence of large polypoid endometrial mass lesions

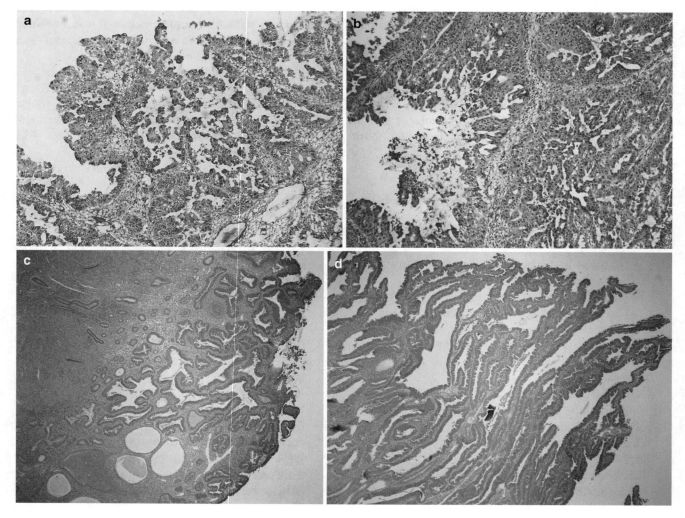

Fig. 4.22 Microscopic growth patterns of endometrial serous carcinoma. Various histological patterns may be seen, including papillary (**a**), slit-like (**b**), glandular (**c**), and villoglandular pattern (**d**)

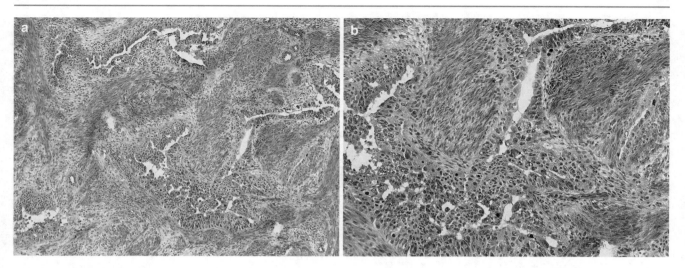

Fig. 4.23 Myometrial invasion by serous carcinoma. Note the characteristic gaping glandular pattern infiltrating the myometrium (**a**, **b**)

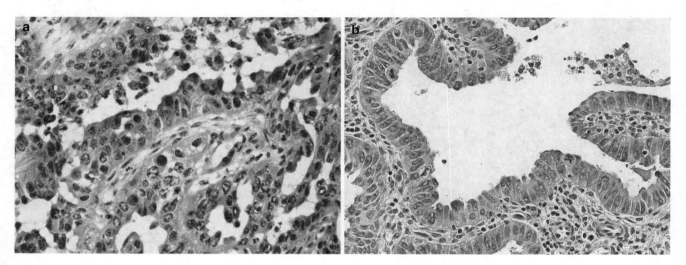

Fig. 4.24 Endometrial serous carcinoma with characteristic scalloping or undulating glandular surface as a result of uneven stratification of high-grade tumor cells (**a**, **b**)

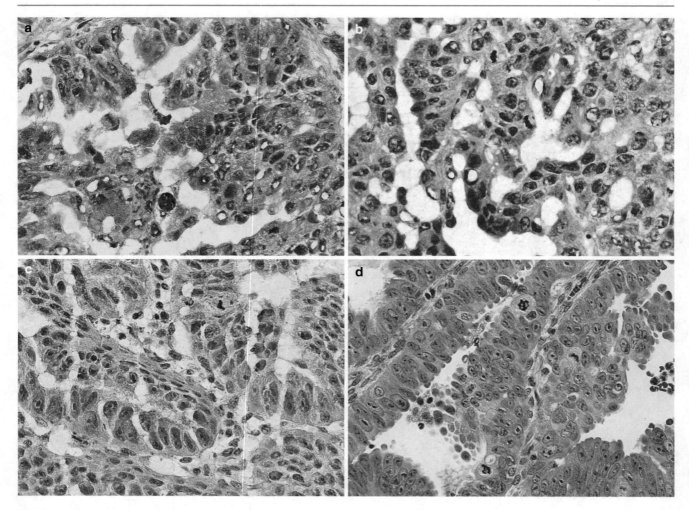

Fig. 4.25 Cytological features of endometrial serous carcinoma. Note the marked nuclear atypia, including high nuclear to cytoplasmic ratio, nucleomegaly, hyperchromasia, macronucleoli, and ubiquitous mitotic figures (**a–d**)

Table 4.2 Frozen section diagnosis of major subtypes of endometrial carcinomas

	Endometrioid	Serous	Clear cell
Patient characteristics	Peri- or postmenopausal, often obese	Postmenopausal	Postmenopausal
Background endometrium	Atypical hyperplasia	Endometrial polyp or atrophic	Atrophic
Histological features	Glandular, villoglandular, or cribriforming growth pattern	Complex, short blunt, stroma-poor papillae, cell buds, and floating clusters	Tubulocystic, glandular, papillary, or solid growth patterns
	Columnar cells with common apical border and smooth luminal surface of tumor glands	Gaping irregular glands with scalloped luminal surface	Polygonal or hobnail cells with clear or eosinophilic cytoplasm forming scalloped luminal surface
	Variable degree of cytological atypia and mitotic activity	Grade 3 nuclei, high nuclear to cytoplasmic ratio, macronucleoli, numerous mitoses, and atypical mitoses	Uniform to highly pleomorphic tumor cells with variable mitotic activity
	Frequent squamous differentiation	Frequent stromal inflammatory cells	Hyalinized stromal cores of tumor papillae and extracellular hyaline bodies
Extent of surgical staging	Varies, depending on tumor grade and extent of invasion	Complete surgical staging	Complete surgical staging

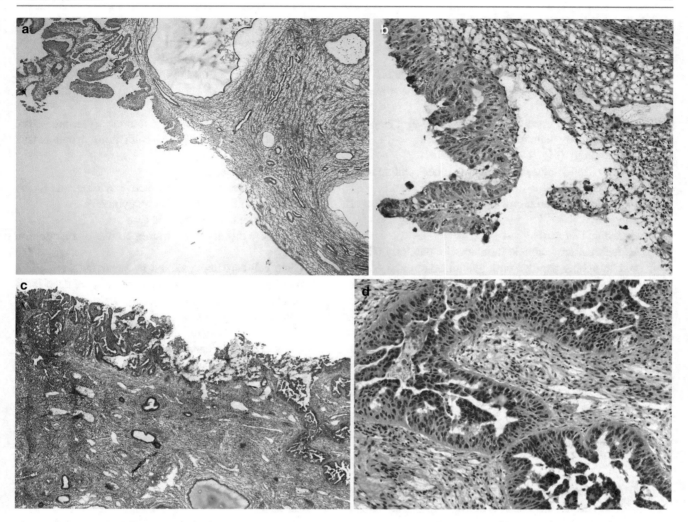

Fig. 4.26 Serous endometrial intraepithelial carcinoma involving an endometrial polyp. Note the high-grade tumor cells replacing the endometrial surface and glandular epithelium without stromal invasion (**a–d**)

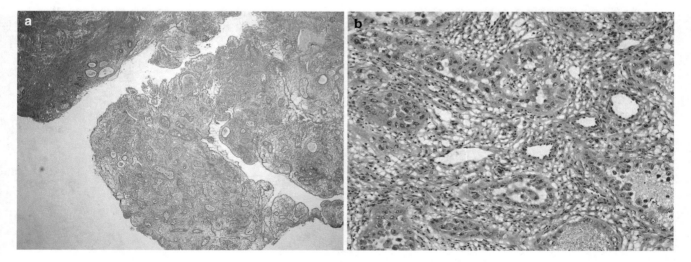

Fig. 4.27 Minimal invasive serous carcinoma involving an endometrial polyp. In addition to serous endometrial intraepithelial carcinoma, areas of the lesion show stromal invasion, but the overall size of the lesion is less than 1 cm (**a, b**)

Clear Cell Carcinoma (CCC) [41, 42]

- Clinical features
  - Represents less than 5 % of endometrial cancers.
  - Most patients are postmenopausal at the time of presentation.
  - Vaginal bleeding is the most common symptom although many patients are asymptomatic.
- Gross pathology (Fig. 4.28)
  - Grossly indistinguishable from other endometrial adenocarcinomas.
  - Early clear cell carcinoma may involve an endometrial polyp.
- Microscopic features
  - Growth patterns include tubulocystic, papillary (short and branching papillae with hyalinized stromal cores) and solid; often admixture of the above patterns (Fig. 4.29).
  - Presence of extracellular eosinophilic globules or hyaline bodies (Fig. 4.30).
  - Scalloped/serrated glandular or luminal surfaces as a result of markedly uneven stratification of tumor cells.
  - Intraglandular mucin is often found and cytoplasmic mucin droplets may be seen in some cases.
  - Characteristic cytological features (Fig. 4.31)
    - Polygonal tumor cells with optically clear to eosinophilic cytoplasm and hobnailing.
      - Cytoplasmic clearing may be difficult to appreciate on frozen section slides.
    - Cells with abundant oxyphilic cytoplasm or flattened small clear cells with psammomatous calcification can be seen.
    - High-grade nuclear atypia including high nuclear/cytoplasmic (N/C) ratio, marked nuclear pleomorphism, nucleomegaly, hyperchromasia, and presence of bizarre nuclei or multinucleation.
    - Most but not all tumors have numerous mitoses and atypical mitotic figures.

- Differential diagnosis
  - Serous carcinoma
  - Endometrioid carcinomas, particularly secretory subtype and those with clear cell squamous differentiation
  - Epithelioid leiomyosarcoma
  - Gestational trophoblastic tumors (placental site trophoblastic tumor and epithelioid trophoblastic tumor)
  - Arias-Stella reaction
  - Clear cell metaplasia with reactive cytological atypia
  - Adenomatoid tumor involving myometrium
  - Mesothelioma of epithelioid type
- Diagnostic pitfalls/key intraoperative consultation issues
  - Clear cell carcinoma should be separated from endometrioid carcinomas due to its tendency for deep myometrial invasion, high frequency of metastases, and unfavorable prognosis.
  - Clear cell changes in squamous differentiation of endometrioid carcinoma merge with typical squamous areas, particularly at the periphery of the tumor nests.
  - Mucinous carcinoma shows abundant cytoplasmic mucin production in at least 50 % of the tumor cells, compared to the cytoplasmic water-clear glycogen in clear cell carcinoma cells.
  - The presence of tubulocystic or solid growth patterns, hyalinized stromal cores, or extracellular hyaline globules is in favor of clear cell carcinoma over serous carcinoma.
  - Presence of sarcomatous elements establishes the diagnosis of malignant mixed Mullerian tumor.
  - Arias-Stella reaction may simulate the cytological changes of clear cell carcinoma (hobnailing, karyomegaly, and hyperchromasia); however, the overall endometrial architecture is preserved and mitotic activity is absent.

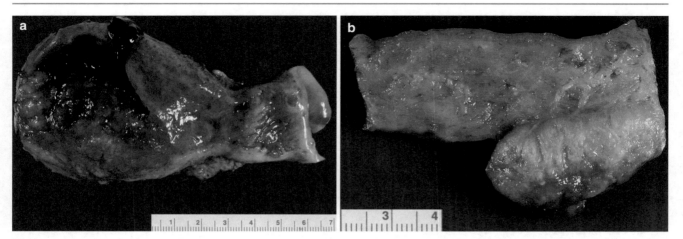

Fig. 4.28 Clear cell carcinoma. Friable solid mass lesions involving the endo-myometrium with necrosis and hemorrhage (**a**, **b**)

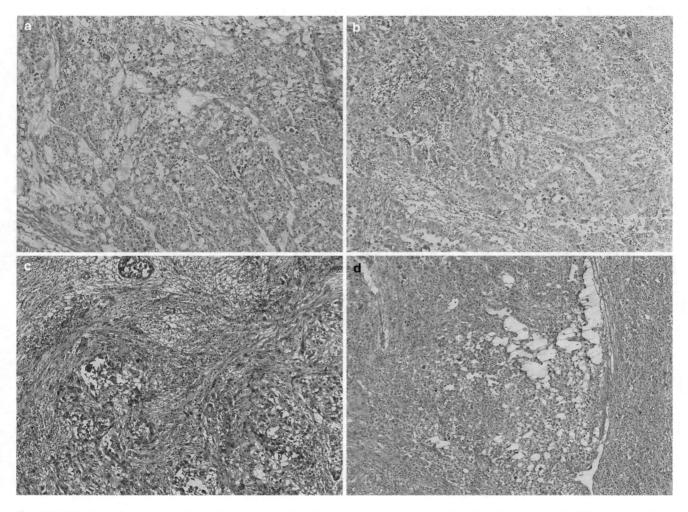

Fig. 4.29 Histological patterns of clear cell carcinoma. Note the presence of tubular (**a**), glandular (**b**, **c**), and solid (**d**) patterns in these examples

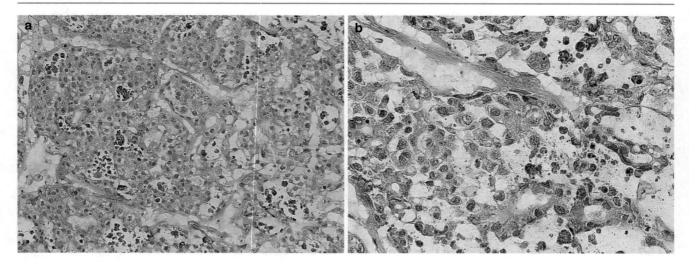

Fig. 4.30 Intra- and extracellular eosinophilic globules or hyaline bodies in endometrial clear cell carcinoma (**a**, **b**)

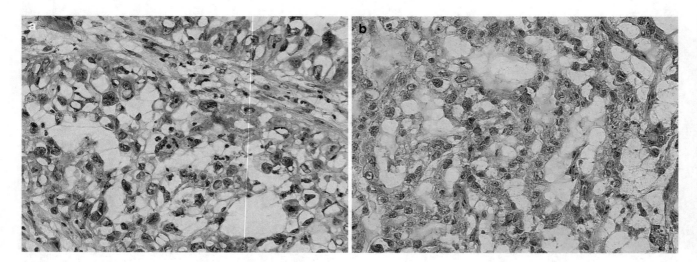

Fig. 4.31 Cytological features of endometrial clear cell carcinoma. Note the presence of polygonal tumor cells with clear to eosinophilic cytoplasm, hobnailing, and marked nuclear atypia (**a**). Uniformly high-grade tumor cells can be seen in some cases (**b**)

Undifferentiated Carcinoma and Dedifferentiated Carcinoma [4, 43–45]

- Median age of patients with undifferentiated carcinoma is 55 years.
- Histologically diffuse proliferation of discohesive cells arranged in sheets (Fig. 4.32).
- The tumor cells are monotonous, round, or polygonal with scant cytoplasm, large vesicular nuclei, prominent nucleoli, and dense chromatin. Mitotic figures are numerous.
- No evidence of lineage differentiation (solid growth without any pattern or glandular formation).
- Tumor necrosis may be abundant and stromal infiltrating lymphocytes are common.
- Dedifferentiated carcinoma is defined by the presence of both undifferentiated carcinoma and well-differentiated endometrioid carcinoma (Fig. 4.33).
  - The two components are histologically distinct and occupy separate tumor areas.
  - The well-differentiated endometrioid carcinoma component is usually a mucosal lesion and the undifferentiated tumor is often myoinvasive and biologically more aggressive.
  - The undifferentiated component must represent at least 20 % of the entire tumor to qualify for such diagnosis.
  - On frozen section, dedifferentiated carcinoma should be separated from endometrioid carcinoma by its

distinct solid undifferentiated component, which may be mistakenly interpreted as a solid growth for the overall grading of an endometrioid carcinoma (Table 4.3), therefore underestimating tumor grade.

Neuroendocrine Carcinomas [46–48]

- Small cell neuroendocrine carcinoma: histologically similar to small cell carcinoma of the lung with small discohesive tumor cells of high N/C ratio, dark chromatin, nuclear molding, numerous mitoses, and presence of necrosis.
- Large cell neuroendocrine carcinoma: high-grade large tumor cells in nests or cords with peripheral palisading and geographic necrosis.
- Frozen section diagnosis of high-grade carcinoma is sufficient for guiding subsequent surgical staging.

Rare endometrial tumor types include giant cell carcinoma, lymphoepitheliomatous carcinoma, hepatoid carcinoma, and poorly differentiated carcinoma with trophoblastic differentiation. Primary endometrial squamous cell carcinoma is very rare, and the diagnosis requires absence of connection to cervical squamous epithelium, lack of any glandular components, and absence of invasive squamous cell carcinoma of the cervix.

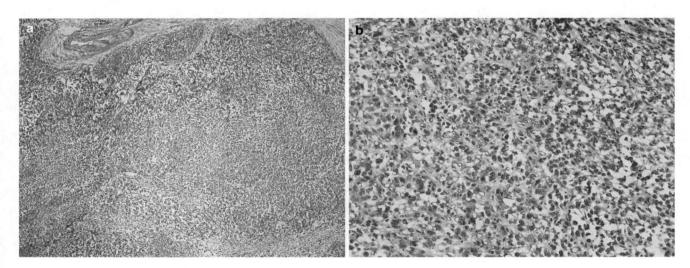

Fig. 4.32 Undifferentiated endometrial carcinoma. Note the presence of discohesive, high-grade carcinoma cells forming large solid sheets (**a**, **b**)

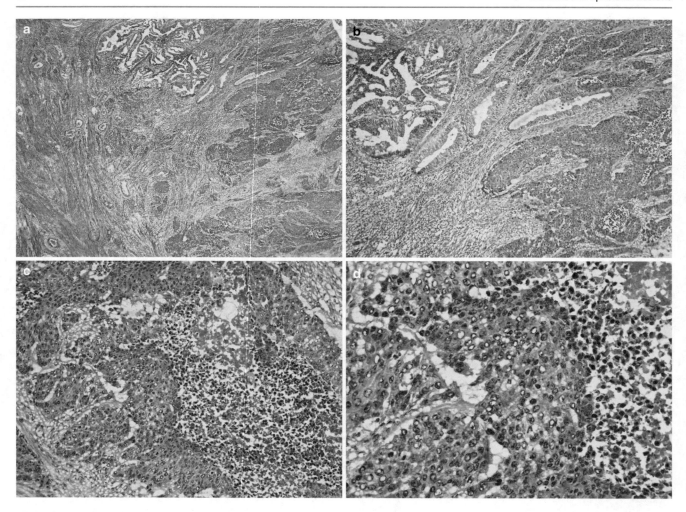

Fig. 4.33 Dedifferentiated endometrial carcinoma. Note the presence of two distinct areas of undifferentiated carcinoma (**a–d**) and well-differentiated endometrioid adenocarcinoma (**a, b,** *left side of images*)

Table 4.3 Differential diagnosis of low-grade endometrioid adenocarcinoma, dedifferentiated carcinoma, and undifferentiated carcinoma

	Endometrioid carcinoma	Dedifferentiated carcinoma	Undifferentiated carcinoma
Overall histology	Relatively uniform histology	Separate glandular and solid areas	Uniform histology
Growth pattern	Endometrioid glandular pattern	Endometrioid glandular and undifferentiated solid patterns	Undifferentiated solid pattern
Cytological atypia	Variable; grade dependent	Low-grade atypia in glandular and high-grade atypia in solid areas	Uniformly high grade
Prognosis	Grade dependent	Aggressive	Aggressive

Mixed Carcinomas [4, 49]

- Represent 10 % of endometrial cancer.
- Defined by the presence of more than one histological subtype of carcinoma, at least one of which falls in type 2 category (serous or clear cell carcinoma) (Fig. 4.34).
- Each component comprises at least 5 % of the entire tumor [4].

- Recognition of mixed carcinoma at the time of intraoperative consultation is clinically relevant, as complete surgical staging should follow. This may be one of the reasons that surgeons request frozen section evaluation of a hysterectomy specimen even when the patient's preoperative diagnosis is endometrioid adenocarcinoma.

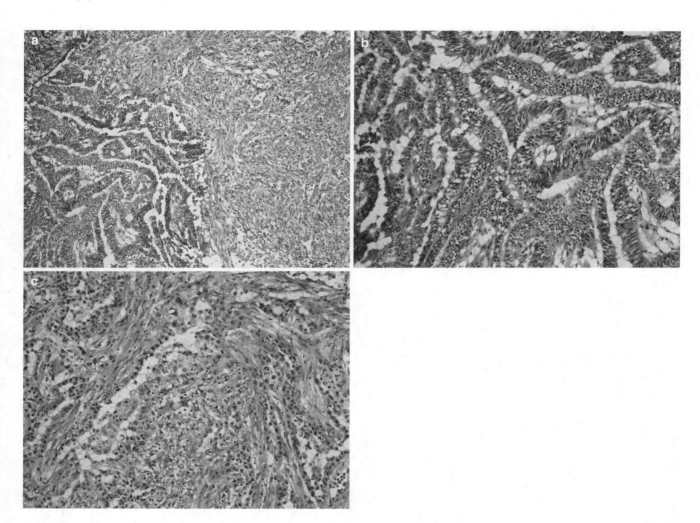

Fig. 4.34 Mixed endometrial carcinoma. Note the presence of admixed endometrioid (**a**, *left side of image*; **b**) and clear cell carcinoma components in this example (**a**, *right side of image*; **c**)

Metastatic Carcinomas [50, 51]

- Secondary endometrial involvement by carcinomas from other sites generally represents systemic dissemination. However, not infrequently, the history of prior malignancy is not available at the time of intraoperative consultation.
- It is important at the time of frozen section diagnosis to recognize metastatic carcinoma to avoid unnecessary gynecologic surgical staging.
- The most frequent sources of metastatic carcinoma involving the endometrium are breast and gastrointestinal primaries.
    - Endometrial involvement by breast lobular carcinoma may be very subtle on frozen sections (Fig. 4.35).
    - Metastatic ductal carcinoma of the breast may simulate endometrioid or even clear cell carcinoma (Fig. 4.36).

- Signet-ring cell carcinoma is the most common metastatic carcinoma from the gastrointestinal tract.
- Diagnostic pitfalls/key intraoperative consultation issues
    - Metastatic carcinoma should be suspected:
        - When the histological findings are unusual for endometrial carcinoma.
        - There is absence of background endometrial atypical hyperplasia.
        - Abundant lymphovascular involvement should raise suspicion for metastatic carcinoma, and the findings should be communicated to the operating surgeon.
        - Presence of a large fibrotic endometrial polyp should raise the possibility of prior breast cancer and tamoxifen treatment.
- Morphologic comparison with the patient's known primary tumor should be pursued whenever possible.

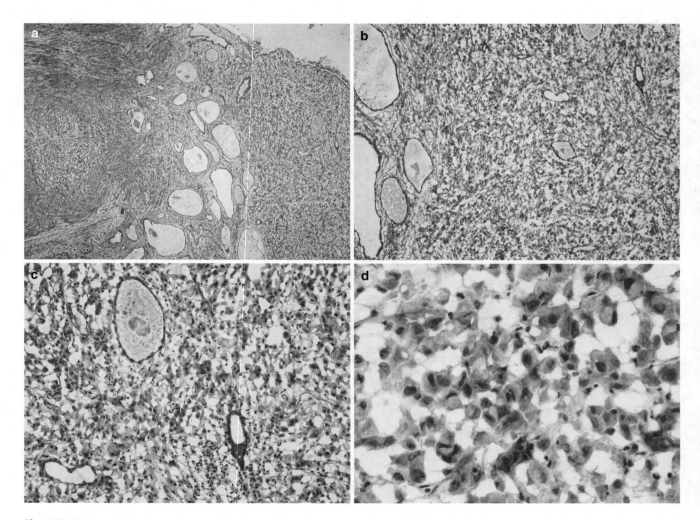

Fig. 4.35 Metastatic lobular carcinoma of the breast. Note the presence of carcinoma cells arranged in singles or cords involving the endomyometrium (**a**, **b**), surrounding and sparing the entrapped benign endometrial glands (**b**, **c**). Some tumor cells have signet-ring morphology with eccentric nuclei and intracytoplasmic mucin (**c**, **d**)

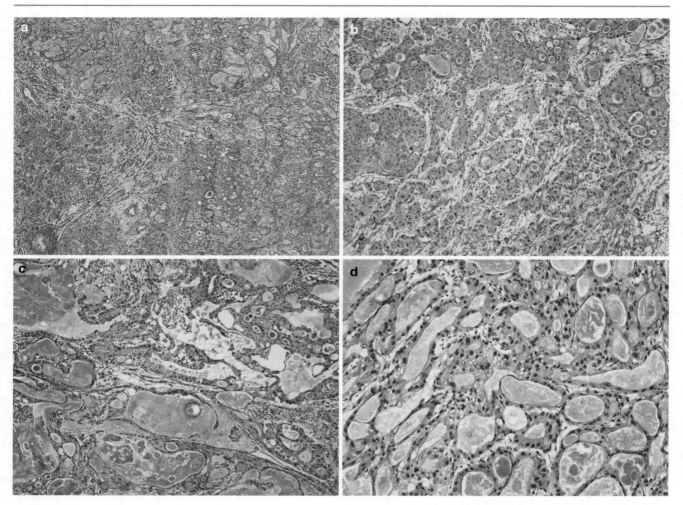

Fig. 4.36 Metastatic ductal carcinoma of the breast. Note the presence of glandular and tubulocystic growth patterns (**a**, **b**) with marked nuclear atypia, hobnailing, and clearing (**c**, **d**), simulating endometrial clear cell carcinoma in this example

References

1. Siegel R, Naishadham D, Jemal A. Cancer statistics, 2013. CA Cancer J Clin. 2013;63:11–30.
2. Ferlay J, Shin HR, Bray F, Forman D, Mathers C, Parkin DM. Estimates of worldwide burden of cancer in 2008: GLOBOCAN 2008. Int J Cancer. 2010;127:2893–917.
3. Sherman ME. Theories of endometrial carcinogenesis: a multidisciplinary approach. Mod Pathol. 2000;13:295–308.
4. Kurman RJ, Carcanglu ML, Herrington CS, Young RH. WHO classification of tumours of female reproductive organs. 4th ed. Lyon: International Agency for Research on Cancer (IARC); 2014; 121–135.
5. Acs G. Intraoperative consultation in gynecologic pathology. Semin Diagn Pathol. 2002;19:237–54.
6. Hanggi W, Katz M, Fravi R, Konig C, Dreher E. [Discrepancy in histopathological findings of curettage material and hysterectomy specimens in malignant tumors of the uterine body]. Schweiz Rundsch Med Prax. 1990;79:1387–9. *[Article in German]*.
7. Soothill PW, Alcock CJ, MacKenzie IZ. Discrepancy between curettage and hysterectomy histology in patients with stage 1 uterine malignancy. BJOG. 1989;96:478–81.
8. Kumar S, Bandyopadhyay S, Semaan A, Shah JP, Mahdi H, Morris R, et al. The role of frozen section in surgical staging of low risk endometrial cancer. PLoS One. 2011;6, e21912.
9. Rahimi S, Marani C, Renzi C, Natale M, Giovannini P, Zeloni R. Endometrial polyps and the risk of atypical hyperplasia on biopsies of unremarkable endometrium: a study on 694 patients with benign endometrial polyps. Int J Gynecol Pathol. 2009;28:522–8.
10. Bakour SH, Khan KS, Gupta JK. The risk of premalignant and malignant pathology in endometrial polyps. Acta Obstet Gynecol Scand. 2000;79:317–20.
11. Hui P, Kelly M, O'Malley DM, Tavassoli F, Schwartz PE. Minimal uterine serous carcinoma: a clinicopathological study of 40 cases. Mod Pathol. 2005;18:75–82.
12. Clement PB, Young RH. Endometrioid carcinoma of the uterine corpus: a review of its pathology with emphasis on recent advances and problematic aspects. Adv Anat Pathol. 2002;9:145–84.
13. Hendrickson MR, Kempson RL. Endometrial epithelial metaplasias: proliferations frequently misdiagnosed as adenocarcinoma. Report of 89 cases and proposed classification. Am J Surg Pathol. 1980;4:525–42.
14. Ip PP, Irving JA, McCluggage WG, Clement PB, Young RH. Papillary proliferation of the endometrium: a clinicopathologic study of 59 cases of simple and complex papillae without cytologic atypia. Am J Surg Pathol. 2013;37:167–77.
15. Nucci MR, Prasad CJ, Crum CP, Mutter GL. Mucinous endometrial epithelial proliferations: a morphologic spectrum of changes with diverse clinical significance. Mod Pathol. 1999;12:1137–42.
16. Arias-Stella J. The Arias-Stella reaction: facts and fancies four decades after. Adv Anat Pathol. 2002;9:12–23.
17. Huettner PC, Gersell DJ. Arias-Stella reaction in nonpregnant women: a clinicopathologic study of nine cases. Int J Gynecol Pathol. 1994;13:241–7.
18. Kurman RJ, Norris HJ. Evaluation of criteria for distinguishing atypical endometrial hyperplasia from well-differentiated carcinoma. Cancer. 1982;49:2547–59.
19. Wheeler DT, Bristow RE, Kurman RJ. Histologic alterations in endometrial hyperplasia and well-differentiated carcinoma treated with progestins. Am J Surg Pathol. 2007;31:988–98.
20. McKenney JK, Longacre TA. Low-grade endometrial adenocarcinoma: a diagnostic algorithm for distinguishing atypical endometrial hyperplasia and other benign (and malignant) mimics. Adv Anat Pathol. 2009;16:1–22.
21. Trimble CL, Kauderer J, Zaino R, Silverberg S, Lim PC, Burke 2nd JJ, et al. Concurrent endometrial carcinoma in women with a biopsy diagnosis of atypical endometrial hyperplasia: a Gynecologic Oncology Group study. Cancer. 2006;106:812–9.
22. Nofech-Mozes S, Ghorab Z, Ismiil N, Ackerman I, Thomas G, Barbera L, et al. Endometrial endometrioid adenocarcinoma: a pathologic analysis of 827 consecutive cases. Am J Clin Pathol. 2008;129:110–4.
23. Creasman W. Revised FIGO staging for carcinoma of the endometrium. Int J Gynaecol Obstet. 2009;105:109.
24. Zaino RJ, Kurman RJ, Diana KL, Morrow CP. The utility of the revised international federation of gynecology and obstetrics histologic grading of endometrial adenocarcinoma using a defined nuclear grading system. A Gynecologic Oncology Group study. Cancer. 1995;75:81–6.
25. Hendrickson MR, Kempson RL. Ciliated carcinoma–a variant of endometrial adenocarcinoma: a report of 10 cases. Int J Gynecol Pathol. 1983;2:1–12.
26. Tobon H, Watkins GJ. Secretory adenocarcinoma of the endometrium. Int J Gynecol Pathol. 1985;4:328–35.
27. Longacre TA, Chung MH, Jensen DN, Hendrickson MR. Proposed criteria for the diagnosis of well-differentiated endometrial carcinoma. A diagnostic test for myoinvasion. Am J Surg Pathol. 1995;19:371–406.
28. Zaino RJ, Silverberg SG, Norris HJ, Bundy N, Morrow CP, Okagaki T. The prognostic value of nuclear versus architectural grading in endometrial adenocarcinoma: a Gynecologic Oncology Group study. Int J Gynecol Pathol. 1994;13:29–36.
29. Murray SK, Clement PB, Young RH. Endometrioid carcinomas of the uterine corpus with sex cord-like formations, hyalinization, and other unusual morphologic features: a report of 31 cases of a neoplasm that may be confused with carcinosarcoma and other uterine neoplasms. Am J Surg Pathol. 2005;29:157–66.
30. Zaloudek C, Hayashi GM, Ryan IP, Powell CB, Miller TR. Microglandular adenocarcinoma of the endometrium: a form of mucinous adenocarcinoma that may be confused with microglandular hyperplasia of the cervix. Int J Gynecol Pathol. 1997;16: 52–9.
31. Zaino RJ, Kurman RJ, Brunetto VL, Morrow CP, Bentley RC, Cappellari JO, Bitterman P. Villoglandular adenocarcinoma of the endometrium: a clinicopathologic study of 61 cases: a gynecologic oncology group study. Am J Surg Pathol. 1998;22:1379–85.
32. Murray SK, Young RH, Scully RE. Uterine endometrioid carcinoma with small nonvillous papillae: an analysis of 26 cases of a favorable-prognosis tumor to be distinguished from serous carcinoma. Int J Surg Pathol. 2000;8:279–89.
33. Stewart CJ, Brennan BA, Leung YC, Little L. MELF pattern invasion in endometrial carcinoma: association with low grade, myoinvasive endometrioid tumours, focal mucinous differentiation and vascular invasion. Pathology. 2009;41:454–9.
34. Hertel JD, Huettner PC, Pfeifer JD. Lymphovascular space invasion in microcystic elongated and fragmented (MELF)-pattern well-differentiated endometrioid adenocarcinoma is associated with a higher rate of lymph node metastasis. Int J Gynecol Pathol. 2014;33:127–34.
35. Hanley KZ, Dustin SM, Stoler MH, Atkins KA. The significance of tumor involved adenomyosis in otherwise low-stage endometrioid adenocarcinoma. Int J Gynecol Pathol. 2010;29:445–51.
36. Melhem MF, Tobon H. Mucinous adenocarcinoma of the endometrium: a clinico-pathological review of 18 cases. Int J Gynecol Pathol. 1987;6:347–55.

37. Carcangiu ML, Chambers JT. Uterine papillary serous carcinoma: a study on 108 cases with emphasis on the prognostic significance of associated endometrioid carcinoma, absence of invasion, and concomitant ovarian carcinoma. Gynecol Oncol. 1992;47:298–305.

38. Brinton LA, Felix AS, McMeekin DS, Creasman WT, Sherman ME, Mutch D, et al. Etiologic heterogeneity in endometrial cancer: evidence from a Gynecologic Oncology Group trial. Gynecol Oncol. 2013;129:277–84.

39. Semaan A, Mert I, Munkarah AR, Bandyopadhyay S, Mahdi HS, Winer IS, et al. Clinical and pathologic characteristics of serous carcinoma confined to the endometrium: a multi-institutional study. Int J Gynecol Pathol. 2013;32:181–7.

40. Wheeler DT, Bell KA, Kurman RJ, Sherman ME. Minimal uterine serous carcinoma: diagnosis and clinicopathologic correlation. Am J Surg Pathol. 2000;24:797–806.

41. Kurman RJ, Scully RE. Clear cell carcinoma of the endometrium: an analysis of 21 cases. Cancer. 1976;37:872–82.

42. Abeler VM, Kjorstad KE. Clear cell carcinoma of the endometrium: a histopathological and clinical study of 97 cases. Gynecol Oncol. 1991;40:207–17.

43. Silva EG, Deavers MT, Bodurka DC, Malpica A. Association of low-grade endometrioid carcinoma of the uterus and ovary with undifferentiated carcinoma: a new type of dedifferentiated carcinoma? Int J Gynecol Pathol. 2006;25:52–8.

44. Tafe LJ, Garg K, Chew I, Tornos C, Soslow RA. Endometrial and ovarian carcinomas with undifferentiated components: clinically aggressive and frequently underrecognized neoplasms. Mod Pathol. 2010;23:781–9.

45. Altrabulsi B, Malpica A, Deavers MT, Bodurka DC, Broaddus R, Silva EG. Undifferentiated carcinoma of the endometrium. Am J Surg Pathol. 2005;29:1316–21.

46. Taraif SH, Deavers MT, Malpica A, Silva EG. The significance of neuroendocrine expression in undifferentiated carcinoma of the endometrium. Int J Gynecol Pathol. 2009;8:142–7.

47. van Hoeven KH, Hudock JA, Woodruff JM, Suhrland MJ. Small cell neuroendocrine carcinoma of the endometrium. Int J Gynecol Pathol. 1995;14:21–9.

48. Chetty R, Clark SP, Bhathal PS. Carcinoid tumour of the uterine corpus. Virchows Arch A Pathol Anat Histopathol. 1993;422:93–5.

49. Quddus MR, Sung CJ, Zhang C, Lawrence WD. Minor serous and clear cell components adversely affect prognosis in "mixed-type" endometrial carcinomas: a clinicopathologic study of 36 stage-I cases. Reprod Sci. 2010;17:673–8.

50. Kumar NB, Hart WR. Metastases to the uterine corpus from extragenital cancers. A clinicopathologic study of 63 cases. Cancer. 1982;50:2163–9.

51. Houghton JP, Ioffe OB, Silverberg SG, McGrady B, McCluggage WG. Metastatic breast lobular carcinoma involving tamoxifen-associated endometrial polyps: report of two cases and review of tamoxifen-associated polypoid uterine lesions. Mod Pathol. 2003;16:395–8.

5

Uterine Mesenchymal Tumors

Introduction

Uterine mesenchymal neoplasms are generally divided into smooth muscle tumors, endometrial stromal tumors, perivascular epithelioid cell tumors, and other mesenchymal tumors of both homologous and heterologous tissue types. In addition, tumors with mixed epithelial and mesenchymal components are also included in this chapter (Table 5.1) [1]. While benign leiomyomas are very common, uterine leiomyosarcoma and endometrial stromal tumors are rare, frequently unexpected lesions at the time of frozen section. The primary function of intraoperative consultation of uterine mesenchymal lesions in a hysterectomy specimen is to rule out malignancy. Careful gross inspection with attention to tumor border infiltration, color, and texture is crucial for adequate sampling of a uterine mesenchymal neoplasm for frozen section evaluation.

© Springer International Publishing Switzerland 2015
P. Hui, N. Buza, *Atlas of Intraoperative Frozen Section Diagnosis in Gynecologic Pathology*,
DOI 10.1007/978-3-319-21807-6_5

Table 5.1 2014 World Health Organization classification of uterine mesenchymal tumors. Data from Kurman et al. [1]

Major heading	Subheading	Subtype	Variant	Variant	Variant
Endometrial stromal tumors	Endometrial stromal nodule		With smooth muscle differentiation		
	Endometrial stromal sarcoma	Low-grade endometrial stromal sarcoma	With smooth muscle differentiation		
		High-grade endometrial stromal sarcoma			
Mixed epithelial and stromal tumors	Adenomyoma	Atypical polypoid adenomyoma (APA)			
	Adenosarcoma	With sarcomatous overgrowth			
	Malignant mixed Mullerian tumor (carcinosarcoma)				
Smooth muscle tumors	Spindle smooth muscle tumor	Leiomyoma	Mitotically active leiomyoma	Leiomyoma with bizarre nuclei	Cellular leiomyoma
		Leiomyosarcoma			
	Epithelioid smooth muscle tumor	Epithelioid leiomyoma	Plexiform tumorlet		
		Epithelioid leiomyosarcoma			
	Myxoid smooth muscle tumor	Myxoid leiomyoma			
		Myxoid leiomyosarcoma			
	Smooth muscle tumor of uncertain malignant potential (STUMP)				
	Smooth muscle tumor with unusual growth pattern or clinical behavior	Diffuse leiomyomatosis			
		Dissecting leiomyoma			
		Intravenous leiomyomatosis			
		Metastasizing leiomyoma			
Perivascular epithelioid cell tumors (PEComa)	Conventional PEComa	PEComatosis			
Other mesenchymal and miscellaneous tumors	Homologous sarcoma	Angiosarcoma			
		Fibrosarcoma			
		Neurogenic sarcoma			
	Heterologous sarcoma	Rhabdomyosarcoma			
		Alveolar soft part sarcoma			
		Rhabdoid tumor			
		Proximal epithelioid sarcoma			
	Undifferentiated uterine sarcoma				
	Uterine tumor resembling ovarian sex-cord tumor				
	Inflammatory myofibroblastic tumor				
	Adenomatoid tumor				

Smooth Muscle Tumors

Smooth muscle tumors of the uterus (see Table 5.1) [1] are categorized into leiomyoma, leiomyosarcoma, smooth muscle tumor of uncertain malignant potential (STUMP), and subsets of histologically mature smooth muscle tumors with either unusual growth patterns or unique clinical behavior (benign metastasizing leiomyoma, intravenous leiomyomatosis, diffuse peritoneal leiomyomatosis, peritoneal parasitic leiomyoma, uterine leiomyomatosis, and dissecting leiomyoma/cotyledonoid leiomyoma).

Conventional Leiomyoma

- Clinical features
    - The most common uterine mesenchymal tumor seen in over 2/3 of hysterectomy specimens.
    - Vaginal bleeding and pelvic pain or pressure are common clinical presentations.
- Gross pathology (Fig. 5.1)
    - Round to oval nodule involving submucosa, myometrium, or subserosa with multiple lesions seen in 2/3 of the cases

- Well-circumscribed, rubbery firm, and solid masses with bulging and whorled cut surface
- Frequent degenerative changes leading to various colors (red, brown, yellow, and hemorrhagic) and texture (edematous, fleshy to obviously necrotic), particularly in a large tumor (Fig. 5.2) and may be quite alarming for possible malignancy (Fig. 5.3)
- Microscopic features
    - Nodular proliferation of fascicles or bundles of mature, elongated smooth muscle cells with eosinophilic cytoplasm, and a centrally located cigar-shaped nucleus (Fig. 5.4).
    - Rich vasculature with characteristic gaping, thick-walled large caliber vessels.
    - Intratumoral hyalinization is common and may be extensive in some cases.
    - Secondary changes
        - Infarction-type necrosis with typical zonal configuration (necrotic smooth muscle cells are surrounded by a rim of granulation or fibrous tissue with varying degrees of hyalinization).
        - Intratumoral hemorrhage or red degeneration (commonly seen after hormonal treatment, with concurrent pregnancy or secondary to uterine artery embolization for symptomatic leiomyomas) (Fig. 5.5).

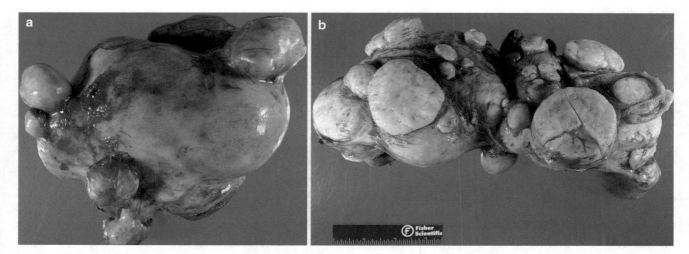

Fig. 5.1 Various gross presentations of uterine leiomyomas. Note the well-circumscribed round to oval nodules (**a**) with bulging, solid, and whorled cut surfaces (**b**)

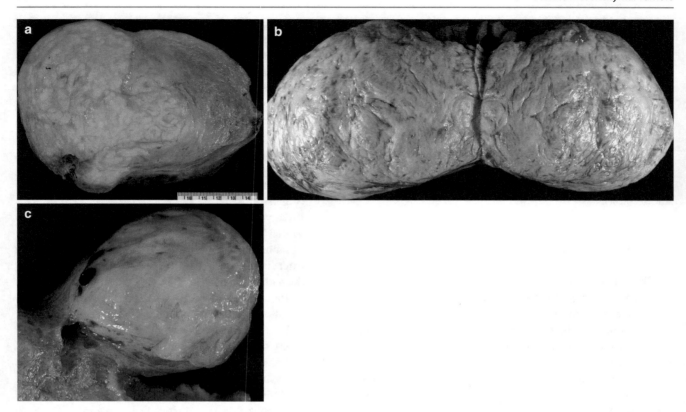

Fig. 5.2 Leiomyomas with degenerative changes. Note the varying colors (*white, brown,* or *yellow*) and texture (firm, fibrotic, or soft, edematous) (**a–c**)

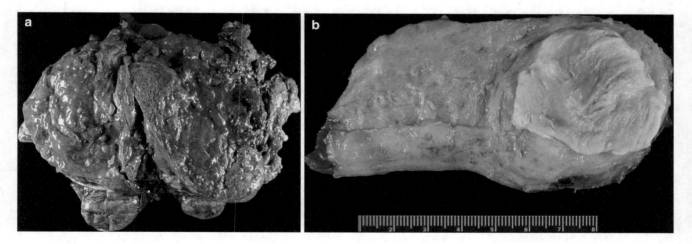

Fig. 5.3 Leiomyomas with a gross appearance suspicious for malignancy. Note the large areas of necrosis and hemorrhage (**a, b**)

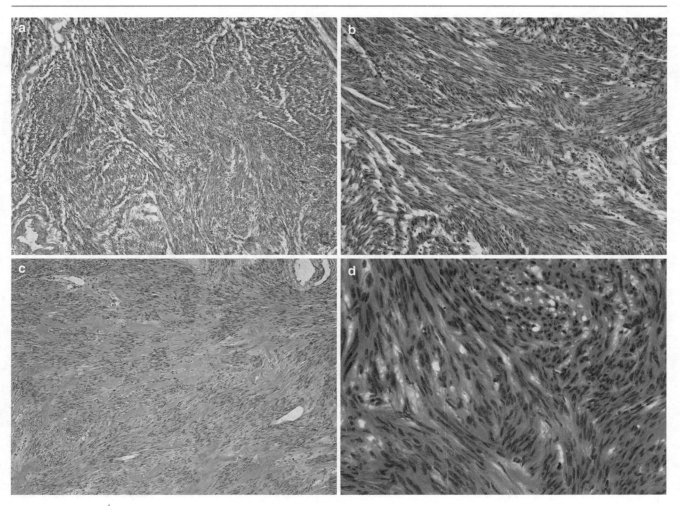

Fig. 5.4 Conventional leiomyoma. Note the mature smooth muscle proliferation in fascicles and bundles with variable stromal hyalinization (**a–c**) and characteristic cigar-shaped nuclei of the tumor cells (**d**)

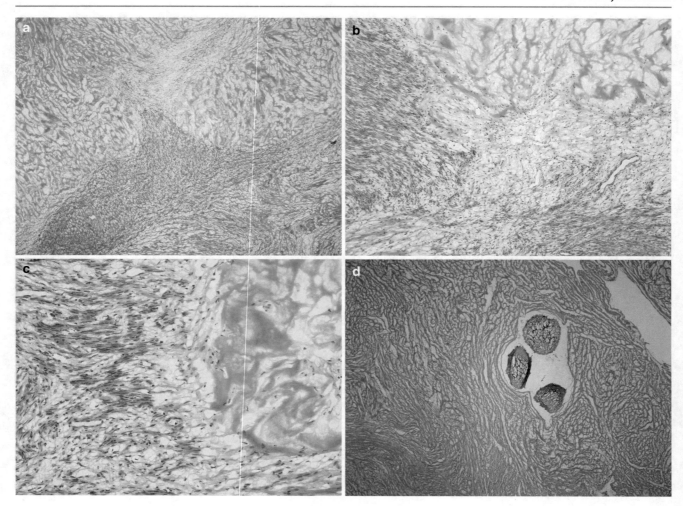

Fig. 5.5 Leiomyoma with hemorrhagic infarction due to therapeutic embolization. Note the characteristic zonal arrangement of the infarcted area, with gradual transition to granulation tissue and to viable smooth muscle cells (**a**–**c**). Intravascular foreign material—used for embolization—is apparent (**d**)

Leiomyoma Variants

- *Cellular leiomyoma* [2]
  - Grossly fleshy tumor nodules.
  - Histologically hypercellular compared to adjacent myometrium, some approaching the cellularity of an endometrial stromal tumor (Fig. 5.6).
  - Cleft-like or gaping, thick-walled vascular spaces are common.
  - Tumor border may show focal irregular extension into the adjacent myometrium.
  - Differential diagnosis
    - Low-grade endometrial stromal sarcoma
    - Smooth muscle tumor of uncertain malignant potential (STUMP)
    - Leiomyosarcoma
- Diagnostic pitfalls/key intraoperative consultation issues
  - The presence of fascicular growth pattern and large, gaping vessels favors a leiomyoma over an endometrial stromal tumor.
  - In contrast to STUMP and leiomyosarcoma, cellular leiomyoma has minimal mitotic activity and absence of coagulative tumor cell necrosis and cytological atypia.
  - When in doubt, interpretation of "smooth muscle tumor, classification is deferred for permanent sections" is recommended for conservative surgical management.
- *Leiomyoma with bizarre nuclei or symplastic leiomyoma* [1, 3]
  - The salient microscopic finding is the focal or diffuse presence of scattered, large atypical smooth muscle cells with abundant eosinophilic cytoplasm and bizarre nuclear shapes and multinucleation.
  - The bizarre tumor cells have hyperchromatic nuclei with frequent intranuclear inclusions.
  - Low mitotic count of less than 5 per 10 high-power fields (HPF)
  - Differential diagnosis (Table 5.2)
    - Leiomyosarcoma
  - Diagnostic pitfalls/key intraoperative consultation issues
    - In contrast to leiomyosarcoma, leiomyoma with bizarre nuclei lacks diffuse moderate to severe cytological atypia, mitotic activity, and coagulative tumor cell necrosis.
    - Chromatin condensation and fragmentation should not be misinterpreted as mitoses or atypical mitotic figures.
    - When in doubt, interpretation of "smooth muscle tumor with atypical features, classification is deferred for permanent sections" may be communicated for conservative surgical management.

- *Mitotically active leiomyoma*
  - The tumor may be associated with high progestin levels (secretory phase, pregnancy, or exogenous hormones) [1, 4, 5].
  - Histologically typical leiomyoma or cellular leiomyoma with 4–15 mitoses per 10 HPF.
  - Significant nuclear atypia and coagulative tumor cell necrosis are absent.
  - Differential diagnosis (see Table 5.2)
    - Leiomyosarcoma
  - Diagnostic pitfalls/key intraoperative consultation issues
    - In contrast to leiomyosarcoma, mitotically active leiomyoma lacks diffuse cytological atypia and coagulative tumor cell necrosis.
    - When in doubt, interpretation of "smooth muscle tumor with increased mitotic activity, classification is deferred for permanent sections" is recommended for conservative surgical management.
- *Apoplectic leiomyoma* (Fig. 5.7) [6, 7]
  - Patient with history of progestin treatment for symptomatic leiomyoma.
  - Grossly typical leiomyoma with foci of hemorrhage.
  - Histologically cellular leiomyoma with areas of hemorrhage and necrosis surrounded by zones of cellular smooth muscle proliferation that may have increased mitotic activity (Fig. 5.8), but no more than 8 per 10 HPF [7].
  - Granulation tissue, hyalinization, and myxoid degeneration may occur.
  - Differential diagnosis
    - Leiomyosarcoma
  - Diagnostic pitfalls/key intraoperative consultation issues
    - The tumor lacks nuclear atypia and coagulative tumor cell necrosis.
    - When in doubt, interpretation of "smooth muscle tumor with atypical features, classification is deferred for permanent sections" is recommended for conservative surgical management.
- *Myxoid leiomyoma* (Fig. 5.9)
  - Rare variant of leiomyoma that may be associated with a concurrent pregnancy.
  - Marked hypocellularity with small spindle or stellate cells embedded in a myxoid matrix [8].
  - Some myxoid leiomyomas may have an infiltrative border.
  - Nuclear atypia, coagulative tumor cell necrosis, and mitotic activity are absent (Fig. 5.10).
  - Differential diagnosis
    - Leiomyosarcoma

– Diagnostic pitfalls/key intraoperative consultation issues
  • For any myxoid tumor with an infiltrative tumor border or any level of noticeable mitotic activity, an interpretation of "myxoid smooth muscle tumor cannot rule out malignancy or defer to permanent section" is recommended for conservative surgical management.

• *Epithelioid leiomyoma (leiomyoblastoma)* [9] (Fig. 5.11)
  – Grossly indistinguishable from conventional leiomyoma.
  – Histological proliferation of polygonal to round cells in sheets, nests, or cords (Fig. 5.12).
  – Admixture with conventional spindled smooth muscle cells is common.
  – Tumor cells have eosinophilic or clear cytoplasm.
  – Absence of cytological atypia, necrosis, and mitotic activity.
  – Its microscopic variant, plexiform tumorlet is generally an incidental microscopic finding [10], most often solitary but may also be multiple.

• *Diffuse leiomyomatosis* [11]
  – Presence of numerous cellular leiomyomatous nodules merging into each other and diffusely involving the myometrium, leading to diffuse and symmetrical enlargement of the uterus.

– Histologically the tumor is identical to conventional leiomyoma.

• *Lipoleiomyoma*
  – Grossly yellow to tan nodular lesion (Fig. 5.13).
  – Leiomyoma with intermixed mature adipocytes (Fig. 5.14).
  – Focal chondroid or other heterologous components may be seen [12].
  – Differential diagnosis includes adenomatoid tumor. However, separation of the two benign entities is not crucial at the time of frozen section diagnosis.

• *Hydropic leiomyoma* (Fig. 5.15)
  – Leiomyoma with focal or zonal edema [13].
  – Edema separates bundles or nodules of smooth muscle. Pseudocyst formation may be seen within the hydropic area.
  – Differential diagnosis
    • Leiomyosarcoma
  – Diagnostic pitfalls/key intraoperative consultation issues
    • In contrast to leiomyosarcoma, hydropic leiomyoma has a zonal hydropic change, non-infiltrative border, and benign cytological features.

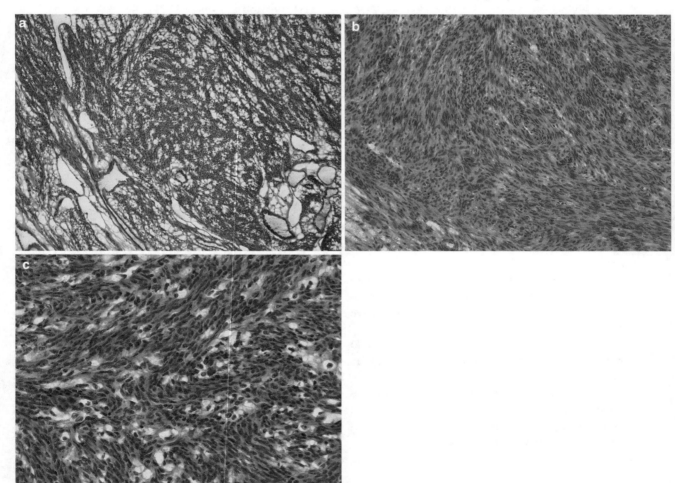

Fig. 5.6 Cellular leiomyoma. Note the marked hypercellularity compared to the adjacent myometrium (**a**) and lack of significant nuclear atypia and mitotic activity (**b**, **c**)

Table 5.2 Uterine smooth muscle tumors with spindled morphology (excluding epithelioid and myxoid variants)

Coagulative tumor cell necrosis[a]	Moderate to severe atypia	Mitoses/10 HPF	Interpretation
None	None	<5	Leiomyoma
		5 to 14	Mitotically active leiomyoma
		≥15	STUMP
	Focal or diffuse	<5	Leiomyoma with bizarre nuclei
		5–9	STUMP
		≥10	Leiomyosarcoma
Present	None	<10	STUMP
		≥10	Leiomyosarcoma
	Focal or diffuse	Any	Leiomyosarcoma
Uncertain	None	Any	STUMP

STUMP smooth muscle tumor of uncertain malignant potential; *HPF* high-power field

[a]Rule out GnRH analogue treatment-induced necrosis, which may be morphologically indistinguishable from true tumor cell necrosis

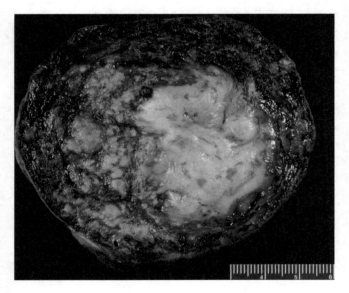

Fig. 5.7 Apoplectic leiomyoma. Note the presence of diffuse hemorrhage

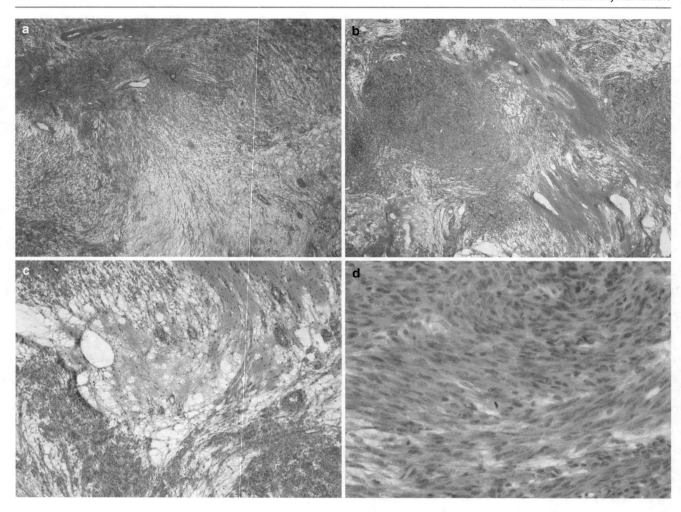

Fig. 5.8 Apoplectic leiomyoma. Cellular leiomyoma with hemorrhage, edema (**a–c**), and increased mitotic activity (**d**)

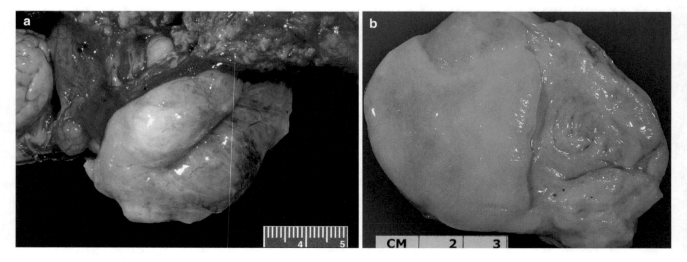

Fig. 5.9 Myxoid leiomyoma. Note the gelatinous gross appearance in these two examples (**a**, **b**)

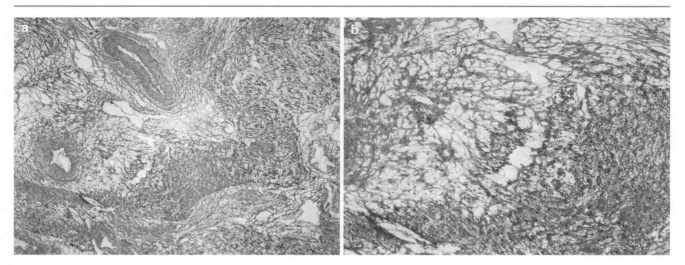

Fig. 5.10 Myxoid leiomyoma. Note the myxoid hypocellular areas in transition to a conventional leiomyoma area (**a**, **b**)

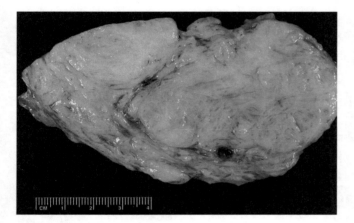

Fig. 5.11 Epithelioid leiomyoma presents as tan nodular lesions

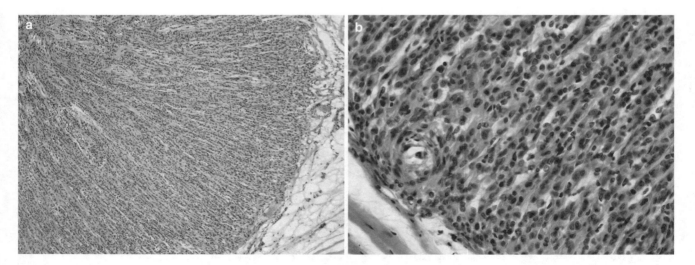

Fig. 5.12 Epithelioid leiomyoma. Note the polygonal to round, uniform epithelioid cells with eosinophilic cytoplasm arranged in cords (**a**, **b**)

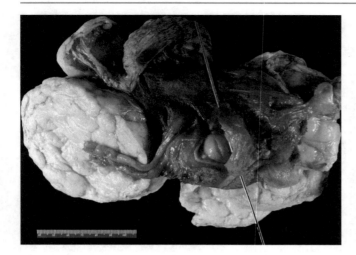

Fig. 5.13 Lipoleiomyoma. Note the presence of well-circumscribed, yellow-tan intramural nodules

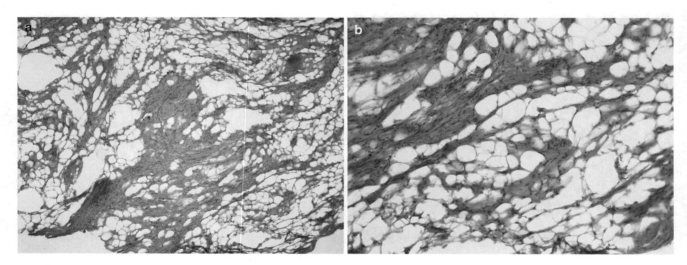

Fig. 5.14 Lipoleiomyoma. Note the variable amount of mature adipocytes admixed within bundles of smooth muscle cells (**a**, **b**)

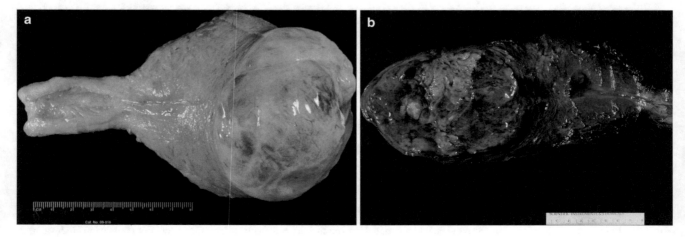

Fig. 5.15 Hydropic leiomyoma. Note semitransparent edematous nodules (**a**) with focal cystic changes (**b**)

Leiomyomas with Unusual Growth Pattern and/or Clinical Behavior

- *Intravenous leiomyomatosis (IVL)* [14, 15] [16]
  - Clinical symptoms are similar to conventional leiomyoma.
  - Some patients have history of multiple myomectomies.
  - Grossly multiple, irregular myometrial nodular or wormlike lesions, some of which may be grossly intravascular.
  - Tumor may extend into parametrial or pelvic vessels and occasionally further into the vena cava and right atrium and ventricle (Fig. 5.16).
  - Microscopically proliferation of serpentine smooth muscle bundles tracking and plugging vasculature at the tumor periphery and beyond (Fig. 5.17a, b).
  - Intravascular tumor plugs are
    - Covered by endothelium
    - Frequently smooth muscle cell poor, along with tissue molding, clefting, hyalinization, fibrosis, and vascularization [17] (Fig. 5.17c, d)
  - Differential diagnosis (Table 5.3)
    - Conventional leiomyomas with irregular tumor borders
    - Leiomyoma with focal vascular invasion
    - Entrapped arteries within myometrial veins (vessel within vessel phenomenon)
    - Low-grade endometrial stromal sarcoma
    - Intravenous growth of leiomyosarcoma
  - Diagnostic pitfalls/key intraoperative consultation issues
    - True intravascular growth of smooth muscle separates IVL from its benign mimics.
    - IVL lacks cytological features and characteristic vasculature of low-grade endometrial stromal sarcoma.
    - When in doubt, careful examination of the gross specimen including extrauterine vasculature and additional frozen sections should be performed.
- *Diffuse peritoneal leiomyomatosis (disseminated peritoneal leiomyomatosis)* [18–20]
  - Patients of reproductive age and over 2/3 of them with a concurrent pregnancy.
  - May be an incidental finding at the time of C-section or postpartum tubal ligation.
  - Grossly appears as multiple peritoneal nodules of less than 1 cm in size (Fig. 5.18).
  - Mature smooth muscle cell proliferation with occasional mitoses (less than 3 per 10 high-power fields) without significant cytological atypia and coagulative tumor cell necrosis (Fig. 5.19).
  - Generally a self-limiting disease with regression after pregnancy. Recurrence may be seen in subsequent pregnancies, however, and malignant transformation to leiomyosarcoma has been reported in rare cases.
  - Differential diagnosis
    - Leiomyosarcoma
  - Diagnostic pitfalls/key intraoperative consultation issues
    - In contrast to leiomyosarcoma, diffuse peritoneal leiomyomatosis lacks cytological atypia and coagulative tumor cell necrosis.
- Benign metastasizing leiomyoma [21]
  - Conventional uterine leiomyoma with concurrent or subsequent (post-myomectomy) extrauterine tumors of similar histology
  - Frequent involvement of lung and rarely retroperitoneal and mediastinal lymph nodes, bone, and soft tissue
  - Differential diagnosis
    - Leiomyosarcoma
  - Diagnostic pitfalls/key intraoperative consultation issues
    - In contrast to leiomyosarcoma, metastasizing leiomyoma lacks diffuse cytological atypia and coagulative tumor cell necrosis.
- *Dissecting leiomyoma* [22, 23]
  - Grossly lobulated myometrial lesion with ill-defined tumor border.
  - Histologically dissecting growth of bundles of mature smooth muscle cells protruding and splitting uterine myometrium.
  - In extremely rare cases, the dissecting smooth muscle bundles may extend into the broad ligament, forming a large mushroomlike mass (cotyledonoid variant).
  - The gross appearance may be quite alarming at the time of frozen section diagnosis. Leiomyosarcoma should be ruled out by careful microscopic examination.

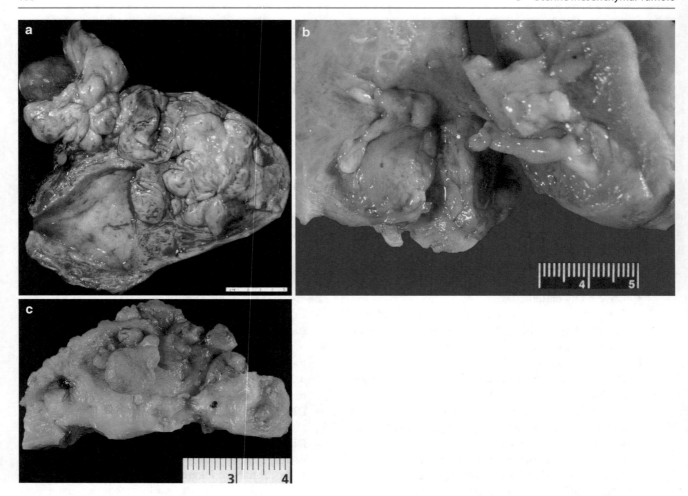

Fig. 5.16 Intravenous leiomyomatosis. Note the presence of multiple, irregular, nodular myometrial, and wormlike intravascular lesions (**a–c**). Note the extrauterine extension of the tumor (**a**, *upper left corner*)

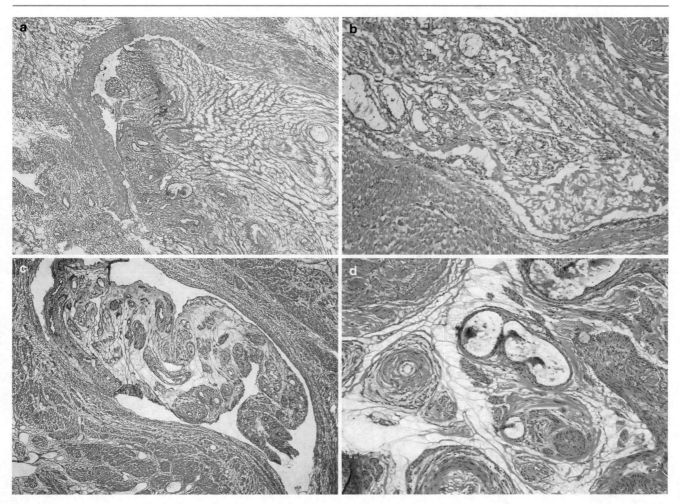

Fig. 5.17 Intravenous leiomyomatosis (IVL). Note the smooth muscle bundles tracking and plugging large caliber vasculature (**a, b**) and the presence of tissue molding, clefting, hyalinization, and vascularization along with diminished smooth muscle cells (**c, d**)

Table 5.3 Frozen section diagnosis of mesenchymal tumors with intravascular growth pattern

	Intravenous leiomyomatosis	Low-grade endometrial stromal sarcoma	Leiomyosarcoma
Patient age	Any age	Mostly <50 years of age	Mostly > 40 years of age
Gross pathology	Multinodular, white, rubbery masses with surrounding wormlike vascular plugging	Infiltrative endo-myometrial soft tan mass with wormlike vascular plugging	Large mass with irregular border and fleshy, necrotic cut surface, may show intravascular mass lesions
Growth pattern	Intravenous growth of leiomyoma, may be cellular; often hyalinized or shows abundant prominent thick-walled vessels	Infiltrative border and tonguelike tumor growth involving adjacent myometrium and lymphovascular spaces. Starburst hyaline plaques and sex-cord differentiation may be seen	Spindle smooth muscle cells with coagulative tumor cell necrosis and hemorrhage
Cytological features	Bland, elongated spindle smooth muscle cells	Monotonous small oval to short spindle cells with scant cytoplasm	Spindle smooth muscle cells with diffuse moderate to severe nuclear atypia
Mitotic activity	None	Low	Frequent (>10 mitoses/10 HPF)
Intratumoral vasculature	Large gaping vessels	Evenly distributed small arterioles	Variably sized vasculature
Extrauterine disease	Often present involving venous structures with thin wormlike plugging	Often seen involving lymphatics with a wormlike plugging appearance	When present, marked expansion of existing vasculature by tumor nodules

HPF high-power field

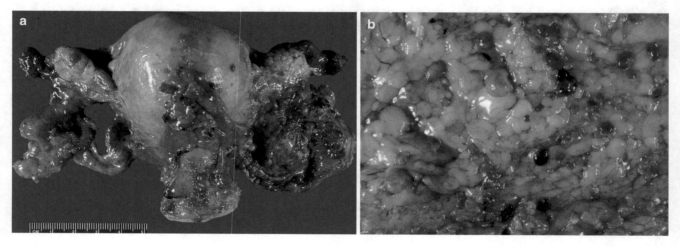

Fig. 5.18 Diffuse peritoneal leiomyomatosis. Note the presence of multiple peritoneal nodules of less than 1 cm on the surface of broad ligaments (**a**) and omentum (**b**)

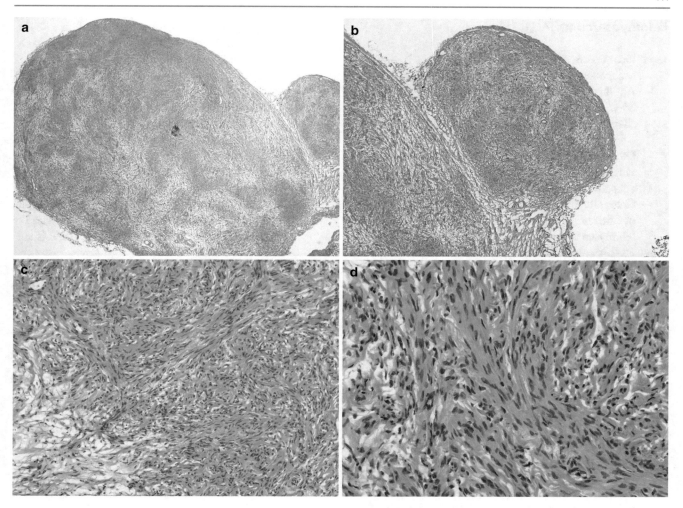

Fig. 5.19 Diffuse peritoneal leiomyomatosis. Nodular proliferation of mature smooth muscle cells (**a**, **b**) without cytological atypia, mitotic activity, or tumor cell necrosis (**c**, **d**)

Leiomyosarcoma [4] [1, 24]

- Clinical features
  - Most common uterine sarcoma.
  - Adult patients over 40 years of age, with a mean age of 55 years.
  - May present with sudden uterine tumor growth in patients not on hormone replacement [25].
  - Other clinical symptoms include vaginal bleeding, pelvic mass, and pelvic pain or pressure.
- Gross pathology (Fig. 5.20)
  - Generally solitary large mass (average size of 10 cm) or the largest mass among multiple conventional leiomyomas.
  - Fleshy, soft, and bulging cut surface with varying colors and textures.
  - Infiltrative tumor border may be grossly apparent.
  - Necrosis and hemorrhage are common.
- Microscopic features (see Table 5.2)
  - Hypercellular spindle cell proliferation forming disorganized fascicles and nodules (Fig. 5.21).
  - Diffuse moderate to severe cytological atypia including marked nuclear pleomorphism and multinucleation (appreciable at low to medium power) (Fig. 5.22).
  - Presence of coagulative tumor cell necrosis.
  - Geographic necrotic pattern showing abrupt transition between viable and necrotic, "ghost" tumor cells.
  - Perivascular cuffing by viable tumor cells surrounded by a necrotic zone is characteristic (Fig. 5.23). In some tumors, the necrosis may be quite subtle (Fig. 5.24).
  - Brisk mitotic activity (10 or more mitoses per 10 HPF), often with abnormal mitotic figures.
- Differential diagnosis
  - Leiomyoma variants and leiomyomas with unusual growth patterns
  - Smooth muscle tumor of uncertain malignant potential (STUMP)
  - Endometrial stromal tumors with smooth muscle differentiation
  - Undifferentiated uterine sarcoma
  - Malignant mixed Mullerian tumor (carcinosarcoma)
- Diagnostic pitfalls/key intraoperative consultation issues
  - The purpose of frozen section diagnosis of smooth muscle tumors is to unequivocally identify leiomyosarcoma (see Table 5.2).
    - Leiomyosarcoma is often a solitary, solid mass and is typically the dominant mass when arising in a background of multiple leiomyomas.

- Careful gross examination with attention to color, texture, and tumor border should guide where the frozen sections are taken from.
- Presence of unequivocal coagulative tumor cell necrosis and at least moderate nuclear atypia are sufficient for diagnosis of leiomyosarcoma regardless of the mitotic activity.
- Tumor cell necrosis can be subtle in some cases. Careful search of the entire frozen section slide or submitting additional tumor blocks may be helpful (see Fig. 5.24).
- In the absence of moderate to severe nuclear atypia, unequivocal tumor cell necrosis combined with the presence of 10 or more mitoses per 10 HPF is sufficient for the diagnosis of malignancy.
- In the absence of tumor cell necrosis, moderate to severe cytological atypia combined with the presence of 10 or more mitoses per 10 HPF is required for the diagnosis of leiomyosarcoma.
  - Overinterpretation of bizarre leiomyoma as leiomyosarcoma due to the presence of nuclear atypia and multinucleation should be avoided. Nuclear fragmentation/karyorrhexis in bizarre leiomyoma should not be misinterpreted as mitotic figures.
  - Apoplectic leiomyoma may show ambiguous necrosis and hemorrhage in a clinical setting of progestin therapy or concurrent pregnancy.
  - Pregnancy may induce red degeneration of leiomyoma resulting in a soft and homogenously necrotic appearance. The patient may present with abdominal pain and fever.
  - Any smooth muscle tumor with a myxoid histology should be considered potentially malignant at the time of frozen section diagnosis (see myxoid leiomyosarcoma).
  - If the histological findings are concerning for malignancy but definitive diagnostic features of leiomyosarcoma are lacking, additional frozen sections from different tumor areas should be evaluated.
  - In any of the above scenarios, if additional frozen sections cannot resolve the uncertainty, a conservative approach should be taken and a frozen diagnosis of "smooth muscle tumor with atypical features, defer to permanent sections to rule out malignancy" is recommended to avoid unnecessary staging surgery, particularly in a young patient who desires preservation of fertility.

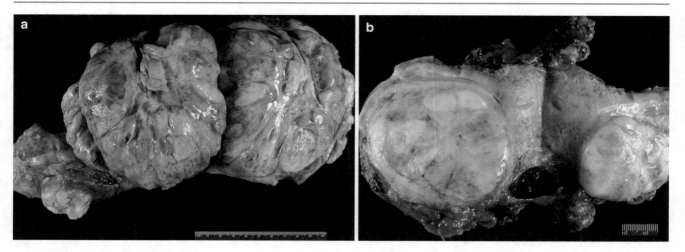

Fig. 5.20 Leiomyosarcoma (spindle cell). Large dominant intramural mass with a fleshy cut surface showing hemorrhage and necrosis (**a**, **b**)

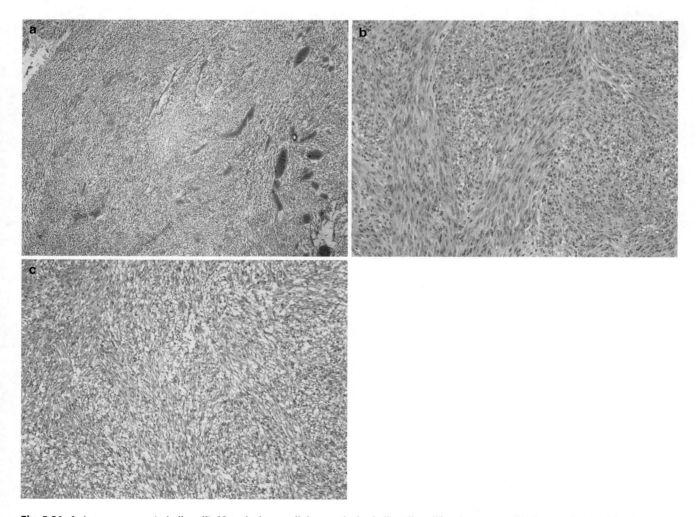

Fig. 5.21 Leiomyosarcoma (spindle cell). Note the hypercellular, atypical spindle cell proliferation, arranged in intersecting fascicles (**a–c**)

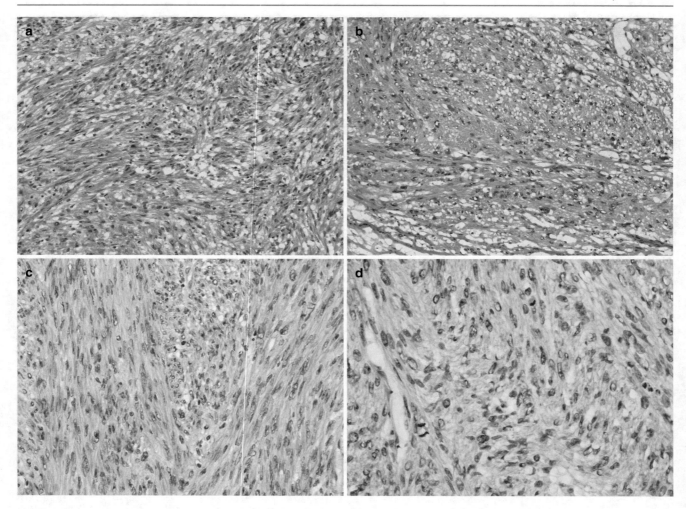

Fig. 5.22 Leiomyosarcoma (spindle cell). Note the diffuse moderate to marked cytological atypia (**a–c**) and brisk mitotic activity (**d**)

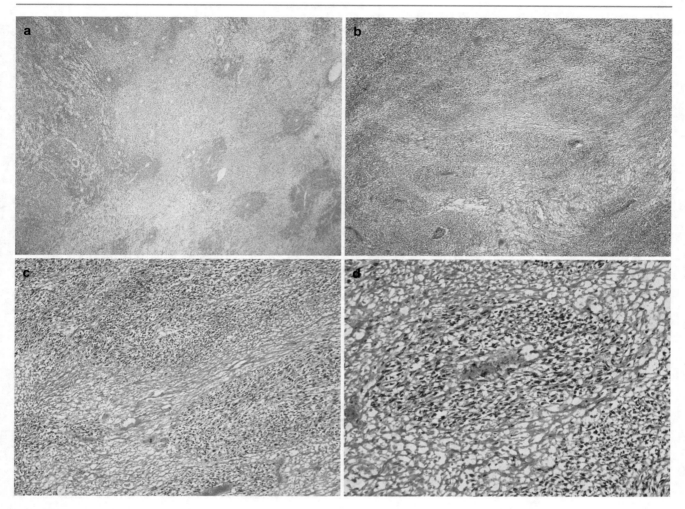

Fig. 5.23 Leiomyosarcoma (spindle cell). Note the geographic coagulative tumor cell necrosis (**a–c**) and characteristic vascular cuffing by viable tumor cells (**d**)

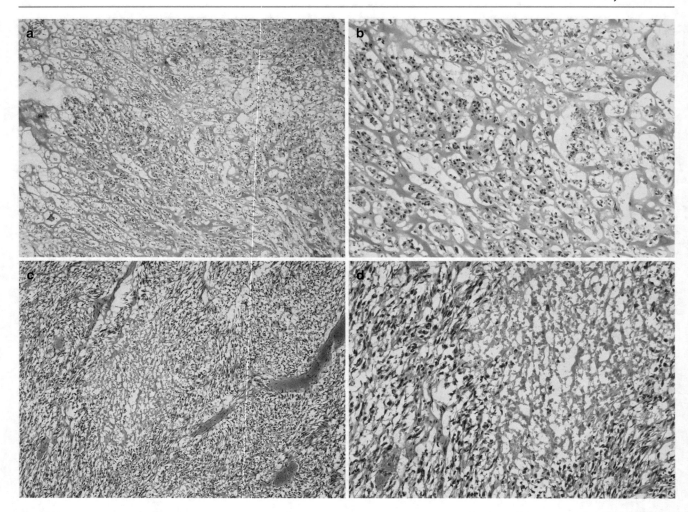

Fig. 5.24 Leiomyosarcoma (spindle cell). Note the presence of subtle and focal coagulative tumor cell necrosis (**a**, **b**) and abrupt transition between the viable and necrotic tumor without an intervening hyalinized zone (**c**, **d**)

Leiomyosarcoma Variants

Epithelioid leiomyosarcoma (Fig. 5.25) [9, 10]

- Diffuse or nested proliferation of polygonal or round epithelioid cells with abundant eosinophilic or clear cytoplasm.
- Spindle smooth muscle component may be seen.
- The presence of moderate to severe cytological atypia, mitotic count of 3 or more per 10 HPF, and coagulative tumor cell necrosis establishes the diagnosis.
- Differential diagnosis
  - Poorly differentiated carcinoma
  - Gestational trophoblastic tumors (placental site trophoblastic tumor and epithelioid trophoblastic tumor)
  - Epithelioid leiomyoma

- Diagnostic pitfalls/key intraoperative consultation issues
  - In contrast to epithelioid leiomyosarcoma, poorly differentiated endometrial carcinoma often shows foci of definitive epithelial differentiation—gland formation or squamous elements.
  - Separation of epithelioid leiomyosarcoma from gestational trophoblastic tumors can be difficult at the time of frozen section diagnosis. Helpful hints in favor of trophoblastic tumors include elevation of serum hCG, stromal deposition of eosinophilic fibrin, and extensive hyalinization.
  - Compared with epithelioid leiomyoma, epithelioid leiomyosarcoma shows obvious cytological atypia, mitotic activity, and coagulative tumor cell necrosis.

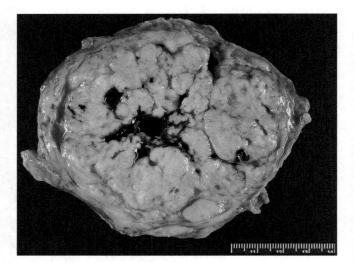

Fig. 5.25 Epithelioid leiomyosarcoma. Note the yellow-tan, fleshy cut surface with focal hemorrhage

Myxoid leiomyosarcoma [26, 27]

- Lobular or irregular gelatinous mass lesion with an infiltrative gross appearance (Fig. 5.26).
- Hypocellular proliferation of small spindle or stellate cells with hyperchromatic nuclei and scant cytoplasm, evenly distributed in a background of abundant myxoid or edematous matrix (Fig. 5.27).
- Coagulative tumor cell necrosis and vascular invasion may be seen.
- Foci of tumor cells with identifiable smooth muscle differentiation are generally seen in non-myxoid areas.
- Presence of coagulative tumor cell necrosis, 2 or more mitoses per 10 HPF and nuclear atypia are diagnostic features.
- Differential diagnosis
  - Myxoid leiomyoma
  - Hydropic leiomyoma
  - Endometrial stromal tumor with myxoid appearance
- Diagnostic pitfalls/key intraoperative consultation issues
  - Frozen sections should be taken from multiple tumor areas.
  - In contrast to myxoid or hydropic leiomyomas, myxoid leiomyosarcoma may show unequivocal features of malignancy in the non-myxoid tumor areas.
  - In cases with equivocal histological features, a conservative approach should be taken and a frozen diagnosis of "smooth muscle tumor with atypical features, defer to permanent sections to rule out malignancy" is recommended.

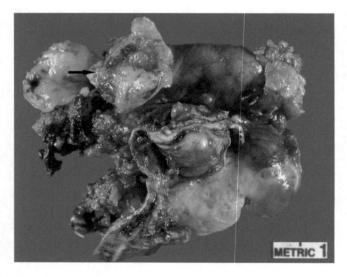

Fig. 5.26 Myxoid leiomyosarcoma. Note the lobular to irregular gelatinous mass lesion (*arrow*)

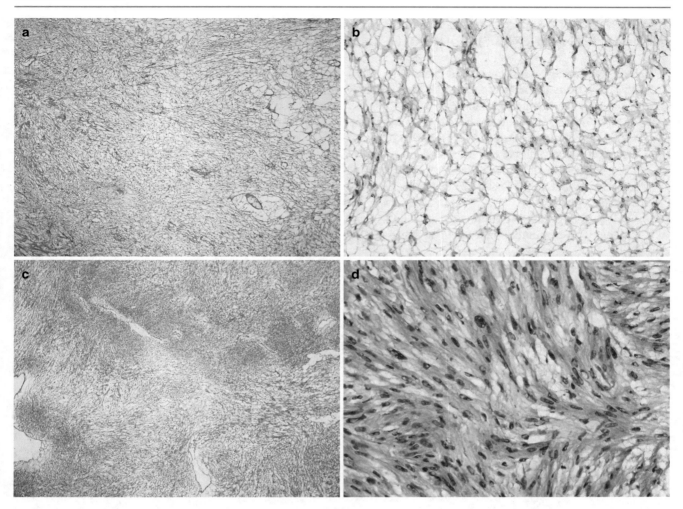

Fig. 5.27 Myxoid leiomyosarcoma. Note the hypocellular, myxoid proliferation of small stellate cells with scant cytoplasm (**a**, **b**), focally merging into an area of atypical spindled smooth muscle proliferation (**c**, **d**)

Smooth Muscle Tumors of Uncertain Malignant Potential (STUMP) [1, 4] [28–31]

- Grossly the tumor may show unusual features (Fig. 5.28).
- Histological features are intermediate between leiomyoma and leiomyosarcoma (see Table 5.2).
    - Focal or diffuse moderate to severe cytological atypia with a mitotic count between 5 and 9 per 10 HPF and lack of coagulative tumor cell necrosis
    - Coagulative tumor cell necrosis with a mitotic count of less than 10 per 10 HPF and lack of significant cytological atypia
    - Otherwise conventional leiomyoma or cellular leiomyoma with a mitotic count of 15 or more per 10 HPF

- Differential diagnosis
    - Leiomyoma variants including cellular, mitotically active, apoplectic, and bizarre leiomyomas
    - Leiomyosarcoma
    - Endometrial stromal tumor
    - Mixed endometrial stromal and smooth muscle tumor
- Diagnostic pitfalls/key intraoperative consultation issues
    - Interpretation of a smooth muscle tumor as STUMP at the time of frozen section consultation is discouraged.
    - If additional frozen sections cannot resolve the uncertainty, a conservative approach should be taken and a frozen diagnosis of "smooth muscle tumor with atypical features, defer to permanent sections for final classification" is recommended.

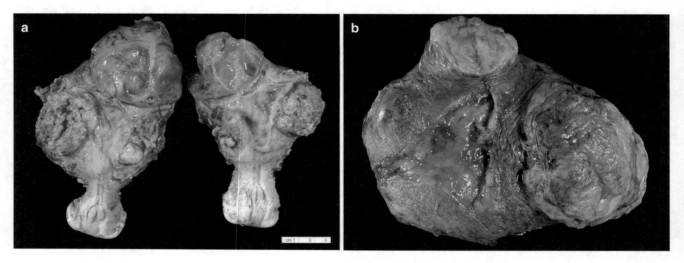

Fig. 5.28 Smooth muscle tumor of uncertain malignant potential (STUMP). Note the unusual gross appearance that may raise concern for leiomyosarcoma (**a, b**)

Endometrial Stromal Tumors

Endometrial stromal tumors are uterine mesenchymal neoplasms with endometrial stromal differentiation. Most tumors have proliferating cells and stromal vasculature histologically resembling the proliferative phase endometrial stroma. While high-grade endometrial stromal sarcoma has obvious malignant features, histological separation of low-grade endometrial stromal sarcoma from a benign endometrial stromal nodule is primarily determined by the presence of infiltrative tumor border, requiring both careful gross and microscopic evaluation at the time of intraoperative consultation (Table 5.4).

Table 5.4 Frozen section diagnosis of endometrial stromal tumors

	ESN	LESS	HESS
Tumor border	Well-circumscribed or only focal myometrial infiltration of <3 mm	Infiltrative tumor with tonguelike projections into myometrium	Polypoid or round mass with or without obvious infiltration
Lymphovascular invasion	Absent	Present—wormlike plugging	Present
Vasculature	Evenly distributed spiral arterioles	Evenly distributed spiral arterioles	Focally evenly distributed spiral arterioles
Tumor cells	Bland oval to short spindled	Bland oval to short spindled	Round high-grade cell proliferation admixed with LESS-like areas
Mitotic activity	Low	Low	High
Tumor cell necrosis	Absent	Generally absent	Present
Collagen deposition	Present in bands or in plaques	Present in bands or in plaques	May be present

ESN endometrial stromal nodule, *LESS* low-grade endometrial stromal sarcoma, *HESS* high-grade endometrial stromal sarcoma

Endometrial Stromal Nodule (ESN) [32, 33]

- Clinical features
  - Reproductive age to postmenopausal women (mean age of 47 years).
  - Vaginal bleeding is the most common symptom.
- Gross pathology (Fig. 5.29)
  - Single round to oval mass, may be polypoid
  - Fleshy, tan to yellow cut surface
  - Sharply demarcated from surrounding endo-myometrium
- Microscopic features
  - Well-circumscribed cellular proliferation with a sharp border to the adjacent endo-myometrium (Fig. 5.30).
  - Proliferation of uniform tumor cells histologically reminiscent of normal endometrial stromal cells at the proliferative phase (Fig. 5.31).
  - Minimal cytological atypia with round to oval nuclei, fine chromatin, and inconspicuous nucleoli.
  - Mitotic activity is usually present, but low.
  - Characteristic spiral arterioles, evenly distributed within the tumor.
  - Fibroblastic areas with marked collagen deposition—hyalinized plaques (starburst configuration)—and foamy macrophages are commonly present.
  - Smooth muscle differentiation can be seen, which is often hypercellular with large caliber, gaping vasculature.
  - Other variable findings include fibromyxoid changes, sex-cord differentiation, epithelioid tumor cells, and focal endometrial glandular differentiation.

- Differential diagnosis
  - Cellular leiomyoma
  - Low-grade endometrial stromal sarcoma
  - Endometrial polyp with cellular stroma
  - Uterine tumor resembling ovarian sex-cord tumor
- Diagnostic pitfalls/key intraoperative consultation issues
  - Gross and histological examination of the tumor border is essential.
    - Focal fingerlike protrusions or isolated satellite tumor foci less than 3 mm from the main tumor—and no more than 3 of such foci—are compatible with the diagnosis of endometrial stromal nodule.
    - Tumors with less than 9 mm border protrusion have been diagnosed as endometrial stromal tumor with limited infiltration, but the behavior of such lesions is uncertain.
    - Infiltrative growth pattern beyond the above-described extent is seen in low-grade endometrial stromal sarcoma.
  - Presence of uniform small arterioles, fibromyxoid changes (particularly starburst hyaline plaques), and absence of large thick-walled vasculature separate endometrial stromal nodule from cellular leiomyoma.
  - In contrast to endometrial stromal tumor, uterine tumor resembling ovarian sex-cord tumor has uniform epithelioid tumor cells forming nests, cords, tubules, or retiform pattern without endometrial stromal cell proliferation.

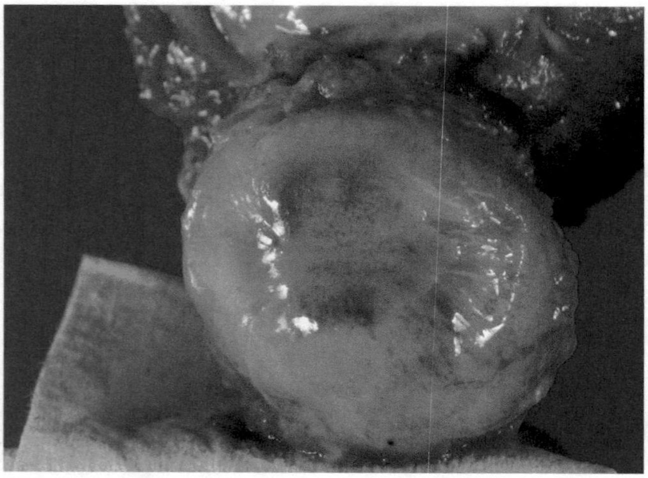

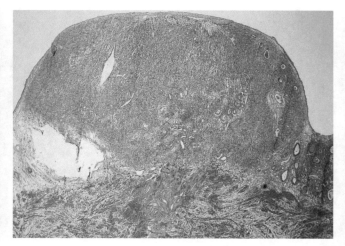

Fig. 5.29 Endometrial stromal nodule. Note the well-circumscribed tumor border

Fig. 5.30 Endometrial stromal nodule. Well-defined tumor border is present in this intramucosal endometrial stromal nodule

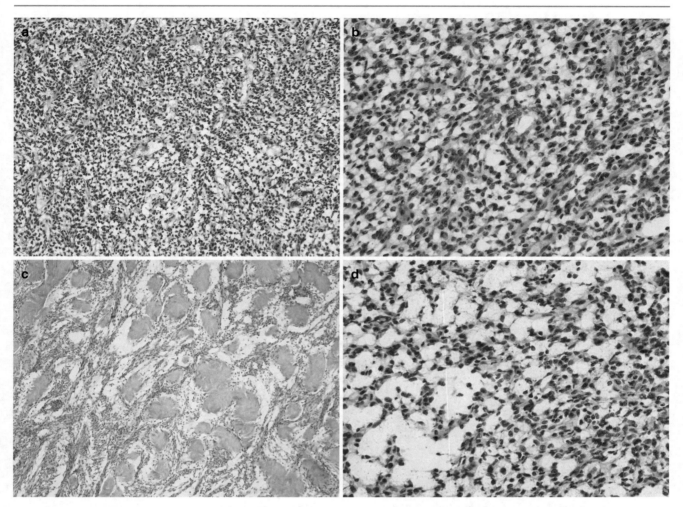

Fig. 5.31 Endometrial stromal nodule. Note the proliferation of uniform small, round to oval stromal cells and characteristic spiral arterioles evenly distributed within the lesion (**a**, **b**). Hyaline plaques (**c**) and foamy macrophages (**d**) are also present

Low-Grade Endometrial Stromal Sarcoma [32, 34–36] [37]

- Clinical features
  - Most common in women younger than 50 years of age.
  - Vaginal bleeding and/or pelvic pain are common symptoms.
- Gross pathology (Fig. 5.32)
  - Infiltrative, soft, tan endo-myometrial lesion
    - May show polypoid protrusion into the endometrial cavity
  - Grossly obvious myometrial and lymphovascular invasion in the form of wormlike plugs, which may extend into extrauterine vessels
- Microscopic features
  - Infiltrative border and tonguelike tumor growth involving adjacent myometrium and lymphovascular spaces (Fig. 5.33).
  - Except the infiltrative tumor border, LESS shares all the histological and cytological features of ESN (see above).
  - Sex-cord differentiation is seen in about 1/5 of the cases (Fig. 5.34).
  - Unusual histological findings:
    - Endometrial glandular differentiation
    - Fibromyxoid changes and hyaline plaques
    - Sex-cord differentiation
    - Epithelioid tumor cells
    - Foamy macrophages
    - Papillary and pseudopapillary changes
    - Smooth muscle differentiation (mixed endometrial stromal and smooth muscle tumor if more than 30 % smooth muscle component is present)
- Differential diagnosis (see Tables 5.3 and 5.4)
  - Endometrial stromal nodule
  - High-grade endometrial stromal sarcoma
  - Intravenous leiomyomatosis
  - Leiomyosarcoma
  - Adenosarcoma
  - Gland-poor adenomyosis
- Diagnostic pitfalls/key intraoperative consultation issues
  - Gross examination is crucial for appropriate sampling for frozen section diagnosis, to demonstrate the infiltrative growth pattern and separate benign endometrial stromal nodule from low-grade endometrial stromal sarcoma.
  - For tumors without grossly obvious infiltrative growth pattern, it may not be practical to evaluate the entire tumor border microscopically at the time of intraoperative consultation, and the diagnosis of "endometrial

stromal tumor, final classification is deferred to permanent sections" can be communicated.
  - High-grade endometrial stromal sarcoma has areas of markedly atypical round cell component with high mitotic activity.
  - Intravenous leiomyomatosis (IVL) lacks cytological features and the characteristic vasculature of low-grade endometrial stromal sarcoma.
  - In contrast to LESS, adenosarcoma is characterized by relatively uniform glandular distribution, periglandular stromal cell cuffing, and intraglandular papillary infoldings.
  - In contrast to LESS, gland-poor adenomyosis does not form a mass lesion, and additional sections may reveal typical foci of adenomyosis.

High-Grade Endometrial Stromal Sarcoma [38]

- Clinical features
  - Most common in patients over 50 years of age.
  - Vaginal bleeding and pelvic mass are common symptoms.
- Gross pathology
  - Endo-myometrial mass lesion with an infiltrative growth pattern
    - May show a polypoid intraluminal component
  - Tan-yellow, fleshy cut surface with frequent necrosis and hemorrhage
  - Frequent extrauterine extension
- Microscopic features
  - Hypercellular nests or sheets of markedly atypical, round tumor cells with a destructive growth pattern.
  - Low-grade endometrial stromal sarcoma-like component may be present.
  - Focal rhabdoid or discohesive pseudopapillary pattern.
  - Conspicuous lymphovascular invasion.
  - Necrosis is common.
  - High mitotic count (>10/10 HPF).
- Differential diagnosis (see Table 5.4)
  - Low-grade endometrial stromal sarcoma
  - Undifferentiated uterine sarcoma
  - Epithelioid leiomyosarcoma
  - Poorly differentiated carcinoma
- Diagnostic pitfalls/key intraoperative consultation issues
  - Separation from the above differential diagnoses may be difficult and is generally not crucial at the time of frozen section diagnosis; interpretation as "high-grade malignant uterine neoplasm" should suffice for the surgical management of the patient.

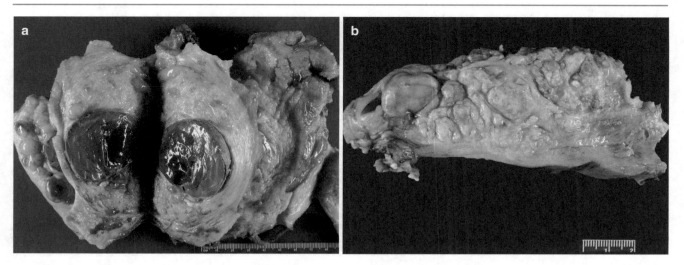

Fig. 5.32 Low-grade endometrial stromal sarcoma (LESS). Note the ill-defined tumor border with satellite nodules, presence of necrosis (**a**), and wormlike myometrial infiltration and lymphovascular plugging (**b**)

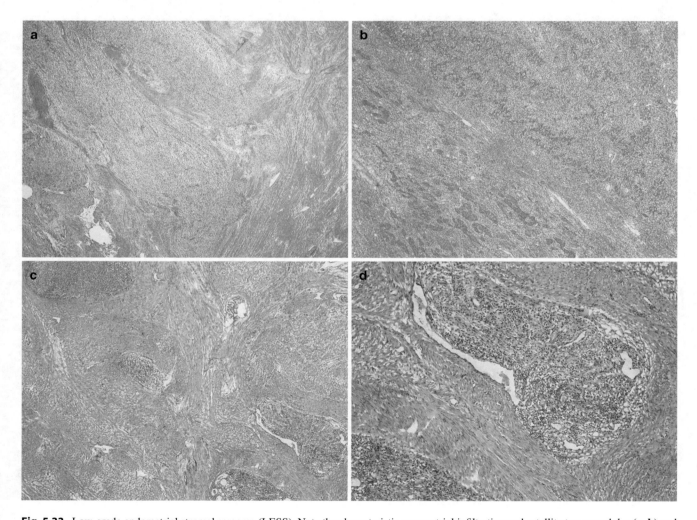

Fig. 5.33 Low-grade endometrial stromal sarcoma (LESS). Note the characteristic myometrial infiltration and satellite tumor nodules (**a**, **b**) and lymphovascular invasion (**c**, **d**)

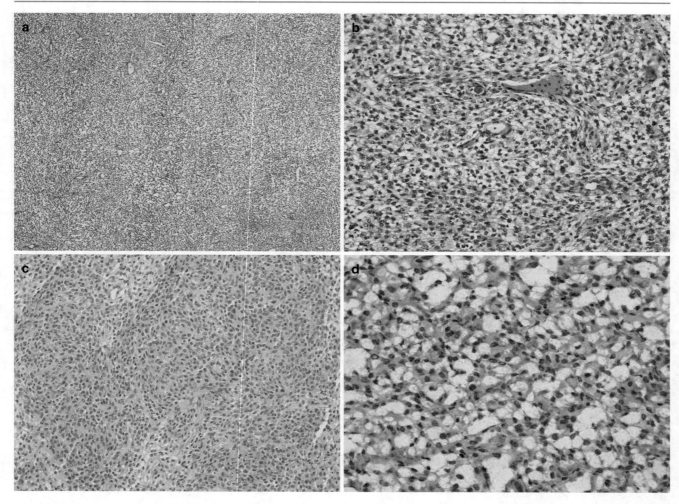

Fig. 5.34 Low-grade endometrial stromal sarcoma (LESS). Similar to endometrial stromal nodule, LESS consists of uniform, small oval cells and characteristic spiral arterioles evenly distributed within the lesion (**a**, **b**). Sex-cord differentiation (**c**) and foamy macrophages (**d**) are also common

Mixed Epithelial and Mesenchymal Tumors

Adenomyoma [39, 40]

- Polypoid submucosal lesion.
- Nodular smooth muscle proliferation with scattered proliferative endometrial glands, some of which are surrounded by thin mantles of endometrial stroma.
- Important differential diagnosis is atypical polypoid adenomyoma (APA, see below).

Atypical Polypoid Adenomyoma (APA) [41, 42]

- Clinical features
  - Most often seen in premenopausal women between 30 and 40 years of age—may rarely occur in postmenopausal patients
  - Typically presents with abnormal vaginal bleeding
- Gross pathology
  - Solitary pedunculated or sessile polypoid mass.
  - Frequently involves the lower uterine segment (Fig. 5.35), less often the uterine corpus and cervix.
- Microscopic features (Figs. 5.36 and 5.37)
  - Irregular, hyperplastic endometrial glands embedded in smooth muscle-rich stroma.

- The glandular epithelium may show mild to moderate cytological atypia including nuclear enlargement, hyperchromasia, loss of polarity, and cytoplasmic eosinophilia.
- Squamous differentiation in the form of immature squamous metaplasia to well-developed squamous morules is common.
  - May simulate a cribriform glandular pattern.
  - Frequently shows focal keratinization and central necrosis.
- Cytologically benign smooth muscle fibers forming bundles or fascicles.
- Differential diagnosis
  - Endometrial polyp
  - Polypoid adenomyoma
  - Mullerian adenosarcoma
- Diagnostic pitfalls/key intraoperative consultation issues
  - In contrast to APA, endometrial polyp and polypoid adenomyoma do not have glandular epithelial atypia.
  - In contrast to adenosarcoma, APA has benign smooth muscle component and absence of periglandular stromal condensation or mitotic activity.
  - Presence of hyperplastic glands in APA should not be overinterpreted as endometrioid adenocarcinoma. However, endometrioid adenocarcinoma may arise in association with an APA (see Fig. 4.18).

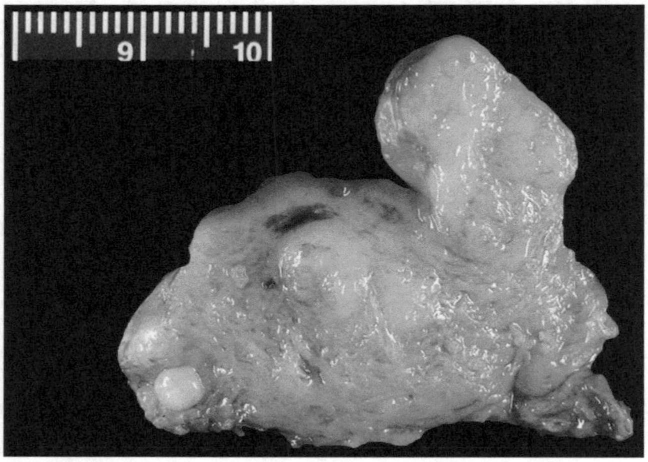

Fig. 5.35 Atypical polypoid adenomyoma (APA). Note the polypoid endometrial lesion

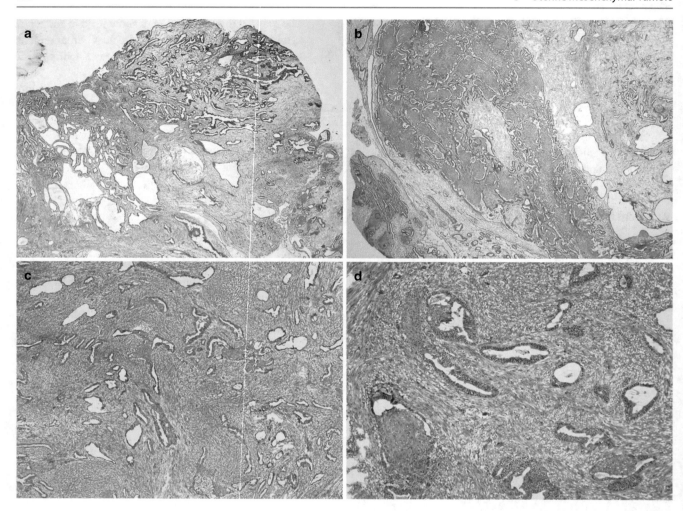

Fig. 5.36 Atypical polypoid adenomyoma (APA). Polypoid lesion consisting of irregular, hyperplastic endometrial glands with prominent squamous differentiation (**a**, **b**) and smooth muscle-rich stroma (**c**, **d**)

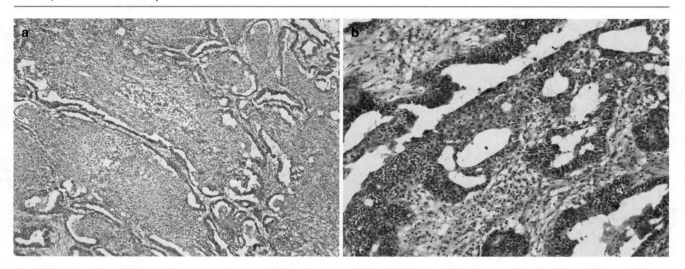

Fig. 5.37 Atypical polypoid adenomyoma (APA). Note the presence of necrosis within the squamous morules (**a**) and mild to moderate cytological atypia of the glandular epithelium (**b**)

Mullerian Adenosarcoma [43–48]

- Clinical features
  - Adult patients with a mean age of 58 years
  - Vaginal bleeding and pelvic pain are the most common presenting symptoms.
  - History of recurrent "polyp" in some cases.
- Gross pathology
  - Polypoid endometrial mass with an average size of 6.5 cm.
  - Most cases are limited to the uterus at presentation.
  - Presence of extrauterine disease signifies the possibility of sarcomatous overgrowth (Fig. 5.38).
- Microscopic features (Fig. 5.39)
  - Biphasic tumor with cystic glandular and sarcomatous components in a broad based polypoid configuration.
  - Mullerian-type glandular epithelium (proliferative endometrial, tubal, or endocervical) with mild to moderate cytological atypia.
  - Low-grade stromal cells condensing or cuffing around cystically dilated glands, frequently with intraglandular papillary intrusions showing a phyllodes-like architecture.
  - Mitotic figures may be difficult to find, although most cases show >4 mitoses/10 HPF.
  - The tumor is frequently heterogenous with hypocellular areas or marked hyalinization. Sex-cord differentiation and heterologous elements including cartilage, adipose tissue, and rhabdomyoblasts may be seen.
  - Sarcomatous overgrowth is diagnosed when the high-grade pure sarcoma element comprises at least 25 % of the tumor.
  - Low-grade sarcomatous overgrowth may also occur.
- Differential diagnosis
  - Adenofibroma
  - Atypical polypoid adenomyoma
  - Endometrial polyp
  - Malignant mixed Mullerian tumor
- Diagnostic pitfalls/key intraoperative consultation issues
  - Adenofibroma is extremely rare.
    - May have intraglandular papillary stromal infoldings but lacks stromal cell condensation and mitotic activity.
  - Endometrial polyp is separated from adenosarcoma by absence of periglandular stromal cell condensation, lack of cytological atypia, and stromal cell mitotic activity.
  - In contrast to adenosarcoma, APA has a benign smooth muscle component and absence of periglandular stromal condensation and mitotic activity.
  - Malignant mixed Mullerian tumor has a malignant epithelial component, which is not seen in adenosarcoma.
  - Extrauterine metastases should raise the possibility of sarcomatous overgrowth in adenosarcoma.
  - Surgical management of adenosarcomas typically requires a complete staging procedure; however, the extent of staging and the role of lymphadenectomy is controversial [49].

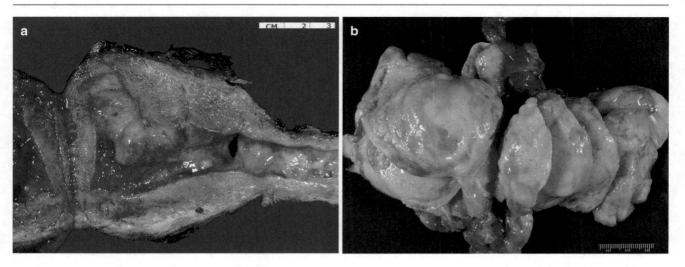

Fig. 5.38 Mullerian adenosarcoma. Fleshy polypoid mass lesions (**a**, **b**)

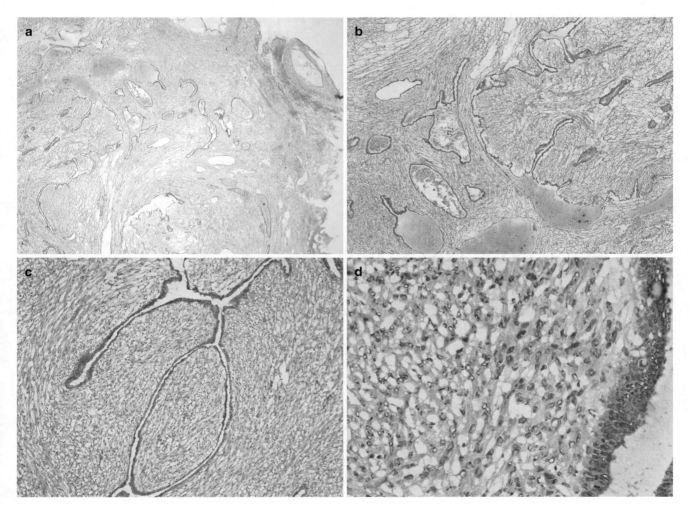

Fig. 5.39 Mullerian adenosarcoma. Note the biphasic proliferation of glandular and stromal components in a broad-based polypoid configuration (**a**) and characteristic periglandular condensation and intraglandular papillary protrusion (**b**, **c**) of mildly atypical stromal cells (**d**)

Malignant Mixed Mullerian Tumor (MMMT)/ Carcinosarcoma [50, 51]

- Clinical features
  - Almost always seen in postmenopausal women.
  - Presents with vaginal bleeding, uterine enlargement, or pelvic mass.
  - One-third of patients have extrauterine disease at presentation.
- Gross pathology (Fig. 5.40)
  - Large polypoid intrauterine mass, frequently occupying the entire endometrial cavity and protruding through the cervical os in 50 % of the cases.
  - Fleshy cut surface with extensive hemorrhage, necrosis, and cystic changes.
  - Gross myometrial and/or cervical involvement is common.
- Microscopic features
  - Intimately admixed but histologically distinct carcinomatous and sarcomatous components in various proportions.
  - The carcinomatous element is usually serous or endometrioid adenocarcinoma (Fig. 5.41), but clear cell, mucinous, or undifferentiated carcinoma may also occur.
  - Usually high-grade sarcoma component of either homologous (high-grade endometrial stromal sarcoma, leiomyosarcoma) or heterologous (rhabdomyosarcoma, chondrosarcoma, osteosarcoma, or liposarcoma) in nature (Fig. 5.42).
- Differential diagnosis
  - Endometrial carcinomas including endometrioid adenocarcinoma with spindle cell morphology
  - Endometrioid adenocarcinoma with focal benign heterologous mesenchymal differentiation
  - Dedifferentiated endometrial carcinoma
  - Mullerian adenosarcoma
  - Endometrial stromal sarcoma with sex-cord differentiation
  - Undifferentiated uterine sarcoma
- Diagnostic pitfalls/key intraoperative consultation issues
  - The carcinomatous component of MMMT may be dominant and well differentiated without myometrial invasion, and the sarcomatous component may be very focal.
    - Additional frozen sections may be submitted to confirm the presence of a sarcomatous component, as MMMT requires extensive, complete surgical staging, in contrast to the potentially less extensive staging surgery of non-myoinvasive well-differentiated endometrioid carcinoma.
  - MMMTs with unusual carcinomatous components such as pure squamous cell carcinoma or adenoid basal cell carcinoma are generally cervical primaries.
  - In postmenopausal patients, a heterologous sarcomatous lesion in the absence of an obvious carcinomatous element is likely a MMMT. Additional frozen sections may show unequivocal carcinomatous component, although it is typically not crucial for surgical management at the time of intraoperative consultation.
  - Endometrioid carcinoma with spindle cells should be separated from MMMT by finding histological transition between typical endometrioid carcinoma glands to low-grade spindled areas and by lack of heterologous mesenchymal elements.
  - MMMT has a malignant epithelial component, which is absent in adenosarcoma.
  - Undifferentiated uterine sarcoma lacks carcinomatous elements.

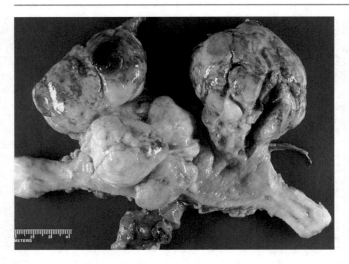

Fig. 5.40 Malignant mixed Mullerian tumor (MMMT). Note the large polypoid intrauterine mass lesions with fleshy, hemorrhagic, and necrotic cut surfaces

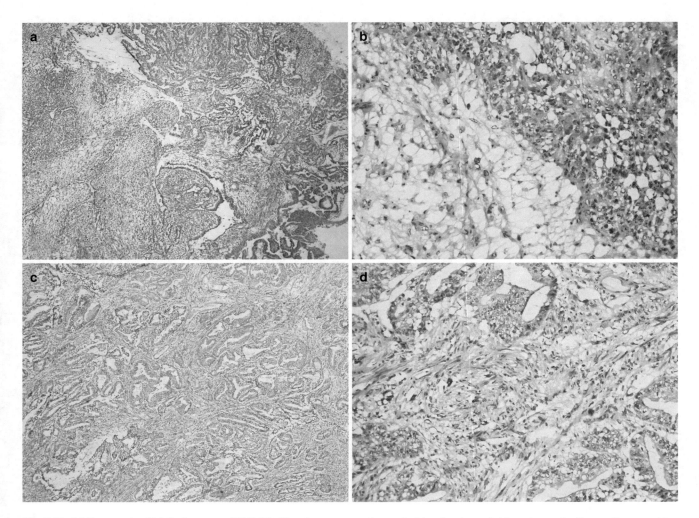

Fig. 5.41 Malignant mixed Mullerian tumor (MMMT). Note the serous carcinoma (**a**, **b**) and endometrioid carcinoma (**c**, **d**) as malignant epithelial components in these two examples of MMMT

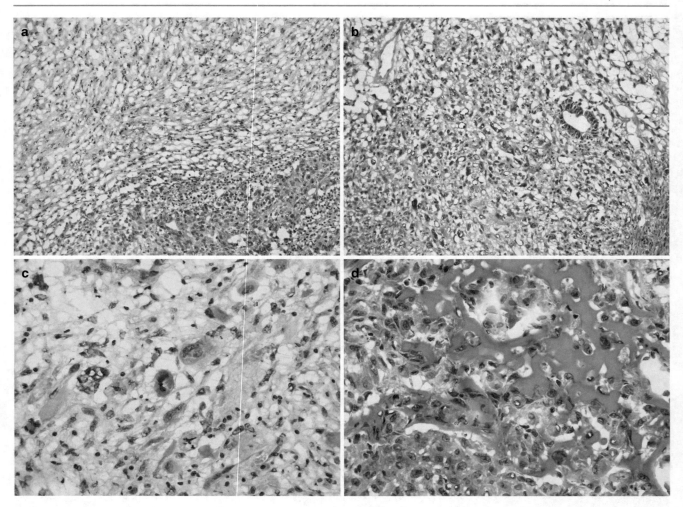

Fig. 5.42 Malignant mixed Mullerian tumor (MMMT). Note the high-grade homologous (fibrosarcoma (**a**, **b**)) or heterologous (rhabdomyosarcoma (**c**) and osteosarcoma (**d**)) sarcoma components in these examples of MMMT

Other Mesenchymal and Miscellaneous Uterine Tumors

Uterine tumor resembling ovarian sex-cord tumor (UTROSCT), inflammatory myofibroblastic tumor (IMT), and perivascular epithelioid cell tumors (PEComa) are relatively distinct and well-documented entities of uterus. Various other soft tissue tumors may rarely occur including vascular tumors, fibrohistiocytic tumors, neurogenic tumors and rhabdomyosarcoma, malignant rhabdoid tumor, epithelioid sarcoma, and alveolar soft part sarcoma.

Undifferentiated Uterine Sarcoma [52]

- High-grade sarcoma arising from the endo-myometrium.
- Frequently high stage at the time of presentation.

- Polypoid mass of >10 cm in size with fleshy, necrotic, and hemorrhagic cut surface (Fig. 5.43).
- Markedly atypical spindle cell proliferation with storiform or herringbone growth patterns (Fig. 5.44).
- No recognizable endometrial stromal or smooth muscle differentiation.
- Rhabdoid or myxoid changes are common.
- Differential diagnosis includes poorly differentiated carcinoma, high-grade endometrial stromal sarcoma, adenosarcoma with sarcomatous overgrowth, MMMT, and leiomyosarcoma.

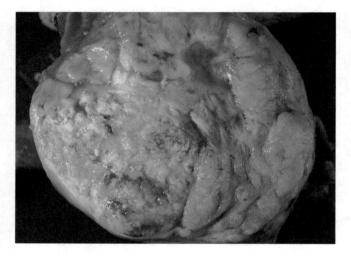

Fig. 5.43 Undifferentiated uterine sarcoma. Mass lesion with a fleshy, tan-yellow, and necrotic cut surface

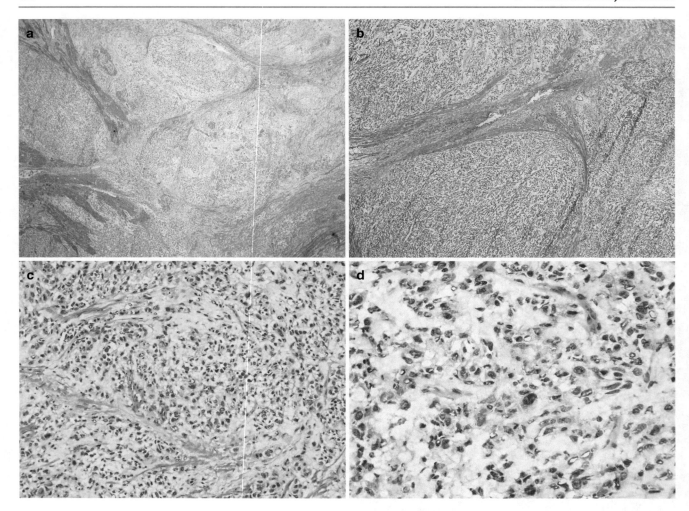

Fig. 5.44 Undifferentiated uterine sarcoma. High-grade spindle cell proliferation without lineage histological differentiation (**a–d**)

Uterine Tumor Resembling Ovarian Sex-Cord Tumor (UTROSCT) [53, 54]

- Uncommon tumor in patients with a mean age of 40 years
- May present with vaginal bleeding or pelvic pain, but often an incidental finding
- Well-circumscribed myometrial lesion or polypoid endometrial mass with solid, yellow to tan cut surface
- Monotonous small round epithelioid cells forming anastomosing cords, nests, tubules, or a retiform pattern
- Minimal cytological atypia and rare mitotic activity
- Differential diagnosis
  - Endometrial stromal tumors with sex-cord differentiation
  - Endometrioid adenocarcinoma with sertoliform pattern
  - Mesonephric adenocarcinoma
  - Epithelioid smooth muscle tumor
- Diagnostic pitfalls/key intraoperative consultation issues
  - In contrast to endometrial stromal tumors, UTROSCT has uniform epithelioid tumor cells arranged in nests, cords, tubules, or a retiform pattern and without endometrial stromal cell proliferation.
  - Presence of tumor areas merging with conventional endometrioid carcinoma and the presence of atypical endometrial hyperplasia are seen in sertoliform endometrioid adenocarcinoma and are not features of UTROSCT.
  - Mesonephric adenocarcinoma generally arises from the lateral wall of cervix and may extend into the myometrium, whereas URTOSCT arises from the uterine corpus.
  - Epithelioid smooth muscle tumors are composed of epithelioid cells without tubule formation or retiform growth pattern.

Inflammatory Myofibroblastic Tumor (IMT) [55]

- Patient age ranges from 4 to 46 years.
- Polypoid or intramural mass lesion involving the lower uterine segment or endo-myometrium.

- Tan to yellow fleshy cut surface.
- Histologically well circumscribed to infiltrative mass composed of fascicles or lobules of spindle myofibroblasts admixed with a lymphoplasmacytic infiltrate and extravasated red cells.
- Myxoid or hyalinized stroma.
- Mitoses may be present (0–2 per 10 HPF)
- No cytological atypia or necrosis.
- Differential diagnosis includes myxoid leiomyosarcoma.
  - In contrast to IMT, myxoid leiomyosarcoma may show obvious malignant smooth muscle differentiation (with cytological atypia, mitoses, and tumor cell necrosis) in the non-myxoid tumor areas.

Perivascular Epithelioid Cell Tumor (PEComa) [56, 57]

- Perimenopausal patients with a mean age of 49 years.
- May be associated with tuberous sclerosis complex.
- Well-circumscribed or infiltrative mass lesion.
- Admixture of variable amounts of sheets or fascicles of spindle to epithelioid cells with clear to eosinophilic cytoplasm.
- Nuclear atypia is usually minimal.
- Prominent delicate capillary network is characteristic.
- Features of malignant PEComa include more than 5 cm in size, infiltrative border, marked cytological atypia, necrosis, and more than 1 mitosis per 50 HPF.
- Differential diagnosis
  - Epithelioid smooth muscle tumors
- Diagnostic pitfalls/key intraoperative consultation issues
  - Diagnosis of PEComa and the distinction between PEComa and epithelioid smooth muscle tumors may be difficult if not impossible on frozen section. A conservative approach should be taken, and frozen diagnosis of "spindle cell tumor, defer to permanent sections for final classification" is recommended to avoid unnecessary staging surgery.

Adenomatoid Tumor [58, 59]

- Generally an incidental finding in adult patients.
- Solitary lesion of less than 4 cm, most often located in the outer myometrium or subserosal region of uterus.
- The cut surface may be solid or partially cystic, tan-yellow with ill-defined borders.
- Histologically characterized by proliferation of anastomosing glands, tubules, cystic spaces, or solid tumor nests composed of mesothelial cells (Fig. 5.45a, b).
- The cells are round, cuboidal, or flattened with eosinophilic cytoplasm.
- Absence of cytological atypia and mitotic activity.
- Intraglandular cytoplasmic bridging is characteristic (Fig. 5.45c, d).

- Nodular smooth muscle hypertrophy is frequently present in the surrounding myometrium.
- Differential diagnosis
  - Metastatic adenocarcinoma (signet ring cell carcinoma)
  - Mesothelioma
  - Lipoleiomyoma
  - Hemangioma and lymphangioma
- Diagnostic pitfalls/key intraoperative consultation issues
  - Absence of cytological atypia and mitotic activity separates adenomatoid tumor from metastatic carcinoma and mesothelioma.
  - Distinction from lipoleiomyoma, hemangioma, and lymphangioma may be difficult and is not crucial at the time of intraoperative consultation.

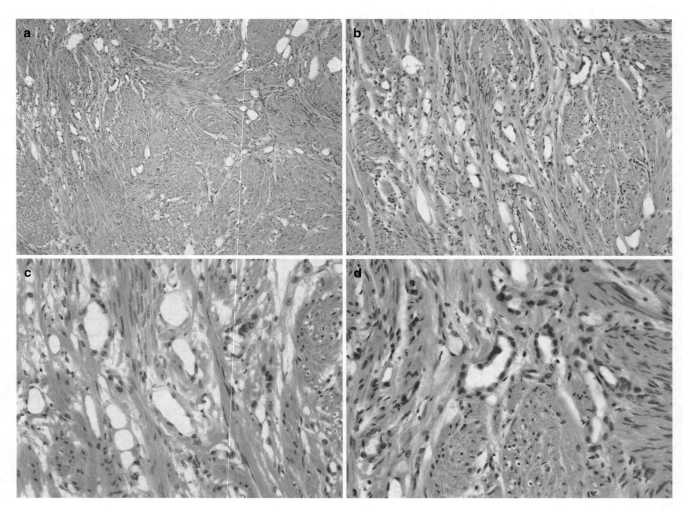

Fig. 5.45 Adenomatoid tumor. Note the anastomosing glands or tubules (**a**, **b**) lined by flattened epithelioid cells within the myometrium with characteristic intraglandular cytoplasmic bridging and absence of significant nuclear atypia or mitotic activity (**c**, **d**)

References

1. Kurman RJ, Carcanglu ML, Herrington CS, Young RH. WHO classification of tumours of female reproductive organs. 4th ed. Lyon: International Agency for Research on Cancer (IARC); 2014; 135–52.

2. Oliva E, Young RH, Clement PB, Bhan AK, Scully RE. Cellular benign mesenchymal tumors of the uterus. A comparative morphologic and immunohistochemical analysis of 33 highly cellular leiomyomas and six endometrial stromal nodules, two frequently confused tumors. Am J Surg Pathol. 1995;19:757–68.

3. Downes KA, Hart WR. Bizarre leiomyomas of the uterus: a comprehensive pathologic study of 24 cases with long-term follow-up. Am J Surg Pathol. 1997;21:1261–70.

4. Bell SW, Kempson RL, Hendrickson MR. Problematic uterine smooth muscle neoplasms. A clinicopathologic study of 213 cases. Am J Surg Pathol. 1994;18:535–58.

5. Perrone T, Dehner LP. Prognostically favorable "mitotically active" smooth-muscle tumors of the uterus. A clinicopathologic study of ten cases. Am J Surg Pathol. 1988;12:1–8.

6. Norris HJ, Hilliard GD, Irey NS. Hemorrhagic cellular leiomyomas ("apoplectic leiomyoma") of the uterus associated with pregnancy and oral contraceptives. Int J Gynecol Pathol. 1988;7:212–24.

7. Hock YL, Goswami P, Rollason TP. Mitotically active haemorrhagic cellular (apoplectic) leiomyoma. Eur J Gynaecol Oncol. 2000;21:28–9.

8. Mazur MT, Kraus FT. Histogenesis of morphologic variations in tumors of the uterine wall. Am J Surg Pathol. 1980;4:59–74.

9. Kurman RJ, Norris HJ. Mesenchymal tumors of the uterus. VI. Epithelioid smooth muscle tumors including leiomyoblastoma and clear-cell leiomyoma: a clinical and pathologic analysis of 26 cases. Cancer. 1976;37:1853–65.

10. Prayson RA, Goldblum JR, Hart WR. Epithelioid smooth-muscle tumors of the uterus: a clinicopathologic study of 18 patients. Am J Surg Pathol. 1997;21:383–91.

11. Mulvany NJ, Ostor AG, Ross I. Diffuse leiomyomatosis of the uterus. Histopathology. 1995;27:175–9.

12. Blandamura S, Florea G, Chiarelli S, Rondinelli R, Ninfo V. Myometrial leiomyoma with chondroid lipoma-like areas. Histopathology. 2005;46:596–8.

13. Clement PB, Young RH, Scully RE. Diffuse, perinodular, and other patterns of hydropic degeneration within and adjacent to uterine leiomyomas. Problems in differential diagnosis. Am J Surg Pathol. 1992;16:26–32.

14. Clement PB. Intravenous leiomyomatosis of the uterus. Pathol Annu. 1988;23(Pt 2):153–83.

15. Carr RJ, Hui P, Buza N. Intravenous leiomyomatosis revisited: an experience of 14 cases at a single medical ce. Int J Gynecol Pathol. 2015;34:169–76.

16. Merchant S, Malpica A, Deavers MT, Czapar C, Gershenson D, Silva EG. Vessels within vessels in the myometrium. Am J Surg Pathol. 2002;26:232–6.

17. Clement PB, Young RH, Scully RE. Intravenous leiomyomatosis of the uterus. A clinicopathological analysis of 16 cases with unusual histologic features. Am J Surg Pathol. 1988;12:932–45.

18. Clement PB, Young RH. Diffuse leiomyomatosis of the uterus: a report of four cases. Int J Gynecol Pathol. 1987;6:322–30.

19. Tavassoli FA, Norris HJ. Peritoneal leiomyomatosis (leiomyomatosis peritonealis disseminata): a clinicopathologic study of 20 cases with ultrastructural observations. Int J Gynecol Pathol. 1982;1:59–74.

20. Sharma P, Chaturvedi KU, Gupta R, Nigam S. Leiomyomatosis peritonealis disseminata with malignant change in a postmenopausal woman. Gynecol Oncol. 2004;95:742–5.

21. Kayser K, Zink S, Schneider T, Dienemann H, André S, Kaltner H, et al. Benign metastasizing leiomyoma of the uterus: documentation of clinical, immunohistochemical and lectin-histochemical data of ten cases. Virchows Arch. 2000;437:284–92.

22. Roth LM, Reed RJ, Sternberg WH. Cotyledonoid dissecting leiomyoma of the uterus. The Sternberg tumor. Am J Surg Pathol. 1996;20:1455–61.

23. Roth LM, Reed RJ. Dissecting leiomyomas of the uterus other than cotyledonoid dissecting leiomyomas: a report of eight cases. Am J Surg Pathol. 1999;23:1032–9.

24. Abeler VM, Royne O, Thoresen S, Danielsen HE, Nesland JM, Kristensen GB. Uterine sarcomas in Norway. A histopathological and prognostic survey of a total population from 1970 to 2000 including 419 patients. Histopathology. 2009;54:355–64.

25. Parker WH, Fu YS, Berek JS. Uterine sarcoma in patients operated on for presumed leiomyoma and rapidly growing leiomyoma. Obstet Gynecol. 1994;83:414–8.

26. King ME, Dickersin GR, Scully RE. Myxoid leiomyosarcoma of the uterus. A report of six cases. Am J Surg Pathol. 1982;6:589–98.

27. Burch DM, Tavassoli FA. Myxoid leiomyosarcoma of the uterus. Histopathology. 2011;59:1144–55.

28. Giuntoli 2nd RL, Gostout BS, DiMarco CS, Metzinger DS, Keeney GL. Diagnostic criteria for uterine smooth muscle tumors: leiomyoma variants associated with malignant behavior. J Reprod Med. 2007;52:1001–10.

29. Ip PP, Cheung AN, Clement PB. Uterine smooth muscle tumors of uncertain malignant potential (STUMP): a clinicopathologic analysis of 16 cases. Am J Surg Pathol. 2009;33:992–1005.

30. Veras E, Zivanovic O, Jacks L, Chiapetta D, Hensley M, Soslow R. "Low-grade leiomyosarcoma" and late-recurring smooth muscle tumors of the uterus: a heterogenous collection of frequently misdiagnosed tumors associated with an overall favorable prognosis relative to conventional uterine leiomyosarcomas. Am J Surg Pathol. 2011;35:1626–37.

31. Ly A, Mills AM, McKenney JK, Balzer BL, Kempson RL, Hendrickson MR, Longacre TA. Atypical leiomyomas of the uterus: a clinicopathologic study of 51 cases. Am J Surg Pathol. 2013;37:643–9.

32. Chang KL, Crabtree GS, Lim-Tan SK, Kempson RL, Hendrickson MR. Primary uterine endometrial stromal neoplasms. A clinicopathologic study of 117 cases. Am J Surg Pathol. 1990;14:415–38.

33. Dionigi A, Oliva E, Clement PB, Young RH. Endometrial stromal nodules and endometrial stromal tumors with limited infiltration: a clinicopathologic study of 50 cases. Am J Surg Pathol. 2002;26:567–81.

34. Norris HJ, Taylor HB. Mesenchymal tumors of the uterus. I. A clinical and pathological study of 53 endometrial stromal tumors. Cancer. 1966;19:755–66.

35. Oliva E, Clement PB, Young RH, Scully RE. Mixed endometrial stromal and smooth muscle tumors of the uterus: a clinicopathologic study of 15 cases. Am J Surg Pathol. 1998;22:997–1005.

36. Clement PB, Scully RE. Endometrial stromal sarcomas of the uterus with extensive endometrioid glandular differentiation: a report of three cases that caused problems in differential diagnosis. Int J Gynecol Pathol. 1992;11:163–73.

37. McCluggage WG, Young RH. Endometrial stromal sarcomas with true papillae and pseudopapillae. Int J Gynecol Pathol. 2008;27:555–61.

38. Lee CH, Mariño-Enriquez A, Ou W, Zhu M, Ali RH, Chiang S, et al. The clinicopathologic features of YWHAE-FAM22 endometrial stromal sarcomas: a histologically high-grade and clinically aggressive tumor. Am J Surg Pathol. 2012;36:641–53.

39. Gilks CB, Clement PB, Hart WR, Young RH. Uterine adenomyomas excluding atypical polypoid adenomyomas and adenomyomas

of endocervical type: a clinicopathologic study of 30 cases of an underemphasized lesion that may cause diagnostic problems with brief consideration of adenomyomas of other female genital tract sites. Int J Gynecol Pathol. 2000;19:195–205.

40. Tahlan A, Nanda A, Mohan H. Uterine adenomyoma: a clinicopathologic review of 26 cases and a review of the literature. Int J Gynecol Pathol. 2006;25:361–5.

41. Longacre TA, Chung MH, Rouse RV, Hendrickson MR. Atypical polypoid adenomyofibromas (atypical polypoid adenomyomas) of the uterus. A clinicopathologic study of 55 cases. Am J Surg Pathol. 1996;20:1–20.

42. Young RH, Treger T, Scully RE. Atypical polypoid adenomyoma of the uterus. A report of 27 cases. Am J Surg Pathol. 1986;86:139–45.

43. Clement PB, Scully RE. Mullerian adenosarcoma of the uterus: a clinicopathologic analysis of 100 cases with a review of the literature. Hum Pathol. 1990;21:363–81.

44. Gallardo A, Prat J. Mullerian adenosarcoma: a clinicopathologic and immunohistochemical study of 55 cases challenging the existence of adenofibroma. Am J Surg Pathol. 2009;33:278–88.

45. Kaku T, Silverberg SG, Major FJ, Miller A, Fetter B, Brady MF. Adenosarcoma of the uterus: a Gynecologic Oncology Group clinicopathologic study of 31 cases. Int J Gynecol Pathol. 1992;11:75–88.

46. Clarke BA, Mulligan AM, Irving JA, McCluggage WG, Oliva E. Mullerian adenosarcomas with unusual growth patterns: staging issues. Int J Gynecol Pathol. 2011;30:340–7.

47. Wu RI, Schorge JO, Dal Cin P, Young RH, Oliva E. Mullerian adenosarcoma of the uterus with low-grade sarcomatous overgrowth characterized by prominent hydropic change resulting in mimicry of a smooth muscle tumor. Int J Gynecol Pathol. 2014;33:573–80.

48. Howitt BE, Quade BJ, Nucci MR. Uterine polyps with features overlapping with those of Mullerian adenosarcoma: a clinicopathologic analysis of 29 cases emphasizing their likely benign nature. Am J Surg Pathol. 2015;39:116–26.

49. Carroll A, Ramirez PT, Westin SN, Soliman PT, Munsell MF, Nick AM, et al. Uterine adenosarcoma: an analysis on management, outcomes, and risk factors for recurrence. Gynecol Oncol. 2014;135:455–61.

50. Silverberg SG, Major FJ, Blessing JA, Fetter B, Askin FB, Liao SY, Miller A. Carcinosarcoma (malignant mixed mesodermal tumor) of the uterus. A Gynecologic Oncology Group pathologic study of 203 cases. Int J Gynecol Pathol. 1990;9:1–19.

51. Ferguson SE, Tornos C, Hummer A, Barakat RR, Soslow RA. Prognostic features of surgical stage. I uterine carcinosarcoma. Am J Surg Pathol. 2007;31:1653–61.

52. Kurihara S, Oda Y, Ohishi Y, Iwasa A, Takahira T, Kaneki E, et al. Endometrial stromal sarcomas and related high-grade sarcomas: immunohistochemical and molecular genetic study of 31 cases. Am J Surg Pathol. 2008;32:1228–38.

53. Irving JA, Carinelli S, Prat J. Uterine tumors resembling ovarian sex cord tumors are polyphenotypic neoplasms with true sex cord differentiation. Mod Pathol. 2006;19:17–24.

54. Nogales FF, Stolnicu S, Harilal KR, Mooney E, Garcia-Galvis OF. Retiform uterine tumours resembling ovarian sex cord tumours. A comparative immunohistochemical study with retiform structures of the female genital tract. Histopathology. 2009;54:471–7.

55. Rabban JT, Zaloudek CJ, Shekitka KM, Tavassoli FA. Inflammatory myofibroblastic tumor of the uterus: a clinicopathologic study of 6 cases emphasizing distinction from aggressive mesenchymal tumors. Am J Surg Pathol. 2005;29:1348–55.

56. Folpe AL, Mentzel T, Lehr HA, Fisher C, Balzer B, Weiss SW. Perivascular epithelioid cell neoplasms of soft tissue and gynecologic origin: a clinicopathologic study of 26 cases and review of the literature. Am J Surg Pathol. 2005;29:1558–75.

57. Lim GS, Oliva E. The morphologic spectrum of uterine PEC-cell associated tumors in a patient with tuberous sclerosis. Int J Gynecol Pathol. 2011;30:121–8.

58. Nogales FF, Isaac MA, Hardisson D, Bosincu L, Palacios J, Ordi J, et al. Adenomatoid tumors of the uterus: an analysis of 60 cases. Int J Gynecol Pathol. 2002;21:34–40.

59. Hes O, Perez-Montiel DM, Alvarado Cabrero I, Zamecnik M, Podhola M, Sulc M, et al. Thread-like bridging strands: a morphologic feature present in all adenomatoid tumors. Ann Diagn Pathol. 2003;7:273–7.

Intrauterine Pregnancy and Gestational Trophoblastic Disease

6

Introduction

This chapter covers the frozen section evaluation of uterine contents for confirmation of intrauterine pregnancy and gestational trophoblastic disease (GTD). The latter encompasses a spectrum of proliferative disorders of placental trophoblast ranging from nonneoplastic hydatidiform moles (partial and complete mole) to malignant trophoblastic tumors [1] (Table 6.1). The most aggressive form of trophoblastic neoplasia, gestational choriocarcinoma, has become uncommon nowadays. Two distinct tumors of the intermediate trophoblast (placental site trophoblastic tumor and epithelioid trophoblastic tumor) are rare but frequently pose a diagnostic challenge when encountered. In addition, two reactive conditions (exaggerated placental site reaction and placental site nodule) are also classified within GTD due to their potential misdiagnosis as neoplastic processes.

Although rarely requested, possible scenarios for frozen section evaluation include assessment for the presence of persistent trophoblastic disease, particularly invasive mole and metastatic trophoblastic lesions (metastatic mole) and diagnosis of trophoblastic tumors.

Table 6.1 2014 World Health Organization classification of gestational trophoblastic disease

Classification	Subtypes	Trophoblastic cell of origin
Hydatidiform mole	Complete mole	Villous trophoblast
	Partial mole	Villous trophoblast
	Invasive mole	Villous trophoblast
Trophoblastic tumors	Gestational choriocarcinoma	Villous trophoblast
	Placental site trophoblastic tumor	Implantation site intermediate trophoblast
	Epithelioid trophoblastic tumor	Chorionic intermediate trophoblast
Nonneoplastic lesions	Exaggerated placental site reaction	Implantation site intermediate trophoblast
	Placental site nodule	Chorionic intermediate trophoblast
Abnormal villous lesions	Various non-molar lesions histologically simulating partial mole	Villous trophoblast

Data from Kurman et al. [2]

© Springer International Publishing Switzerland 2015
P. Hui, N. Buza, *Atlas of Intraoperative Frozen Section Diagnosis in Gynecologic Pathology*,
DOI 10.1007/978-3-319-21807-6_6

Intrauterine Pregnancy

- Frozen section evaluation may be requested to confirm intrauterine gestation and/or to rule out an ectopic pregnancy.
- Gestational tissue, i.e., chorionic villi and/or fetal parts may be grossly identifiable.
- Histological evidence of intrauterine pregnancy includes chorionic villi, fetal parts, and implantation site intermediate trophoblast (Fig. 6.1).
- Diagnostic pitfalls/key intraoperative consultation issues
    - Intrauterine pregnancy is confirmed by the presence of any of the three gestational tissue types: chorionic villi, fetal parts, or implantation site intermediate trophoblast.
    - Edematous endometrial and endocervical tissue fragments may be misinterpreted as chorionic villi; however, this pitfall can be avoided by recognition of

cytotrophoblast and syncytiotrophoblast on the villous surface.
- Presence of rare syncytiotrophoblast—without other gestational tissues—in an endometrial curettage does not rule out an ectopic pregnancy.

Hydatidiform Mole

Hydatidiform moles are nonneoplastic proliferations of the villous trophoblast, characterized by enlarged hydropic villi along with trophoblastic hyperplasia. They are incompatible with fetal survival and are genetically defined by their unique parental chromosome contributions. The two main subtypes are complete hydatidiform mole (CHM) and partial hydatidiform mole (PHM). Invasive hydatidiform mole is characterized by myometrial invasion. Persistent GTD is a clinical diagnosis and includes invasive mole and metastatic mole that may develop following either CHM or PHM.

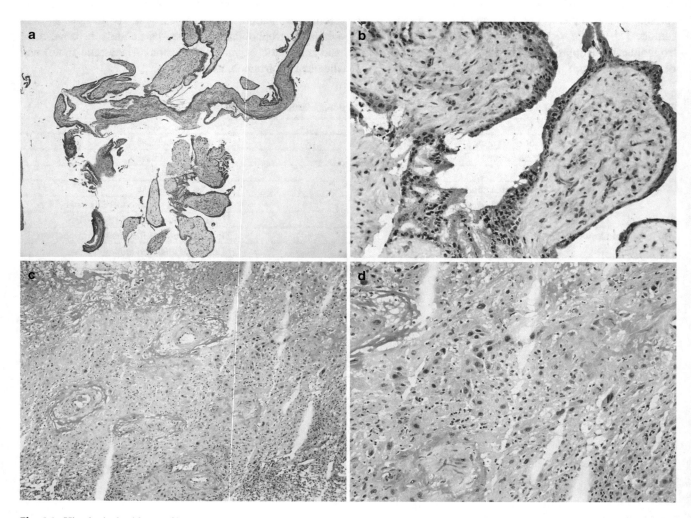

Fig. 6.1 Histological evidence of intrauterine pregnancy. Note the presence of chorionic villi (**a**, **b**) and implantation site intermediate trophoblast (**c**, **d**) in this uterine curettage specimen

Complete Hydatidiform Mole (CHM) [1, 2]

- Clinical features
  - Patients with fully developed CHM present in the second trimester of pregnancy with vaginal bleeding, uterine enlargement, markedly elevated serum human chorionic gonadotropin (hCG), hyperemesis, toxemia, and hyperthyroidism.
  - Very early complete moles are frequently evacuated without clinical suspicion as missed abortion and without abnormally elevated serum hCG.
- Gross pathology
  - Diffuse villous hydrops.
  - No fetal parts present.
  - Early evacuation of complete molar tissue before the second trimester typically lacks a gross lesion.
- Microscopic features (Fig. 6.2)
  - Markedly edematous villi with central cistern formation.
  - Diffuse circumferential trophoblastic hyperplasia involving both cytotrophoblast and syncytiotrophoblast.
  - Presence of cytological atypia.
  - Absence of nucleated fetal red blood cells and fetal parts.
  - *Early complete mole* shows normal-sized chorionic villi with abnormal "cauliflower-like" or polypoid configurations. The villous stroma is characteristically hypercellular, composed of stellate fibroblasts embedded in a bluish myxoid matrix with prominent karyorrhexis. Trophoblastic hyperplasia may be focally present or absent.
- Differential diagnosis
  - Partial mole
  - Hydropic non-molar abortion
- Diagnostic pitfalls/key intraoperative consultation issues
  - Well-developed CHM presents with diffusely hydropic villi, which is not present in PHM and non-molar conditions.
  - Separation of very early complete mole from hydropic non-molar gestations, early gestational sac, and PHM is often challenging but not crucial at the time of intraoperative consultation.

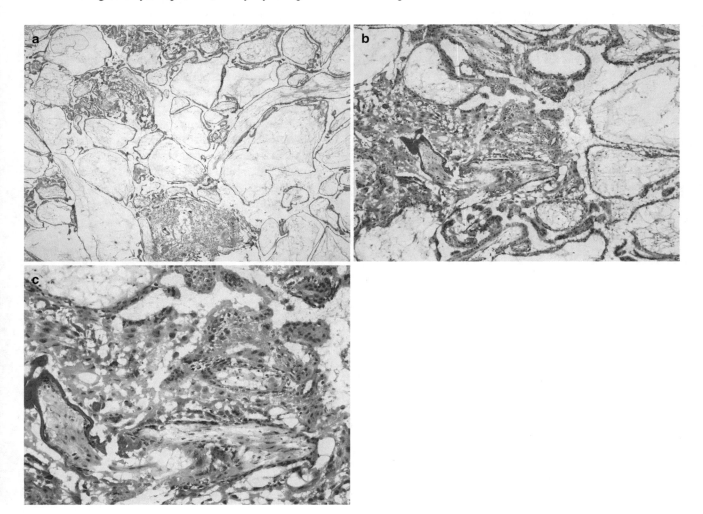

Fig. 6.2 Well-developed complete mole. Note the diffuse villous hydrops with cistern formation (**a**), marked, circumferential villous trophoblastic hyperplasia, (**b**) and nuclear atypia of the trophoblast (**c**)

Partial Hydatidiform Mole (PHM) [1, 3]

- Clinical features
  - Majority of patients present in the late first trimester or early second trimester with missed or incomplete abortion.
  - Uterine size is usually small or appropriate for gestational age.
  - Serum hCG is usually moderately elevated and a fetus may be seen on ultrasound.
- Gross pathology
  - Normal-sized villi admixed with edematous, enlarged ones
  - Frequent gestational sac or fetal parts
- Microscopic features
  - Two populations of villi: large, hydropic, irregular villi in the background of small and fibrotic villi.
  - The larger villi show hydropic changes with central cistern formation, irregular/scalloped contours, and trophoblastic pseudo-inclusions.
  - Trophoblastic hyperplasia is usually mild and focal, and intermediate trophoblasts lack significant nuclear atypia.
  - Fetal blood vessels and nucleated red blood cells are commonly seen.
- Differential diagnosis
  - Complete mole
  - Hydropic non-molar abortion
  - Various chromosomal abnormalities, particularly trisomy syndromes
  - Placental mesenchymal dysplasia
- Diagnostic pitfalls/key intraoperative consultation issues
  - Diagnostic separation from early complete mole, hydropic non-molar gestations, and placental mesenchymal dysplasia is often challenging, but not crucial at the time of intraoperative consultation.

Invasive Hydatidiform Mole [4]

- Generally presents after the initial evacuation with persistent elevation of hCG.
- Frozen section may be requested to diagnose invasive mole and/or to evaluate the extent of disease.
- Both complete and partial hydatidiform moles may progress into invasive or metastatic moles in approximately 15–20 % and 0.5–4 % of cases, respectively.
- When hysterectomy is performed (Fig. 6.3), molar villi invading the myometrium without intervening decidua are diagnostic (Fig. 6.4).
- Rarely molar villi also invade intramyometrial vessels and may spread to vagina, vulva and broad ligament. Lung metastases can also develop.
- Differential diagnosis
  - Noninvasive complete and partial mole
  - Abnormal placentation of non-molar pregnancy— placenta accreta, increta, or percreta
  - Gestational choriocarcinoma
- Diagnostic pitfalls/key intraoperative consultation issues
  - Noninvasive mole shows no histological evidence of villous tissue in direct contact with myometrial smooth muscle and does not involve lymphovascular spaces.
  - Placenta accreta, increta, and percreta show normal (non-molar) chorionic villi invading the myometrium without intervening decidua.
  - Exuberant trophoblastic proliferation should not be misinterpreted as choriocarcinoma in the presence of molar villi.

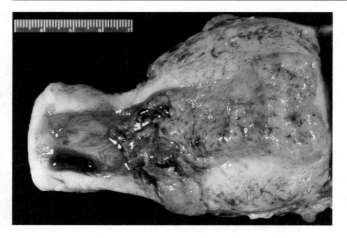

Fig. 6.3 Invasive complete mole. Note hydropic molar tissue diffusely involving the endometrium with focal invasion into the myometrium at the lower uterine segment area

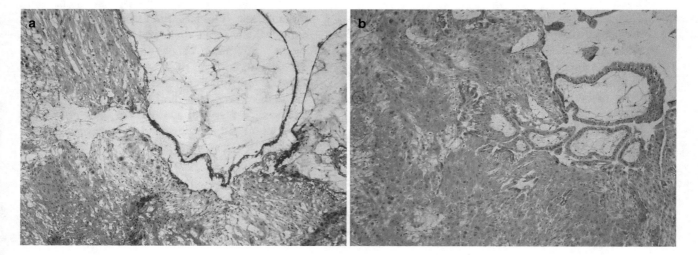

Fig. 6.4 Invasive complete mole. Note attachment of molar villi to the myometrial smooth muscle without intervening decidua (**a**, **b**)

Gestational Trophoblastic Tumors

Gestational Choriocarcinoma (CC) [5, 6]

- Clinical features
  - Presents during reproductive years (average age of 30 years).
  - Clinical symptoms include vaginal bleeding and/or extrauterine hemorrhage as a result of metastases to lung, brain, liver, kidney, and gastrointestinal tract.
  - Develops following normal gestation, hydatidiform mole, or abortion in 50 %, 22.5 %, and 20 % of the cases, respectively.
  - Markedly elevated serum hCG.
- Gross pathology
  - Bulky, extensively hemorrhagic, and necrotic mass lesion with destructive invasive border
- Microscopic features (Fig. 6.5)
  - Triphasic or biphasic growth pattern composed of distinct populations of villous intermediate trophoblast, cytotrophoblast, and syncytiotrophoblast.
  - Abundant tumor necrosis and hemorrhage.
  - Marked nuclear atypia, often with bizarre nuclei.
  - Brisk mitotic activity with frequent atypical mitotic figures.
  - Vascular invasion is common.
  - Chorionic villi are absent.

- Differential diagnosis
  - Placental site trophoblastic tumor
  - Epithelioid trophoblastic tumor
  - Carcinoma with trophoblastic differentiation
  - Previllous trophoblasts of early placenta formation
  - Trophoblastic proliferation of complete mole after the initial evacuation
  - Exaggerated placental site reaction
- Diagnostic pitfalls/key intraoperative consultation issues
  - Recent history of gestation, marked elevation of serum hCG, and biphasic or triphasic tumor cell proliferation are important hints for the correct diagnosis at the time of intraoperative consultation.
  - Placental site trophoblastic tumor and epithelioid trophoblastic tumor have low level of serum hCG and develop years after pregnancy.
  - In contrast to choriocarcinoma, carcinoma with trophoblastic differentiation typically occurs in older patients with low level of serum hCG and shows at least focal glandular epithelial differentiation.
  - Presence of molar chorionic villi traditionally precludes the diagnosis of choriocarcinoma.
  - Exaggerated placental site reaction does not form a mass lesion and lacks cytological atypia and marked elevation of serum hCG.

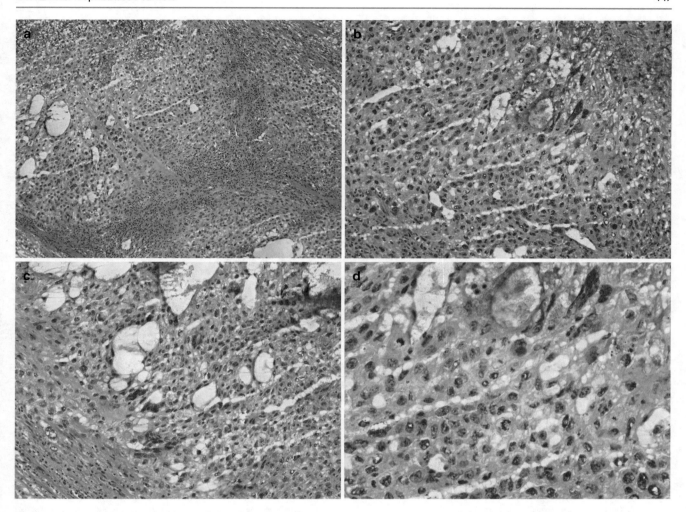

Fig. 6.5 Gestational choriocarcinoma. Note the triphasic proliferation of villous intermediate trophoblast (large mononuclear cells), cytotrophoblast (smaller monocular cells), and syncytiotrophoblast (multinucleate cells) (**a**, **b**) and the presence of marked nuclear atypia and brisk mitotic activity (**c**, **d**)

Placental Site Trophoblastic Tumor (PSTT) [7]

- Clinical features
  - Uncommon neoplasm of implantation site intermediate trophoblast.
  - Patients usually present during their reproductive years, months to several years after an antecedent term pregnancy, abortion, or a hydatidiform mole.
  - Clinical symptoms include irregular vaginal bleeding or amenorrhea and asymmetric uterine enlargement.
  - Most patients have low level of serum hCG.
  - Majority of PSTTs are cured by hysterectomy. 10–15 % of tumors recur or develop metastases, most commonly to the lungs.
- Gross pathology
  - Soft, tan-white or yellow infiltrative mass involving the endo-myometrium
  - Occasionally may have foci of hemorrhage and necrosis
- Microscopic features
  - Infiltrative endo-myometrial growth.
  - Proliferation of atypical intermediate trophoblast as single cells, aggregates, or cords splitting apart individual smooth muscle fibers.
  - The tumor cells are predominantly mononuclear, but binucleated and multinucleated forms are also common.
  - Moderate to severe nuclear atypia and mitotic activity are usually present.
- Differential diagnosis
  - Poorly differentiated carcinoma
  - Epithelioid smooth muscle tumors
  - Epithelioid trophoblastic tumor
  - Exaggerated implantation site
  - Choriocarcinoma
- Diagnostic pitfalls/key intraoperative consultation issues
  - Separation of epithelioid leiomyosarcoma from PSTT can be difficult at the time of frozen section diagnosis. Helpful hints in favor of trophoblastic tumor include elevation of serum hCG, stromal deposition of eosinophilic fibrin, and extensive hyalinization.
  - Unlike PSTT, poorly differentiated endometrial carcinoma may show foci of glandular or squamous differentiation and does not have elevation of serum hCG.
  - PSTT does not have extensive destructive growth and a triphasic growth pattern typical of choriocarcinoma. The serum hCG level in PSTT is much lower than that of choriocarcinoma.
  - In contrast to PSTT, exaggerated placental site is a microscopic finding in a concurrent non-molar or molar pregnancy and does not form an invasive mass lesion.

Epithelioid Trophoblastic Tumor (ETT) [8]

- Clinical features
  - Very rare trophoblastic tumor arising from the intermediate trophoblast of chorion laeve.
  - Patients present during their reproductive years with abnormal vaginal bleeding and mild to moderate elevation of serum hCG.
  - The tumor may develop 1–18 years (mean 6.2) after a full-term delivery, spontaneous abortion, or a molar pregnancy.
  - Most tumors have a benign clinical course, but local recurrence and metastases occur in approximately 25 % of cases.
- Gross pathology
  - Well-defined tan to brown nodule
  - Frequently involves the endocervix or lower uterine segment
- Microscopic features
  - Typically an expansile lesion.
  - Solid nests and sheets of mononuclear intermediate trophoblastic cells.
  - Tumor nests frequently contain eosinophilic, hyalinized material and necrotic debris, resembling keratin. Geographic necrosis is common.
  - The tumor cells are fairly uniform with mild to moderate nuclear atypia and relatively abundant eosinophilic or clear cytoplasm.
  - Mitoses are common and may be numerous.
  - The tumor cells may colonize the cervical mucosal surface, simulating cervical squamous intraepithelial lesion.
  - Decidualized benign stromal cells are frequently found around the tumor nests.
- Differential diagnosis
  - Squamous cell carcinoma of the cervix
  - Choriocarcinoma
  - Placental site trophoblastic tumor
  - Epithelioid smooth muscle tumor
- Diagnostic pitfalls/key intraoperative consultation issues
  - ETT frequently involves the cervix and histologically simulates squamous cell carcinoma (SCC) by its epithelioid tumor nests, presence of keratin-like material within the tumor nests and colonization of cervical mucosa. In contrast to cervical SCC, patients with ETT have low level of serum hCG and lack history of human papillomavirus infection and cervical dysplasia.
  - Unlike choriocarcinoma, ETT has only low level of serum hCG, and it lacks extensive destructive growth and triphasic morphologic pattern.
  - Separation of epithelioid leiomyosarcoma from ETT can be difficult at the time of frozen section diagnosis.

Helpful hints in favor of trophoblastic tumor include elevation of serum hCG, extensive hyalinization, and calcification.

- In contrast to ETT, placental site nodule is an incidental microscopic finding and does not form an invasive mass lesion.

Tumorlike Conditions

Exaggerated Placental Site Reaction (EPS) [9]

- Reactive process, usually seen with a concurrent pregnancy—non-molar or molar, particularly complete mole.
- Generally a microscopic lesion.
- Infiltrative growth pattern of intermediate trophoblasts within the myometrium with presence of extracellular fibrinoid material.
- Evenly distributed multinucleated intermediate trophoblasts.
- The differential diagnosis is PSTT. Unlike PSTT, exaggerated placental site reaction does not form an invasive mass lesion and presents with a concurrent pregnancy.

Placental Site Nodule (PSN) [10, 11]

- Retained placental chorion laeve tissue that persists for months to years after pregnancy.
- Incidental microscopic finding and is not accompanied by serum hCG elevation.
- Histologically, PSN is a nodular or plaque-like lesion that is paucicellular with marked hyalinization and scattered inactive intermediate trophoblast without significant atypia or mitotic activity.

- The main differential diagnosis is ETT. In contrast to ETT, placental site nodule does not form an invasive mass lesion, has an extensive hyalinized matrix, and lacks atypia and mitotic activity.

References

1. Kurman RJ, Carcanglu ML, Herrington CS, Young RH. WHO classification of tumours of female reproductive organs. 4th ed. Lyon: International Agency for Research on Cancer (IARC); 2014; 155–67.
2. Keep D, Zaragoza MV, Hassold T, Redline RW. Very early complete hydatidiform mole. Hum Pathol. 1996;27:708–13.
3. Buza N, Hui P. Partial hydatidiform mole: histologic parameters in correlation with DNA genotyping. Int J Gynecol Pathol. 2013;32(3): 307–15.
4. Gaber LW, Redline RW, Mostoufi-Zadeh M, Driscoll SG. Invasive partial mole. Am J Clin Pathol. 1986;85(6):722–4.
5. Ober WB, Edgcomb JH, Price Jr EB. The pathology of choriocarcinoma. Ann N Y Acad Sci. 1971;172:299–426.
6. Bower M, Brock C, Fisher RA, Newlands ES, Rustin GJ. Gestational choriocarcinoma. Ann Oncol. 1995;6:503–8.
7. Baergen RN, Rutgers JL, Young RH, Osann K, Scully RE. Placental site trophoblastic tumor: a study of 55 cases and review of the literature emphasizing factors of prognostic significance. Gynecol Oncol. 2006;100:511–20.
8. Fadare O, Parkash V, Carcangiu ML, Hui P. Epithelioid trophoblastic tumor: clinicopathological features with an emphasis on uterine cervical involvement. Mod Pathol. 2006;19:75–82.
9. Shih IM, Kurman RJ. The pathology of intermediate trophoblastic tumors and tumor-like lesions. Int J Gynecol Pathol. 2001;20: 31–47.
10. Young RH, Kurman RJ, Scully RE. Placental site nodules and plaques. A clinicopathologic analysis of 20 cases. Am J Surg Pathol. 1990;14:1001–9.
11. Huettner PC, Gersell DJ. Placental site nodule: a clinicopathologic study of 38 cases. Int J Gynecol Pathol. 1994;13:191–8.

Fallopian Tube

7

Introduction

Neoplastic or reactive lesions presenting at the fallopian tube as a primary site of involvement are uncommon. The fallopian tube is most often received for intraoperative frozen section evaluation as part of a salpingo-oophorectomy specimen. The primary disease site may not always be accurately determined by preoperative imaging studies or the surgeon's intraoperative assessment, and the specimen sent to pathology as an ovarian/adnexal mass occasionally may reveal a primary fallopian tube disease process. The most common primary fallopian tube lesions include epithelial neoplasms—benign, borderline, or malignant—embryonal remnants and cysts (e.g., paratubal cyst), endometriosis, inflammatory conditions, and ectopic pregnancy. Frozen section of the fallopian tube is indicated when the lesion is located within the tube or the primary site—ovarian versus tubal—cannot be determined with certainty based on the gross examination. Thorough intraoperative gross evaluation of the fallopian tube is typically sufficient when the main lesion is of primary ovarian or uterine origin. The role and optimal pathology protocol for intraoperative assessment of risk-reducing salpingo-oophorectomy specimens is still evolving, and currently no standardized guidelines exist. This chapter covers the frozen section pathologic features and implications of the most common neoplastic and nonneoplastic tubal lesions and clinicopathologic considerations of intraoperative evaluation of risk-reducing salpingo-oophorectomy specimens.

P. Hui, N. Buza, *Atlas of Intraoperative Frozen Section Diagnosis in Gynecologic Pathology*,
DOI 10.1007/978-3-319-21807-6_7

Primary Tumors of the Fallopian Tube

Serous Adenofibroma

- Most often an incidental finding.
- Small, benign biphasic tumor, typically located at the fimbriated end of the fallopian tube [1].
- May form a grossly recognizable mass.
- Histology is similar to its ovarian counterpart: variably sized irregular glands lined by benign tubal-type epithelium and fibromatous stromal component (Fig. 7.1).
  - No significant nuclear atypia or mitotic activity.
- Differential diagnosis
  - Serous borderline/atypical proliferative tumor (SBT/APST)

- Diagnostic pitfalls/key intraoperative consultation issues
  - Lack of significant cytological atypia and papillary epithelial proliferation separates this entity from SBT/APST.

Serous Borderline/Atypical Proliferative Tumor (SBT/APST)

- Rare tumor, histologically resembling its ovarian counterpart.
- Clinicopathologic implications and prognosis are similar to ovarian SBT/APST.

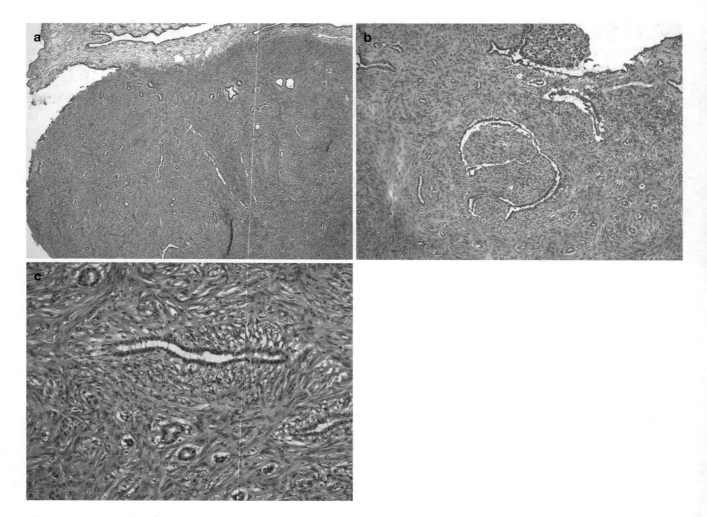

Fig. 7.1 Serous adenofibroma. Variably sized, round, or irregularly shaped glands in a background of fibromatous stroma; note the adjacent tubal fimbria (**a**, *upper left* portion of image). The glands are lined by a single layer of tubal-type epithelium without atypia (**b**, **c**)

Serous Tubal Intraepithelial Carcinoma (STIC)

- Noninvasive serous carcinoma, most often arising in the fimbria or distal end of the fallopian tube.
- The reported incidence of STIC in risk-reducing salpingo-oophorectomy specimens is 0.6–6 % [2–5].
- Most STICs do not form a grossly recognizable mass lesion; however, rare cases of exophytic noninvasive serous carcinoma may be identified on gross examination as a small nodule [6].
- Microscopically STIC demonstrates multilayered epithelium with hyperchromatic, markedly atypical cells (Fig. 7.2).
    - High nuclear to cytoplasmic ratio.
    - Prominent nucleoli.
    - Loss of polarity.
    - Absence of cilia.
    - Mitotic figures are often present.
    - Tumor cells may exfoliate into the tubal lumen.
    - Absence of stromal invasion.
- Differential diagnosis
    - Tangential sectioning of tubal epithelium
    - Benign metaplastic changes—transitional, squamous, or papillary syncytial metaplasia—of the tubal epithelium
    - Tubal epithelial hyperplasia
    - Atypical epithelial lesions falling short of STIC morphologic criteria
    - Invasive tubal high-grade serous carcinoma
    - Secondary tubal spread from other gynecologic—ovarian or uterine—primaries
- Diagnostic pitfalls/key intraoperative consultation issues
    - Atypical epithelial lesions falling short of STIC morphologic criteria do not need to be specified on frozen section as they do not require further surgery.

- Recurrence rate of STIC is low (has been reported in less than 10 % of cases) [7, 8].
- Peritoneal washing is recommended.
- No uniform guidelines on the role and extent of surgical staging; approximately 50 % of patients with STIC in the literature underwent hysterectomy and omental biopsy/omentectomy, and only 24 % had lymph node sampling performed [7].
- The diagnosis of STIC on frozen section (i.e., on morphology alone, without ancillary studies) may be very challenging, and a conservative approach or deferral to permanent sections is reasonable in difficult cases to avoid overdiagnosis.
- Invasive tubal serous carcinoma typically requires surgical staging [8].
- Secondary tubal involvement—by direct spread or metastasis—by other gynecologic primary tumors (ovarian or endometrial) may colonize the tubal epithelium mimicking STIC.
    - If the diagnosis of ovarian or endometrial malignancy is established (previously or intraoperatively), additional tubal involvement (whether secondary or synchronous primary tumor) typically does not have a significant impact on the surgical management.
- Metastatic tumors from non-gynecologic primaries may also mimic STIC, but they usually involve the stroma of fallopian tube and multiple other organs as well.
    - In patients with prior history of non-gynecologic malignancy, morphologic comparison with the prior specimen(s)—if available at the time of frozen section—should be made.

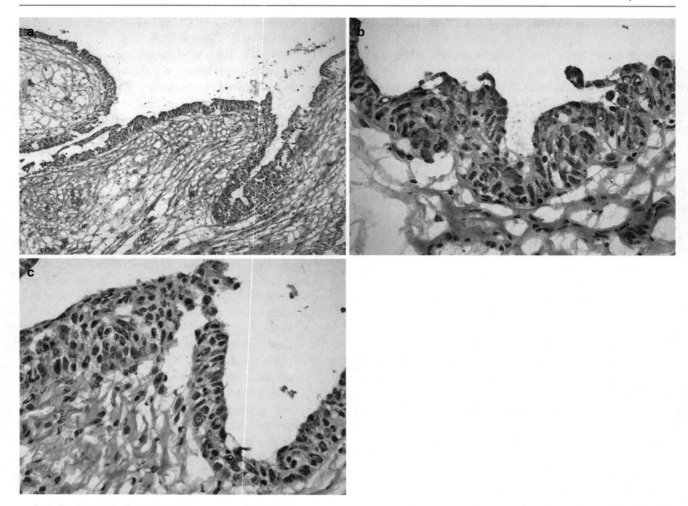

Fig. 7.2 Serous tubal intraepithelial carcinoma (STIC). Multilayered epithelium (**a**) with loss of polarity, hyperchromasia, increased nuclear to cytoplasmic ratio, and severe cytological atypia are characteristic (**b**, **c**). Mitotic figures are common (**c**)

High-Grade Serous Carcinoma (Invasive)

- Most common type of tubal carcinoma.
- May present with abdominal/pelvic pain or may be an incidental finding.
  - Tubal carcinomas (intraepithelial and invasive) have been reported in 5–10 % of risk-reducing salpingo-oophorectomy specimens [2–5].
- May involve bilateral fallopian tubes.
- Histologically resembles high-grade ovarian serous carcinoma (see Chap. 8) (Fig. 7.3).
  - Papillary, solid, or slit-like glandular pattern.
  - Marked nuclear atypia and frequent mitotic figures, including atypical mitoses.
  - Stromal invasion.
  - Necrosis and lymphovascular invasion may be apparent on frozen section.
  - Psammoma bodies may be seen.
- Differential diagnosis
  - Serous tubal intraepithelial carcinoma (STIC)
  - Secondary tubal spread from other gynecologic—ovarian or uterine—or non-gynecologic primaries
- Diagnostic pitfalls/key intraoperative consultation issues
  - Secondary tubal involvement—via direct spread or metastasis—by ovarian or endometrial serous carcinoma is common.
    - If the diagnosis of ovarian or endometrial malignancy is established (previously or intraoperatively), additional tubal involvement (whether secondary or synchronous primary tumor) typically does not have a significant impact on the surgical management.
  - Metastatic tumors from non-gynecologic primaries (most commonly breast or gastrointestinal) may mimic primary tubal carcinoma.
    - In patients with prior history of non-gynecologic malignancy, morphologic comparison with the prior specimen(s)—if available at the time of frozen section—should be made.

Adenomatoid Tumor

- Benign tumor of mesothelial origin.
- Usually small, incidental finding (<2 cm in size).
- May be identified grossly as a solid, white, or yellow mass lesion.
- Microscopic features are similar to its uterine counterpart (see Chap. 5).
  - Proliferation of small, irregular glandular spaces lined by bland mesothelial cells.
  - No significant nuclear atypia or mitotic activity.
  - Basophilic mucoid material may be seen in gland lumens.
- Differential diagnosis
  - Angioma and lymphangioma
  - Metastatic adenocarcinoma, especially of the signet-ring cell type
- Diagnostic pitfalls/key intraoperative consultation issues
  - Significant nuclear atypia, single cell spread, stromal infiltration, and stromal desmoplastic reaction are not features of adenomatoid tumor and should raise suspicion for metastatic adenocarcinoma.
    - If there is a clinical history of malignancy, morphologic comparison with the prior specimen(s) should be made.

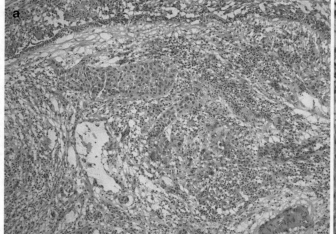
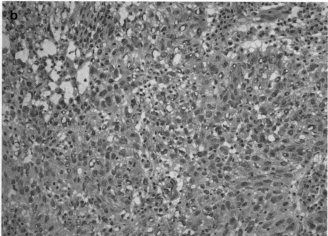
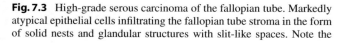

Fig. 7.3 High-grade serous carcinoma of the fallopian tube. Markedly atypical epithelial cells infiltrating the fallopian tube stroma in the form of solid nests and glandular structures with slit-like spaces. Note the overlying tubal epithelium (**a**). High nuclear to cytoplasmic ratio, prominent nucleoli, and frequent mitoses are seen (**b**)

Metastatic Tumors of the Fallopian Tube

Gynecologic Primaries

- The most common secondary fallopian tube involvement—via direct spread or metastasis—is by ovarian or endometrial primaries.
- The pattern of involvement may be:
  - Superficial mucosal, colonizing the tubal epithelium mimicking an in situ lesion
  - Infiltrative, involving the tubal wall
  - Luminal; detached tumor fragments in the tubal lumen
- In cases of known ovarian or endometrial malignancy, additional tubal involvement typically does not have a significant impact on the immediate surgical management.
  - Determination of tumor origin—secondary or synchronous independent primary—can be deferred to permanent sections.

Non-gynecologic Primaries

- Less frequently the tube may harbor metastases from extragenital primary sites—particularly the gastrointestinal tract and breast (Fig. 7.4).
- Lymphovascular invasion is commonly identified.
- No gynecologic staging surgery is performed for metastatic tumors involving the fallopian tube.
- Concurrent ovarian metastasis may also be present; hence, evaluation of ovaries—if available for frozen section—may be helpful.
- In patients with prior history of non-gynecologic malignancy, morphologic comparison with the prior specimen(s) should be made.

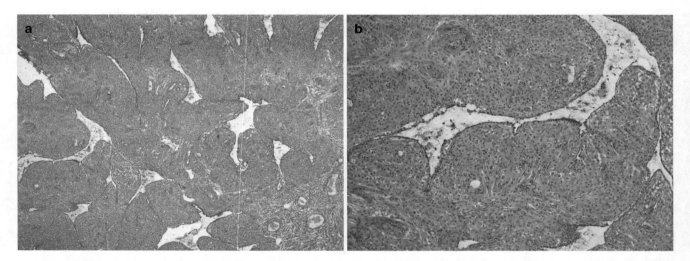

Fig. 7.4 Metastatic lobular carcinoma of the breast involving fallopian tube mucosa. Note the thickened, hypercellular mucosal folds (**a**) infiltrated by relatively uniform discohesive tumor cells (**b**). The overlying thin tubal epithelium is uninvolved (**b**)

Nonneoplastic/Reactive Lesions of the Fallopian Tube

Tubal Epithelial Hyperplasia

- Relatively common benign finding in fallopian tubes.
- Focal proliferation/pseudostratification of tubal epithelium (Fig. 7.5a, b).
- Papillary architecture—papillary tubal hyperplasia—is less common, showing papillary projections of tubal epithelium and round tips of papillae floating in the fallopian tube lumen (Fig. 7.5c–e).
- No significant nuclear atypia or mitotic activity.
- Ciliated cells are typically present.
- Psammomatous calcifications may be seen in papillary tubal hyperplasia.

- Differential diagnosis
  - Serous borderline/atypical proliferative tumor (SBT/APST)
  - Serous tubal intraepithelial carcinoma (STIC)
- Diagnostic pitfalls/key intraoperative consultation issues
  - Papillary tubal hyperplasia may be associated with SBT/APST [9].
  - No impact on intraoperative surgical management.
  - May mimic SBT/APST or STIC on low magnification; high magnification shows lack of significant nuclear atypia or mitotic activity and preserved nuclear polarity.
  - If the histologic features are equivocal, conservative approach or deferral to permanent sections is reasonable to avoid overtreatment.

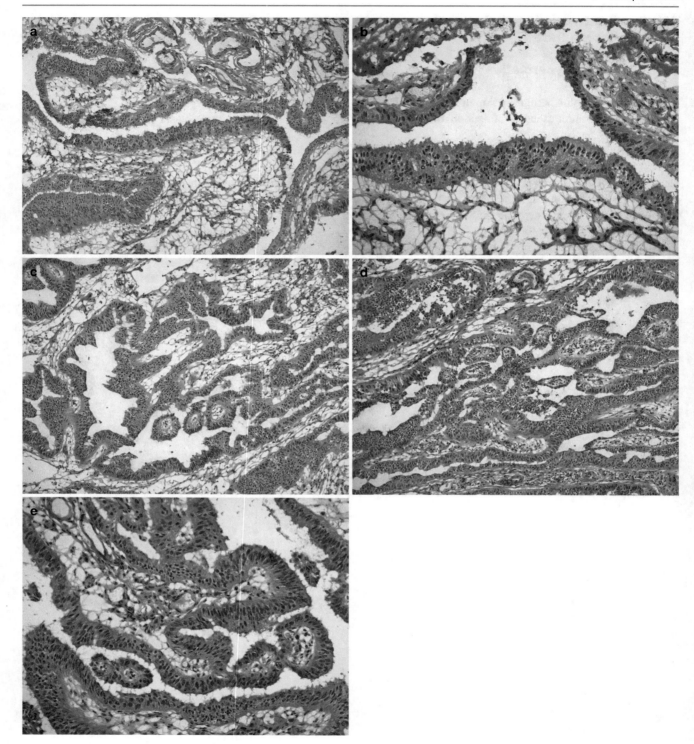

Fig. 7.5 Tubal epithelial hyperplasia shows pseudostratification of tubal epithelium without cytological atypia or loss of polarity (**a, b**). Papillary tubal hyperplasia forms papillary epithelial projections into the tubal lumen with occasional free-floating round tips of papillae (**c–e**)

Embryonic Remnants/Cysts

- *Mesonephric remnants* are commonly encountered adjacent to the fallopian tube and are usually easily recognized as small, round glandular structures lined by a single layer of low columnar or cuboidal epithelial cells (Fig. 7.6).
  - Smooth muscle is typically prominent surrounding the mesonephric remnants.
  - No significant nuclear atypia or mitotic activity.
  - Intraluminal eosinophilic secretion may be seen.
  - Ciliated cells may be present.
- *Walthard nests*—transitional-type epithelial nests, *adrenocortical rests,* and aggregates of *hilus cells* may also be identified near the fallopian tube.
- *Paratubal cysts* may range from less than a cm to several cm in size and are most commonly lined by tubal-type epithelium (Fig. 7.7).
  - May mimic an ovarian lesion clinically and/or radiologically.
  - Lack significant epithelial proliferation, nuclear atypia, or mitotic activity.
  - Rarely SBT/APST may arise in paratubal cysts.

Endometriosis

- Endometriosis may involve the serosal aspect or mucosa of the fallopian tube.
- Similar to other sites, microscopic examination shows variable proportions of endometrial glandular epithelium and endometrial stroma often with hemosiderin-laden macrophages.
- Definitive diagnosis is typically not required on frozen section.

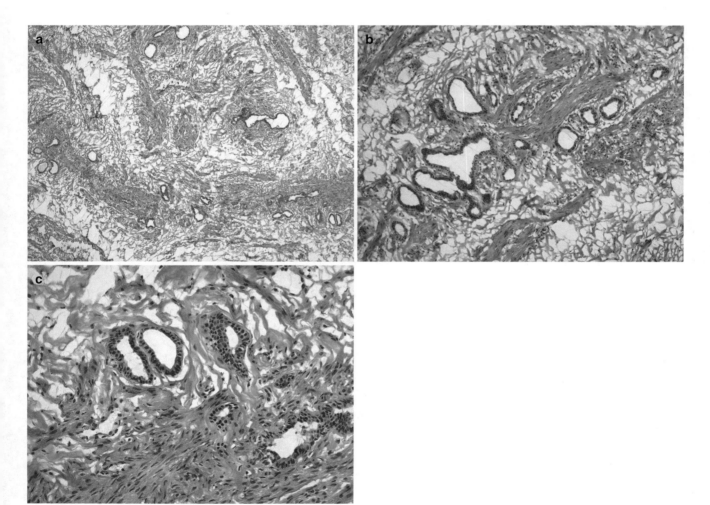

Fig. 7.6 Mesonephric remnants are small glandular structures surrounded by prominent smooth muscle (**a**, **b**). The lining epithelium is a single layer of cuboidal or low columnar cells without atypia (**c**)

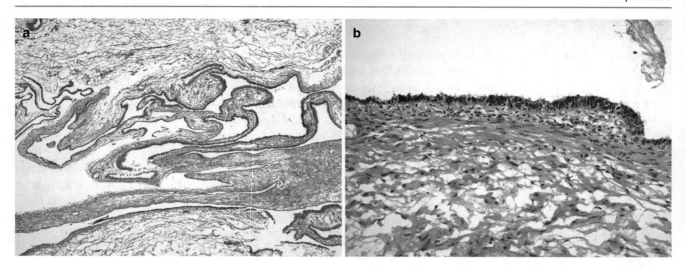

Fig. 7.7 Paratubal cyst with a thin, folded cyst wall (**a**) and tubal-type epithelial lining with ciliated cells (**b**)

Salpingitis: Acute and Chronic

- Acute and chronic inflammation of the fallopian tube may result in significant edema, necrosis, and pelvic- and tubo-ovarian adhesions mimicking a mass lesion clinically and/or radiologically.
- Microscopic examination shows variable amount of acute and/or chronic inflammatory infiltrate often with extensive adhesions, edema, and hemorrhage (Fig. 7.8).

- Necrosis may also be seen.
- Reactive tubal epithelial changes and surface mesothelial hyperplasia may also be present (see Chap. 13).
  - Epithelial atypia should be interpreted with caution in the background of marked acute and/or chronic inflammation to avoid overdiagnosis.

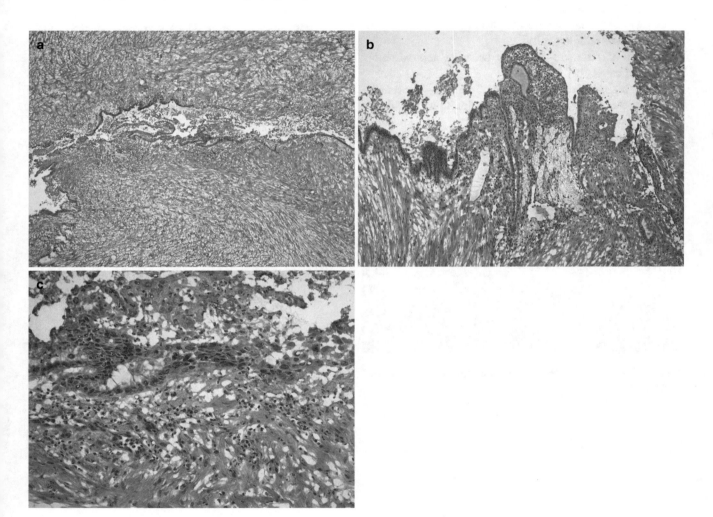

Fig. 7.8 Acute and chronic salpingitis. Note the mixed inflammatory infiltrate involving the tubal mucosa (**a**) with aggregates of foamy macrophages (**b**). Reactive epithelial changes may also be seen (**c**)

Ectopic Pregnancy

- Ectopic pregnancy accounts for approximately 1–2 % of all pregnancies, most of which occur in the fallopian tube [10].
  - Rare cases involve bilateral fallopian tubes, and simultaneous ectopic and intrauterine pregnancies may also occur [11].
- Clinical symptoms include amenorrhea, vaginal bleeding, and abdominal pain.
- Occasionally may mimic neoplastic proliferation clinically and/or radiologically.
- Rupture of fallopian tube may occur in approximately 25 % of cases [12].
- Gross findings include dilatation of the tube—most commonly the ampulla, red-blue discoloration, and dusky serosal surface (Fig. 7.9).
- Microscopically presence of chorionic villi—viable or necrotic—and/or implantation site confirm the diagnosis of tubal pregnancy; fetal parts are less commonly seen (Fig. 7.10).
  - Identification of necrotic/degenerated chorionic villi may be difficult on frozen section.
  - Edematous tubal mucosal folds may mimic chorionic villi.
    - Helpful features confirming chorionic villi (versus tubal mucosa): presence of multinucleated syncytiotrophoblast on villous surface and absence of cilia.
  - Trophoblastic proliferation may be exuberant, sheet-like, raising concern for gestational trophoblastic disease (see Chap. 6).
    - Confirmation of ectopic pregnancy is typically sufficient on frozen section; definitive diagnosis of gestational trophoblastic disease can be deferred to permanent sections.

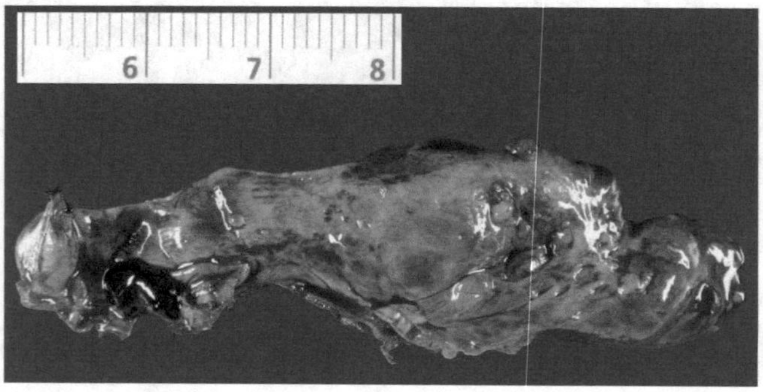

Fig. 7.9 Tubal pregnancy. The fallopian tube is dilated with a *red-blue*, dusky serosal surface

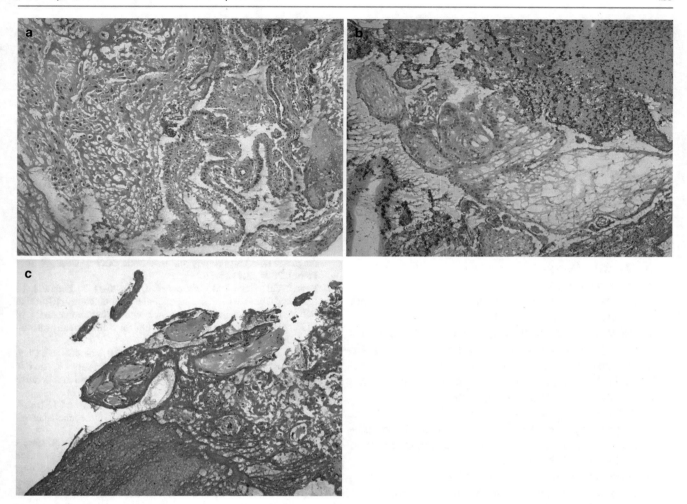

Fig. 7.10 Tubal pregnancy. Edematous tubal mucosal folds may mimic chorionic villi (**a**, *right side* of image). Blood clot with clusters of intervillous intermediate trophoblast (**a**, *left side* of image) and degenerated chorionic villi with multinucleated syncytiotrophoblast (**b**, **c**)

Risk-Reducing Salpingo-oophorectomy Specimens

- Prophylactic bilateral salpingo-oophorectomy is often performed in women who are at increased risk for epithelial ovarian and fallopian tube malignancy.
- Prophylactic bilateral salpingo-oophorectomy has been shown to reduce the risk of ovarian cancer by 90 % and the risk of breast cancer by 50 % in *BRCA* mutation carriers [13].
- In addition to *BRCA1* and *BRCA2* mutation carriers, patients with Lynch syndrome or strong family history of breast and ovarian carcinoma may also undergo risk-reducing salpingo-oophorectomy (RRSO).
- The reported rate of tubal carcinomas (intraepithelial and invasive) in RRSO specimens has ranged between 5 and 10 %, with intraepithelial carcinoma (STIC) only in 0.6–6 % of cases [2–5, 7, 14].
- Most tumors in RRSO specimens are small and may not be detected by gross examination.
- To enhance detection of early lesions in RRSO specimens, a gross examination protocol has been proposed and adopted by many institutions—termed the "sectioning and extensively examining the fimbriated end" (SEE-FIM) protocol [15, 16], which includes:
  - Specimen fixation before grossing
  - Sectioning of the distal 2 cm of fallopian tube longitudinally and the remainder of the tube perpendicular to the lumen at 2–3 mm intervals
  - Sectioning of ovaries at 2–3 mm intervals
  - Microscopic examination of the entire specimen
- No standard pathology guidelines exist for optimal intraoperative evaluation of RRSO specimens.
- Practical considerations at the time of frozen section include:
  - Sectioning of RRSO specimens fresh (without proper formalin fixation) may result in uneven slices and suboptimal tissue quality.
  - Frozen section evaluation may potentially exhaust the lesional tissue.
  - Patients may benefit from an immediate staging procedure if a high-grade serous carcinoma (tubal or ovarian) is diagnosed on frozen section.
  - A recent study recommends a practical algorithmic approach based on the preparedness of the surgical team and the gross findings [6]:
    - If the surgical team is prepared to proceed with staging surgery in case a carcinoma is diagnosed on frozen section, then intraoperative gross evaluation of the specimen should be performed.
      - Any grossly identified nodule >0.5 cm should be submitted for frozen section.
    - If the surgical team is not prepared for staging surgery, immediate formalin fixation followed by the SEE-FIM protocol (see above) is recommended.

References

1. Bossuyt V, Medeiros F, Drapkin R, Folkins AK, Crum CP, Nucci MR. Adenofibroma of the fimbria: a common entity that is indistinguishable from ovarian adenofibroma. Int J Gynecol Pathol. 2008;27:390–7.
2. Carcangiu ML, Peissel B, Pasini B, Spatti G, Radice P, Manoukian S. Incidental carcinomas in prophylactic specimens in BRCA1 and BRCA2 germ-line mutation carriers, with emphasis on fallopian tube lesions: report of 6 cases and review of the literature. Am J Surg Pathol. 2006;30:1222–30.
3. Callahan MJ, Crum CP, Medeiros F, Kindelberger DW, Elvin JA, Garber JE, et al. Primary fallopian tube malignancies in BRCA-positive women undergoing surgery for ovarian cancer risk reduction. J Clin Oncol. 2007;25:3985–90.
4. Rabban JT, Barnes M, Chen LM, Powell CB, Crawford B, Zaloudek CJ. Ovarian pathology in risk-reducing salpingo-oophorectomies from women with BRCA mutations, emphasizing the differential diagnosis of occult primary and metastatic carcinoma. Am J Surg Pathol. 2009;33:1125–36.
5. Powell CB, Chen LM, McLennan J, Crawford B, Zaloudek C, Rabban JT, et al. Risk-reducing salpingo-oophorectomy (RRSO) in BRCA mutation carriers: experience with a consecutive series of 111 patients using a standardized surgical-pathological protocol. Int J Gynecol Cancer. 2011;21:846–51.
6. Rabban JT, Mackey A, Powell CB, Crawford B, Zaloudek CJ, Chen LM. Correlation of macroscopic and microscopic pathology in risk reducing salpingo-oophorectomy: implications for intraoperative specimen evaluation. Gynecol Oncol. 2011;121:466–71.
7. Wethington SL, Park KJ, Soslow RA, Kauff ND, Brown CL, Dao F, et al. Clinical outcome of isolated serous tubal intraepithelial carcinomas (STIC). Int J Gynecol Cancer. 2013;23:1603–11.
8. Powell CB, Swisher EM, Cass I, McLennan J, Morquist B, Garcia RL, et al. Long term follow up of BRCA1 and BRCA2 mutation carriers with unsuspected neoplasia identified at risk reducing salpingo-oophorectomy. Gynecol Oncol. 2013;129:364–71.
9. Kurman RJ, Vang R, Junge J, Hannibal CG, Kjaer SK, Shih IM. Papillary tubal hyperplasia: the putative precursor of ovarian atypical proliferative (borderline) serous tumors, noninvasive implants, and endosalpingiosis. Am J Surg Pathol. 2011;35:1605–14.
10. Farquhar CM. Ectopic pregnancy. Lancet. 2005;366:583–91.
11. Marcus SF, Macnamee M, Brinsden P. Heterotopic pregnancies after in-vitro fertilization and embryo transfer. Hum Reprod. 1995;10:1232–6.
12. Falcone T, Mascha EJ, Goldberg JM, Falconi LL, Mohla G, Attaran M. A study of risk factors for ruptured tubal ectopic pregnancy. J Womens Health. 1998;7:459–63.
13. Roukos DH, Briasoulis E. Individualized preventive and therapeutic management of hereditary breast ovarian cancer syndrome. Nat Clin Pract Oncol. 2007;4:578–90.
14. Finch A, Shaw P, Rosen B, Murphy J, Narod SA, Colgan TJ. Clinical and pathologic findings of prophylactic salpingo-oophorectomies in 159 BRCA1 and BRCA2 carriers. Gynecol Oncol. 2006;100:58–64.
15. Lee Y, Medeiros F, Kindelberger D, Callahan MJ, Muto MG, Crum CP. Advances in the recognition of tubal intraepithelial carcinoma: applications to cancer screening and the pathogenesis of ovarian cancer. Adv Anat Pathol. 2006;13:1–7.
16. Gwin K, Wilcox R, Montag A. Insights into selected genetic diseases affecting the female reproductive tract and their implication for pathologic evaluation of gynecologic specimens. Arch Pathol Lab Med. 2009;133:1041–52.

Ovarian Epithelial Tumors

8

Introduction

Surface epithelial tumors are the most common group of ovarian neoplasms in general and represent approximately 90 % of ovarian malignancy; hence, they are one of the most frequently encountered gynecologic specimens in the frozen section laboratory. Preoperative diagnostic workup of ovarian tumors is usually limited to imaging studies and serum markers, both of which suffer from low sensitivity and specificity. Intraoperative frozen section evaluation therefore is crucial for determining the required extent of surgery: limited cystectomy or unilateral salpingo-oophorectomy for benign tumors—especially in young patients desiring fertility preservation—or extensive staging procedure with bilateral salpingo-oophorectomy, lymph node dissection, omentectomy, and peritoneal biopsies for ovarian carcinomas. Accurate diagnosis and classification of borderline (atypical proliferative) tumors may also allow for conservative surgical management and fertility preservation in the reproductive age group [1, 2]. Misinterpretation of the frozen section, on the other hand, may result in unnecessary extensive surgical procedure or will put the patient at risk for a second surgery.

Combination of careful gross examination, appropriate sampling, and interpretation of morphologic findings along with familiarity of the clinical context is key to the accurate frozen section diagnosis and successful intraoperative consultation on epithelial ovarian tumors. The proportion of solid and cystic areas on gross examination may provide a preliminary impression in this group of neoplasms, as vast majority of completely cystic tumors with a smooth lining and without solid nodules is histologically benign [3]. On the other hand, many of the benign epithelial tumors have a partially or entirely solid cut surface, e.g., adenofibromas or benign Brenner tumors. Serous tumors, both benign and malignant, are often bilateral; however, bilaterality of mucinous tumors—especially those with borderline or overt malignant features—should always raise suspicion for metastasis. In addition, mucinous tumors generally require more extensive sampling even at the time of frozen section, due to their significant histological heterogeneity. Clinical history of any previous malignancy is very important in this setting, but may not be provided by the clinical team unless asked specifically. The patient's age and reproductive status also play a significant role in the frozen section consultation of ovarian epithelial tumors. The distinction between borderline tumors and invasive carcinomas may be difficult at the time of frozen section and a conservative approach may be appropriate, especially in young patients to avoid overdiagnosis of carcinoma.

The differential diagnosis of epithelial ovarian tumors also includes other primary ovarian neoplasms—e.g., sex cord-stromal tumors, germ cell tumors, and other miscellaneous neoplastic or nonneoplastic conditions, which will be separately discussed in detail within the following chapters.

© Springer International Publishing Switzerland 2015
P. Hui, N. Buza, *Atlas of Intraoperative Frozen Section Diagnosis in Gynecologic Pathology*,
DOI 10.1007/978-3-319-21807-6_8

Serous Ovarian Tumors

Serous Cystadenoma

- Clinical features
  - Usually adults; mean age between 40 and 60 years
  - Up to 20 % bilateral
- Gross pathology (Fig. 8.1)
  - Uni- or oligolocular cyst.
  - Up to 30 cm in size, mean: 5–8 cm.
  - Smooth external surface.
  - Typically filled with clear, watery fluid; occasionally appears thicker, mucoid in consistency.
  - Smooth inner lining without solid areas or papillary excrescences.
  - Gross sampling should include multiple fragments or "rolled up" cyst wall in one block.
- Microscopic features (Fig. 8.2)
  - Single layer of cuboidal to columnar cells, resembling tubal-type epithelium; often with pseudostratification of nuclei.
  - Ciliated cells are present.
  - No cytological atypia.
  - No significant epithelial proliferation.
- Differential diagnosis
  - *Serous cystadenoma with focal epithelial proliferation* (<10 % of epithelial lining shows atypical proliferation) [4, 5]
  - Serous borderline tumor (SBT)/atypical proliferative serous tumor (APST)
  - *Mucinous cystadenoma*; especially when cyst contents appear grossly mucinous
  - Endometriosis
  - Other cystic benign, nonneoplastic lesions (e.g., paratubal cyst, hydrosalpinx, cystic follicle/follicular cyst)
- Diagnostic pitfalls/key intraoperative consultation issues
  - *Tangential sectioning* of serous/tubal-type epithelium may mimic epithelial proliferation.
  - *Prominent pseudostratification* of nuclei may mimic epithelial proliferation/atypia.
  - *Serous cystadenoma with focal epithelial proliferation* (<10 % of epithelial lining shows atypical proliferation) [4, 5].
    - Does not meet criteria for SBT/APST, no staging surgery is necessary.
    - Additional frozen section sampling should be pursued to rule out SBT/APST.
    - Surgeon may be advised that additional sampling for permanent sections could increase the percentage of atypical proliferation, especially in large tumors.
  - SBT/APST
    - Epithelial proliferation and tufting in at least 10 % of tumor with mild cytological atypia
  - Mucinous cystadenoma
    - Classification/diagnosis is based on histological cell type, not gross appearance of cyst contents.
    - Surgeon may perform appendectomy if the frozen section diagnosis indicates a mucinous cystadenoma (see mucinous ovarian tumors).
  - Precise distinction from benign, nonneoplastic cystic lesions is typically not required on frozen section.

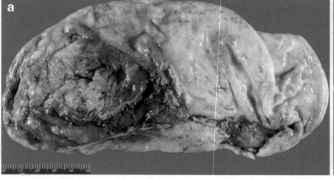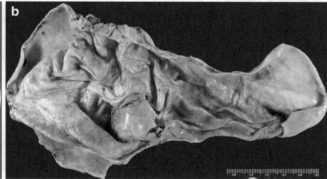

Fig. 8.1 Serous cystadenoma macroscopic appearance: smooth ovarian surface (**a**) and unilocular cyst with thin wall and a smooth cyst lining without papillary excrescences (**b**)

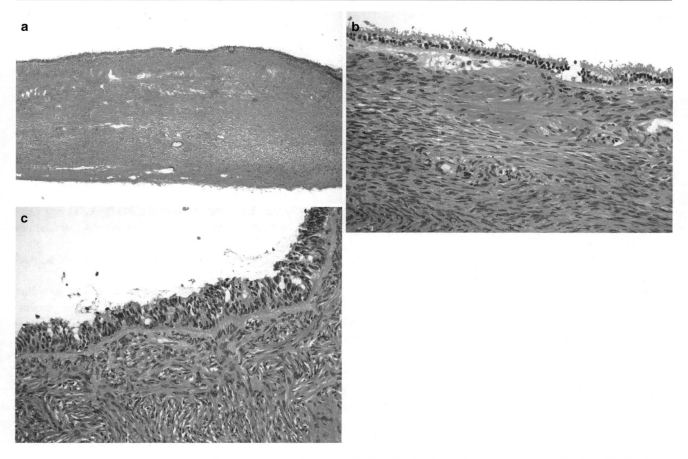

Fig. 8.2 Serous cystadenoma. The cyst is lined by ciliated tubal-type epithelium (**a**, **b**) often with nuclear pseudostratification (**c**). Significant epithelial proliferation, tufting, and cytological atypia are absent

Serous Cystadenofibroma/Adenofibroma

- Clinical features
  - Usually occurs in adults, with a mean age between 40 and 60 years
  - Up to 20 % bilateral
- Gross pathology (Fig. 8.3)
  - Surface may be lobulated or have coarse, firm papillary projections.
  - Variable proportion of cystic and solid areas.
  - Lining of cystic component may have papillary projections, which are typically firm and coarse
  - Serous adenofibromas without a cystic component have a solid, firm cut surface occasionally with visible small lumina ("spongelike" appearance).
  - Gross sampling should be focused on papillary and solid areas, with multiple blocks if necessary.
- Microscopic features (Fig. 8.4a, b)
  - Broad, fibrous papillae lined by a single layer of serous (tubal-type) epithelium, protruding into the cyst lumen (cystadenofibroma) or scattered glands with serous (tubal-type) lining embedded in fibrous stroma (adenofibroma).
  - Ciliated cells are present.
  - No cytological atypia or significant epithelial proliferation.
  - May show focal calcifications (stromal or epithelial).
- Differential diagnosis
  - *Serous cystadenoma with focal epithelial proliferation* (<10 % of epithelial lining shows atypical proliferation) [4, 5]

- Serous borderline tumor (SBT)/atypical proliferative serous tumor (APST)
- Endometriosis
- Endometrioid adenofibroma
- Diagnostic pitfalls/key intraoperative consultation issues
  - *Tangential sectioning* of serous/tubal-type epithelium may mimic epithelial proliferation (Fig. 8.4c).
  - *Prominent pseudostratification* of nuclei may mimic epithelial proliferation/atypia (see Fig. 8.2c).
  - *Serous cystadenofibroma with focal epithelial proliferation* (<10 % of epithelial lining shows atypical proliferation) [4, 5] (Fig. 8.5).
    - Does not meet criteria for SBT/APST, has been shown to have a benign clinical course, and does not require staging surgery.
    - Additional frozen section sampling should be pursued to rule out SBT/APST.
    - Surgeon may be advised that additional sampling for permanent sections could increase the percentage of atypical proliferation, especially in large tumors.
  - SBT/APST
    - Papillary projections of the cyst lining in serous cystadenofibroma are typically firm and coarse, scattered, and few in number—in contrast to the large number of soft, friable papillary intraluminal growth in SBT/APST.

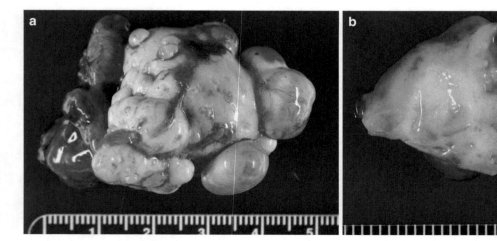

Fig. 8.3 Serous cystadenofibroma. The ovarian surface is often lobulated and may show coarse papillary projections (**a**). The cyst lining may also show coarse, firm papillary protrusions into the lumen (**b**)

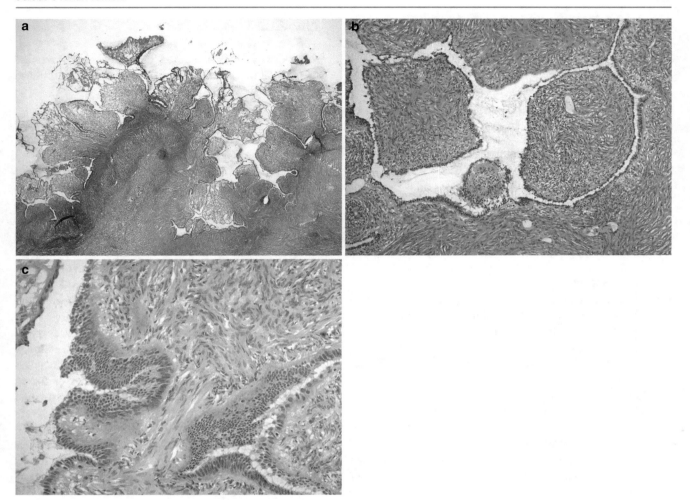

Fig. 8.4 Serous cystadenofibroma. Note the broad, fibrous papillae lined by a single layer of serous (tubal-type) epithelium (**a, b**). Tangential sectioning may result in pseudostratification mimicking epithelial proliferation (**c**)

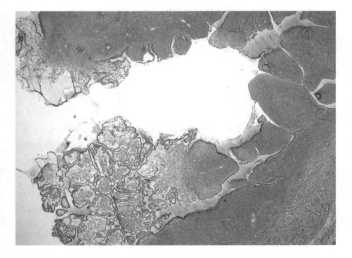

Fig. 8.5 Serous cystadenofibroma with focal epithelial proliferation. Focal papillary epithelial proliferation is seen on low magnification in the left lower portion of this serous cystadenofibroma, comprising less than 10 % of the entire epithelial lining

Serous Borderline Tumor (SBT)/Atypical Proliferative Serous Tumor (APST)

- Clinical features
  - Mean patient age is 42 years [6].
  - Up to 55 % bilateral [7].
- Gross pathology
  - Typically cystic.
  - Can have a wide size range, although usually >5 cm [6].
  - Abundant friable papillary projections on the cyst lining (Fig. 8.6a).
  - Papillary projections may also be present on the ovarian surface.
  - Less commonly the entire tumor presents as a "cauliflower-like" surface mass without a cystic component (Fig. 8.6b).
  - Inking of ovarian surface (at least in the area where frozen sections are submitted from) is helpful in determining surface involvement.
  - Gross sampling should be focused on intracystic and surface papillary and solid areas, with multiple blocks if necessary.
- Microscopic features
  - Hierarchical branching papillae (Fig. 8.7a).
  - Epithelial proliferation in the form of stratification (multiple cell layers, rather than multiple layers of nuclei as seen in "pseudostratification" of benign tumors), budding, and tufting in at least 10 % of tumor (Fig. 8.7b, c).
  - Micropapillary or cribriform architectural pattern may be seen focally (<5 mm) [6].
  - Mild to moderate nuclear atypia with oval to round nuclei (Fig. 8.7d).
  - Nucleoli are usually inconspicuous, but occasionally may be prominent.
  - Low mitotic activity.
  - Ciliated, hobnail, and round eosinophilic cells are often present (Fig. 8.7e).
  - Psammomatous calcifications within the epithelium or stroma (see Fig. 8.7d)
    - Psammomatous calcifications are nonspecific; may also be seen in benign serous tumors, as well as low-grade and high-grade carcinomas
  - Microinvasion (<5 mm in greatest dimension) may be present: round eosinophilic cells (single cells or small clusters) in a desmoplastic stroma (Fig. 8.8).

- Differential diagnosis
  - Serous cystadenoma/cystadenofibroma
  - Serous cystadenoma with focal epithelial proliferation (<10 % of epithelial lining shows atypical proliferation) [4, 5]
  - Mucinous/seromucinous borderline tumor
  - SBT/APST micropapillary variant/noninvasive low-grade serous carcinoma
  - Low-grade serous carcinoma
  - High-grade serous carcinoma
- Diagnostic pitfalls/key intraoperative consultation issues
  - *Serous cystadenoma/cystadenofibroma* may mimic a SBT/APST due to pseudostratification (multiple layers of nuclei, as opposed to multiple layers of cells in true epithelial stratification of SBT/APST) or tangential sectioning of the epithelium. Cystadenoma/cystadenofibroma lacks cytological atypia and has oval or elongated nuclei, rather than the more commonly round nuclei of SBT/APST.
  - *Serous cystadenoma/adenofibroma with focal atypical epithelial proliferation:* It may be difficult to estimate the percentage of epithelial proliferation within a cystic serous tumor based on limited number of frozen sections. If based on both gross and microscopic examination—the epithelial proliferation is relatively focal and there is a chance that it may fall under 10 % after thorough sampling on permanent sections, a conservative frozen section interpretation of "serous cystadenoma with focal epithelial proliferation" may be reported, especially in young patients. The surgeon should be advised that additional sampling might increase the percentage of involvement and result in an upgrade to SBT/APST on the final diagnosis.
  - Definitive diagnosis of *microinvasion or microinvasive carcinoma* in SBT/APST on the frozen sections is typically not necessary for clinical management; frozen section diagnosis of "serous borderline tumor" or "at least serous borderline tumor" is appropriate. Presence of microinvasion does not have a significant impact on survival [5, 8].
  - SBTs/APSTs may display more nuclear irregularity, pleomorphism, and prominent nucleoli, raising the differential of low-grade serous carcinoma. Stromal invasion measuring >5 mm should be classified as invasive low-grade serous carcinoma.
  - The distinction between SBT/APST and *noninvasive (SBT/APST micropapillary variant) or invasive*

low-grade serous carcinoma is typically not crucial at the time of frozen section; frozen section diagnosis of "at least serous borderline tumor" or "serous borderline tumor with micropapillary features" is appropriate.

– *High-grade serous carcinomas (HGSC)* may have a predominantly papillary architecture mimicking SBT/APST on low magnification. However on higher magnification HGSC shows marked nuclear pleomorphism, numerous mitotic figures and often necrosis, none of which are features of SBT/APST. Identification of the more common solid or glandular patterns (with "slit-like" configurations) is also helpful in making the diagnosis of HGSC, and ruling out SBT/APST. HGSC requires complete surgical staging, in contrast to the optional conservative—fertility-preserving—surgery for SBT/APST, which typically affects a younger patient group.

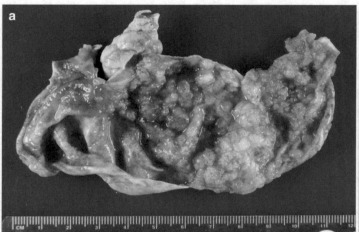 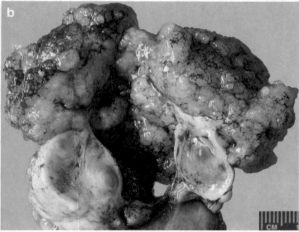

Fig. 8.6 Serous borderline tumor (SBT)/atypical proliferative serous tumor (APST). The cut surface shows a unilocular cyst with abundant, friable tan-pink intraluminal papillary projections (**a**). Occasionally SBT/APST presents as a solid surface growth with a "cauliflower-like" gross appearance (**b**)

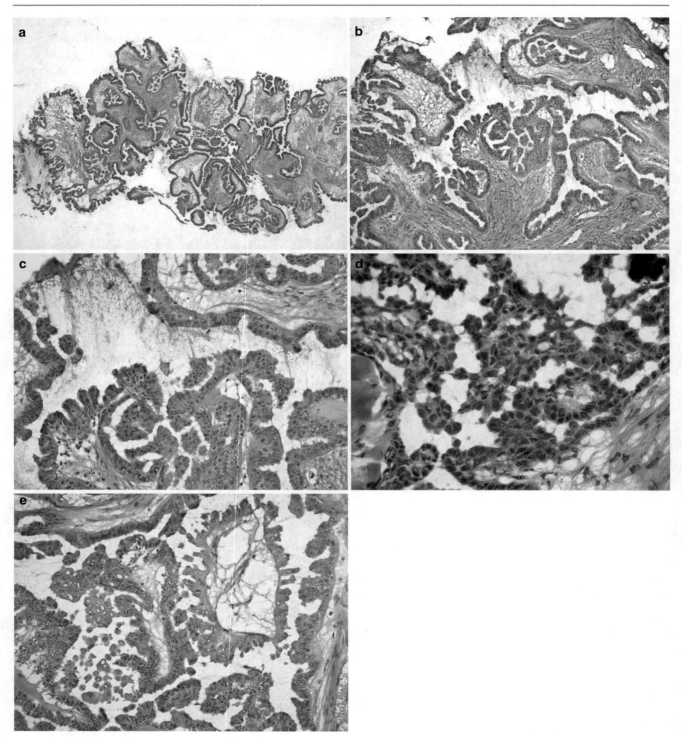

Fig. 8.7 Microscopic features of SBT/APST. Note the hierarchical branching papillae (**a**, **b**) and epithelial proliferation with tufting (**b**, **c**). The tumor cell nuclei are mildly atypical with occasional conspicuous nucleoli (**d**). Psammoma bodies are often present (**d**, *right upper corner*). Hobnail cells and round, eosinophilic cells are also common (**e**)

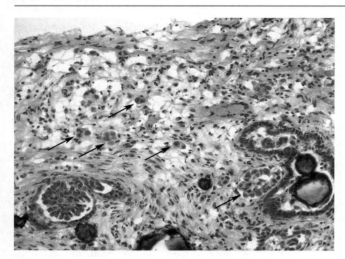

Fig. 8.8 Microinvasion in SBT/APST. Note the small clusters of round, eosinophilic tumor cells in a desmoplastic stroma (*arrows*). Numerous psammoma bodies are also seen

SBT/APST Micropapillary Variant/Noninvasive Low-Grade Serous Carcinoma

- Clinical and gross features
  - Similar to SBT/APST
  - May be more often bilateral [9]
- Microscopic features
  - Non-hierarchical branching micropapillary or cribriform architecture—in at least one confluent area measuring 5 mm [6] (Fig. 8.9).
  - Micropapillae are at least five times taller than wide with scant or no fibrovascular cores.
    - Micropapillae are smoothly contoured.
  - Round or polygonal, uniform nuclei; slightly more nuclear atypia and higher nuclear to cytoplasmic (N/C) ratio than SBT/APST.
  - Ciliated cells are absent.
  - Low mitotic activity (but may be slightly higher than SBT/APST).
- Differential diagnosis
  - SBT/APST with extensive tufting and eosinophilic metaplasia
  - SBT/APST with focal micropapillary features (<5 mm)
  - Low-grade serous carcinoma, invasive
  - High-grade serous carcinoma

- Diagnostic pitfalls/key intraoperative consultation issues
  - Prognostic significance of *micropapillary variant of SBT (noninvasive low-grade serous carcinoma)* is controversial, has been reported to be clinically more aggressive than SBT/APST in some studies [6, 10, 11].
    - May be more frequently associated with surface involvement and invasive implants [7, 9–13].
  - The distinction between SBT/APST and *SBT micropapillary variant (noninvasive low-grade serous carcinoma)* may not be crucial at the time of frozen section depending on the patient's age and fertility status. Frozen section diagnosis of "serous borderline tumor," "at least serous borderline tumor" or "serous borderline tumor with micropapillary features" may be communicated.
    - Fertility-sparing surgery may be performed in younger patients.
  - *High-grade serous carcinoma* (HGSC) shows marked nuclear pleomorphism, numerous mitotic figures, and often necrosis, none of which are features of SBT/APST. One should be very cautious when considering HGSC in the reproductive age group, as it is a highly aggressive tumor, requiring complete surgical staging.

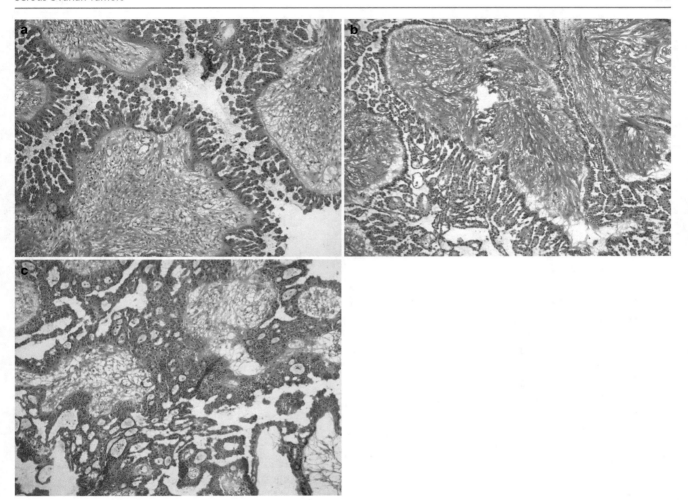

Fig. 8.9 SBT/APST—micropapillary variant/noninvasive low-grade serous carcinoma. Note the non-hierarchical branching of long, slender micropapillae (at least 5 times longer than wide) (**a**, **b**) or cribriform architecture (**c**)

Low-Grade Serous Carcinoma (LGSC), Invasive

- Clinical features
  - Rare, less than 5 % of all serous carcinomas
  - Occurs in younger patients than high-grade serous carcinoma (HGSC) [9, 14]
  - Commonly advanced stage at the time of presentation
  - Often bilateral
- Gross pathology
  - Solid or partially cystic mass with papillary growth (Fig. 8.10).
  - Cut surface may appear gritty, due to calcifications.
  - Necrosis is practically absent.
  - Inking of ovarian surface (at least in the area where frozen sections are submitted from) is helpful in determining surface involvement.
  - Gross sampling for frozen section should be focused on solid and papillary areas, with multiple blocks if necessary.
- Microscopic features (Fig. 8.11)
  - Irregular small nests, micro- or macro-papillae, or single cells.
  - Destructive stromal invasion.
  - Relatively uniform nuclei with mild to moderate atypia.
    - Nuclear pleomorphism is usually slightly increased compared to SBT/APST.
    - Prominent nucleoli may be seen.
  - Low mitotic activity (<12 mitoses/10 high-power field).

- Psammomatous calcifications may be abundant ("psammocarcinoma").
- Necrosis is practically absent.
- Differential diagnosis
  - SBT/APST
  - SBT/APST—micropapillary variant/noninvasive low-grade serous carcinoma
  - High-grade serous carcinoma
  - Malignant mesothelioma (see Chap. 13)
- Diagnostic pitfalls/key intraoperative consultation issues
  - The distinction between *LGSC and SBT/APST* may not be crucial at the time of frozen section. Requesting additional biopsies from any extraovarian lesions or implants—if detected by the surgeon—may be helpful in identifying destructive stromal invasion and establishing the diagnosis of LGSC.
    - Potential role of fertility-preserving surgery in this tumor group is not well documented.
    - Prognosis is stage dependent; 5-year survival rates for advanced stage LGSC have been reported between 40 and 85 % [15, 16].
  - Although *high-grade serous carcinoma (HGSC)* may show focal or predominant papillary architecture mimicking LGSC, presence of other types of growth patterns—solid and glandular with slit-like spaces—is a helpful diagnostic clue for HGSC. In addition, HGSC shows marked nuclear pleomorphism and numerous mitotic figures. Necrosis is also common in HGSC, while it is practically absent in LGSC.

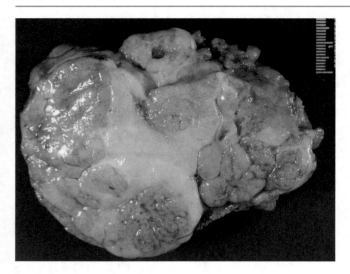

Fig. 8.10 Low-grade serous carcinoma showing a predominantly solid, tan-pink cut surface

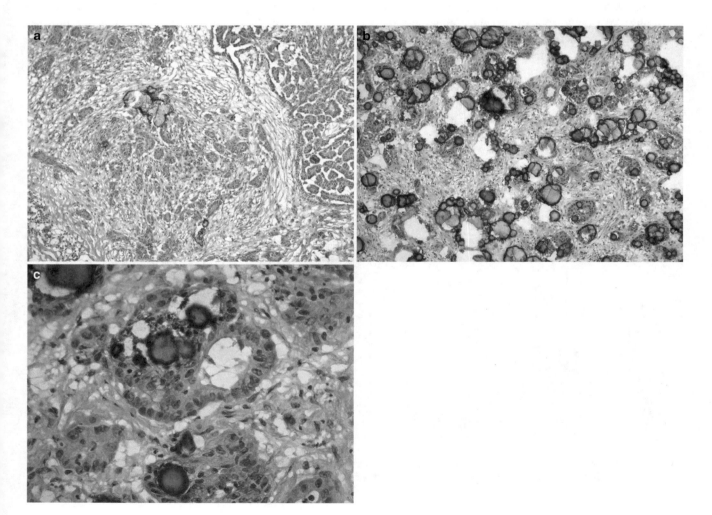

Fig. 8.11 Low-grade serous carcinoma. The tumor cells infiltrate the stroma forming irregular nests or micropapillae with abundant psammoma bodies (**a, b**). Mild to moderate nuclear atypia with conspicuous nucleoli is seen (**c**)

Peritoneal Implants of SBT/APST (Noninvasive)

- Microscopic features
  - Hierarchical branching papillae or detached cell clusters, histologically similar to ovarian SBT/APST (epithelial-type noninvasive implants) (Fig. 8.12).
  - Desmoplastic noninvasive implants are associated with significant desmoplastic reaction without infiltrative growth.
- Differential diagnosis
  - Endosalpingiosis
  - Endometriosis
  - Low-grade serous carcinoma (LGSC) (previously termed "invasive implants") [6]
  - Well-differentiated papillary mesothelioma [see Chap. 13]
  - Malignant mesothelioma, with papillary pattern [see Chap. 13]
- Diagnostic pitfalls/key intraoperative consultation issues
  - *Endosalpingiosis* consists of simple benign glands lined by a single layer of columnar, tubal-type epithelium. No epithelial proliferation, tufting, or atypia is seen. Calcifications may be present.
  - *Low-grade serous carcinoma (LGSC)* (previously termed "invasive implants") shows destructive stromal invasion and generally increased nuclear atypia, compared to (noninvasive) implants of SBT/APST.
    - Distinction between LGSC and noninvasive implants of SBT/APST may not be crucial at the time of frozen section—especially in the older age group—the differential diagnosis may be communicated to the surgeon.
    - Sampling of additional peritoneal lesions or the ovary for frozen section may be helpful if more specific classification is desired.
  - *Well-differentiated papillary mesothelioma* [see also Chap. 13] is a benign entity usually presenting as a small (<2 cm), incidental solitary papillary lesion, without any nuclear atypia or mitotic activity. Clinical correlation with the surgeon regarding the intraoperative findings is important. Extensive or multifocal lesions should raise concern for malignant mesothelioma or other entities in the differential (e.g., serous tumors/implants). Surgical sampling of additional lesions might be helpful.
  - *Malignant mesothelioma* [see Chap. 13] can often have a *papillary pattern*, but it usually coexists with other architectural patters (tubular and solid) that are not typical features of serous implants. The stroma may show prominent myxoid change. Presence of intracytoplasmic and extracellular mucoid material may be helpful in ruling out a serous tumor.
  - HGSC shows marked nuclear pleomorphism and numerous mitotic figures, in contrast to the mild to moderate nuclear atypia and low mitotic activity of SBT/APST implants.
  - *Psammomatous calcifications with no viable tumor cells* should be communicated to the surgeon as such. Additional sampling of any clinically suspicious mass lesions may be helpful to reveal epithelial tumor cells.

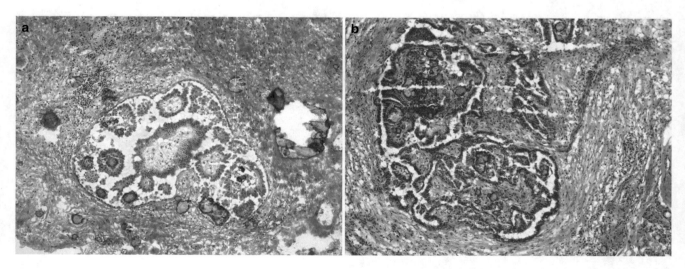

Fig. 8.12 Peritoneal implants of SBT/APST (**a, b**). Noninvasive epithelial implants of SBT/APST show hierarchical branching of atypical papillary epithelial proliferation without stromal invasion. Psammomatous calcifications are often present

Lymph Node Involvement by Serous Tumors

- Microscopic features
  - Epithelial cells forming papillary or glandular structures within the lymph node, histologically similar to the primary ovarian SBT/APST or LGSC (Fig. 8.13).
    - Papillary architecture with proliferation and tufting.
    - Cytological atypia.
    - Psammomatous calcifications are common.
  - Epithelial cells—single or in small clusters—with nuclear atypia and abundant eosinophilic cytoplasm.
- Differential diagnosis
  - Endosalpingiosis
  - Endometriosis
  - Benign mesothelial inclusions
  - Metastatic carcinoma
    - HGSC
    - Other gynecologic or non-gynecologic primaries
- Diagnostic pitfalls/key intraoperative consultation issues
  - *Endosalpingiosis* consists of simple benign glands lined by a single layer of columnar, tubal-type epithelium. No epithelial proliferation, tufting, or atypia is seen. Calcifications may be present (Fig. 8.14).
    - May be located in the lymph node capsule or within the parenchyma
  - Distinction between metastatic carcinoma and involvement by SBT/APST or LGSC may be difficult on frozen section if the tumor focus is small; additional tissue samples and comparison with the primary (ovarian) lesion may be helpful.
    - Clinical history of previous gynecologic and non-gynecologic primaries and morphologic comparison with the patient's previous material (if available) may offer important diagnostic clues

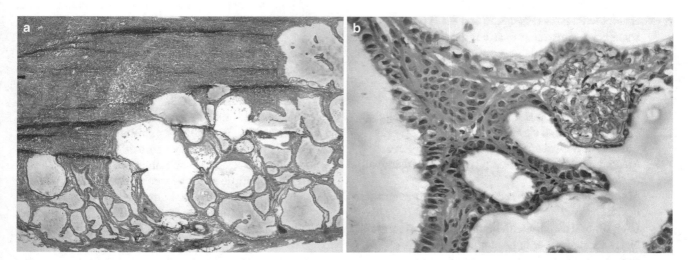

Fig. 8.13 Lymph node involvement by SBT/APST. Note the papillary epithelial clusters of eosinophilic epithelial cells (**a**) with noticeable nuclear atypia (**b**)

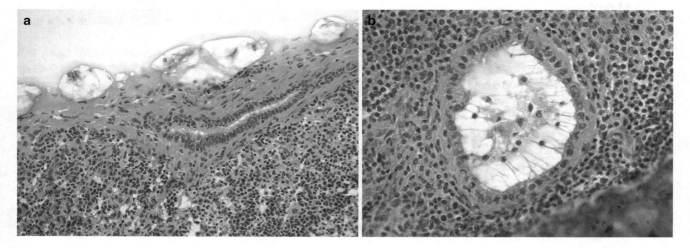

Fig. 8.14 Endosalpingiosis in lymph nodes (**a**, **b**). Note simple, small glands lined by a single layer of columnar, tubal-type epithelium without epithelial proliferation, tufting, or atypia

High-Grade Serous Carcinoma (HGSC)

- Clinical features
  - Most common type of ovarian carcinoma
  - Mean patient age: late 50s to early 60s
  - Over 90 % of cases present at an advanced stage
  - Majority of cases are bilateral
- Gross pathology (Fig. 8.15)
  - Size ranges from <1 to 20 cm.
  - May be entirely solid or partially cystic with a solid component.
  - Ovarian surface is frequently irregular, grossly involved by tumor.
  - Cut surface often shows hemorrhage and necrosis.
  - May show intracystic papillary growth pattern.
  - Sampling of one or two blocks from the solid or papillary viable tumor areas is usually sufficient for frozen section.
    - Sampling of grossly obvious foci of necrosis and hemorrhage should be avoided.
- Microscopic features (Figs. 8.16 and 8.17)
  - Usually an admixture of various morphologic patterns: solid, complex glandular with slit-like spaces, cribriform, and papillary.
    - Rarely may show predominant or exclusive papillary pattern.
    - Undulating bands of epithelial cells resembling transitional cell carcinoma may be seen.
  - Stromal desmoplastic response may be present.
  - Marked nuclear atypia with prominent, eosinophilic nucleoli.
  - Multinucleated tumor cells and bizarre pleomorphic nuclei.
  - High mitotic activity with atypical mitotic figures.
  - Necrosis in small or large confluent foci.
  - Psammomatous calcifications are common.
  - Cytoplasmic vacuolization may be present.
- Differential diagnosis
  - SBT/APST
  - LGSC
  - Other Mullerian (gynecologic) carcinomas:
    - Endometrioid adenocarcinoma, clear cell carcinoma, malignant Brenner tumor, carcinosarcoma (malignant mixed Mullerian tumor)
  - Malignant germ cell tumors (MGCT)
  - Metastatic tumors (gastrointestinal, breast)
  - Malignant mesothelioma, with papillary pattern
- Diagnostic pitfalls/key intraoperative consultation issues
  - Two most important issues regarding the intraoperative diagnosis:
    - Recognize the tumor as a *high-grade epithelial* malignancy.
    - *Rule out metastasis* from other—non-gynecologic—primaries.

- Rarely HGSC may show a predominant papillary growth pattern without obvious stromal invasion, mimicking SBT/APST. However, unlike SBT/APST, HGSC displays marked nuclear atypia and high mitotic activity.
- While the architectural features of HGSC may mimic LGSC on low-power examination, higher magnification shows the obvious differences in nuclear atypia and mitotic index.
- The distinction between HGSC and other high-grade carcinomas of Mullerian origin (e.g., endometrioid and clear cell carcinoma, malignant Brenner tumor) is usually not critical on intraoperative sections. Frozen section diagnosis can be communicated to the surgeon as "high-grade carcinoma, consistent with Mullerian primary."
- HGSC arising from the fallopian tube or peritoneum is morphologically identical to HGSC of ovary—distinction between these primary sites is not critical for intraoperative management.
- Metastatic endometrial serous carcinoma also shares the morphologic features of ovarian HGSC, but it is usually not crucial for intraoperative management to distinguish between the two primaries.
- *Mucinous tumors:* HGSC may show intracytoplasmic vacuoles raising the possibility of mucinous differentiation. In addition, intraluminal necrosis can mimic the type of "dirty necrosis" often seen in metastatic colon adenocarcinomas. It is helpful to find areas (multiple sections may be submitted if necessary) with papillary and slit-like glandular architecture, psammomatous calcifications, and bizarre, markedly atypical nuclei to establish the diagnosis of HGSC.
- MGCTs typically present at a much younger age (children or young adults), than HGSC.
- Metastatic tumors (gastrointestinal and breast).
  - Clinical history and morphologic comparison of patient's previous material (if available) are most helpful.
  - Papillary and slit-like glandular architecture and psammomatous calcifications, although not entirely specific for HGSC, are less often seen in metastatic tumors of the ovary.
- Malignant mesothelioma, with papillary pattern [see Chap. 13].
  - Malignant mesothelioma can closely mimic HGSC. However, it generally has more uniform tumor cells, with lesser degree of nuclear atypia (mild to moderate), and the mitotic activity is not as high as that of HGSC. Psammomatous calcifications may be seen in both tumors.

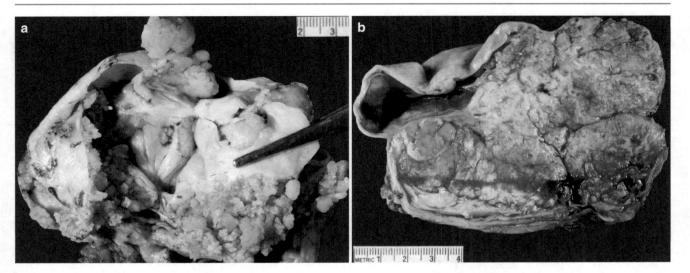

Fig. 8.15 High-grade serous carcinoma on gross examination may be a partially cystic mass lesion with intracystic papillary growth (**a**) or predominantly solid with areas of necrosis and hemorrhage (**b**)

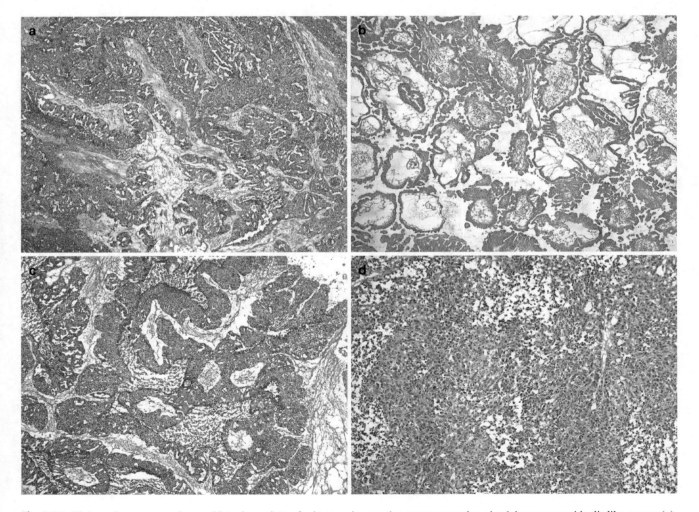

Fig. 8.16 High-grade serous carcinoma. Note the variety of microscopic growth patterns: complex glandular pattern with slit-like spaces (**a**), papillary (**b**), undulating epithelial cell "ribbons" (**c**), and solid sheets of tumor cells (**d**)

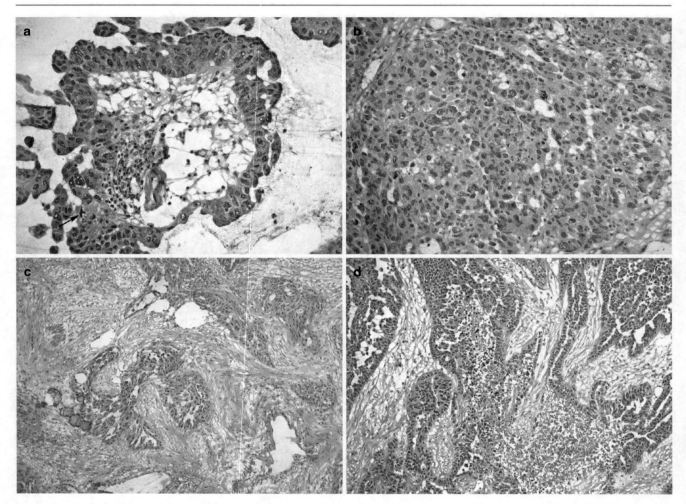

Fig. 8.17 High-grade serous carcinoma, high magnification. Marked nuclear atypia, brisk mitotic activity with atypical mitoses (**a**, *arrow*; **b**), desmoplastic reaction (**c**), and necrosis (**d**) are characteristic

Mucinous Ovarian Tumors

Mucinous Cystadenoma

- Clinical features
  - Most common ovarian mucinous tumor
  - Wide patient age range; mean 50 years [6]
  - Commonly presents with pelvic pain and/or mass
  - Typically unilateral (95 %)
- Gross pathology (Fig. 8.18)
  - Size may vary from 1 to >30 cm (mean 10 cm).
  - Smooth ovarian surface.
  - Cystic, uni- or multilocular cut surface.
    - Rarely may be entirely or partially solid—mucinous adenofibroma or due to associated Brenner tumor or mature teratoma
  - Cyst contents are viscous, glistening mucoid material.
    - Appearance of cyst contents may be helpful to form an initial impression, but only the type of epithelial lining is used in the final histological classification
  - Mucinous tumors often show significant morphologic heterogeneity; therefore, multiple areas should be sampled for frozen section for adequate assessment.
- Microscopic features (Figs. 8.19, 8.20, and 8.21)
  - Epithelial lining is simple, nonstratified, most commonly resembling *gastric foveolar-type or intestinal-type* epithelium with goblet cells.
  - Epithelium may be undulating or may form filiform papillae with fibrovascular cores.
  - Nuclei are basally located, small, uniform without significant atypia.
  - Abundant slightly basophilic cytoplasm.
  - Low nuclear to cytoplasmic ratio.
  - Mitotic figures are rare or absent.
  - Invaginations of cyst lining into ovarian stroma are not uncommon and should not be mistaken for epithelial complexity or invasion.
  - "Spillage" of acellular mucin into the ovarian stroma may be seen ("pseudomyxoma ovarii") and may be associated with histiocytic response.
  - Less commonly *seromucinous* (previously also termed endocervical-type or Mullerian-type) lining may be seen with variable admixture of serous and mucinous (endocervical-type) epithelial cells.
    - Seromucinous tumors are often associated with endometriosis.
  - Intestinal-type mucinous cystadenomas may be associated with Brenner tumor or mature teratoma.

- Differential diagnosis
  - Other benign cystic entities—serous cystadenoma, follicular cyst, simple cyst, and endometriotic cyst
  - Mucinous cystadenoma with focal epithelial proliferation/atypia (<10 % of tumor)
  - Mucinous borderline tumor (MBT)/atypical proliferative mucinous tumor (APMT)
    - Epithelial proliferation and atypia is present in >10 % of the tumor.
  - Metastatic mucinous carcinomas
- Diagnostic pitfalls/key intraoperative consultation issues
  - Distinction between benign mucinous cystadenoma and other benign cysts should be made on frozen section if possible. If the frozen section diagnosis indicates a mucinous ovarian tumor (even benign mucinous cystadenoma), the surgeon may survey the appendix intraoperatively and may elect to perform appendectomy to rule out the possibility of an appendiceal primary.
  - Distinction between intestinal and seromucinous subtypes of mucinous cystadenoma is not critical on frozen sections.
  - Tangential sectioning of epithelium or invaginations of cyst lining into ovarian stroma may mimic epithelial proliferation.
  - *Mucinous cystadenoma with focal proliferation and atypia* (<10 % of epithelial lining shows proliferation or atypia) [5, 17].
    - Does not meet criteria for MBT/APMT; no staging surgery is necessary.
    - Additional frozen section sampling may be helpful.
    - Surgeon may be advised that additional sampling for permanent sections could increase the percentage of atypical proliferation, especially in large tumors.
  - Metastatic mucinous carcinoma.
    - Rarely metastatic mucinous tumors from appendiceal, pancreatobiliary, and endocervical primaries can mimic benign mucinous ovarian cystadenoma ("maturation phenomenon"), especially on limited frozen section sampling
    - Bilaterality, small size (<10 cm) and ovarian surface involvement strongly favor metastasis [18, 19]
    - The surgeon should be inquired about:
      - Patient's clinical history of prior malignancies
      - Any concurrent mass lesions/imaging findings
      - Intraoperative findings

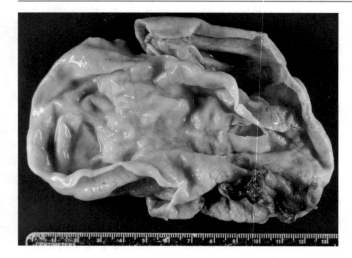

Fig. 8.18 Mucinous cystadenoma often appears as a uni- or multiloculated cyst on gross examination

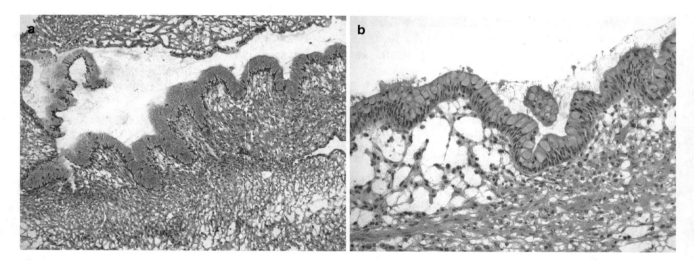

Fig. 8.19 Mucinous cystadenoma is lined by a single layer of nonstratified mucinous epithelium, resembling gastric foveolar-type (**a**) or intestinal-type epithelium with goblet cells (**b**)

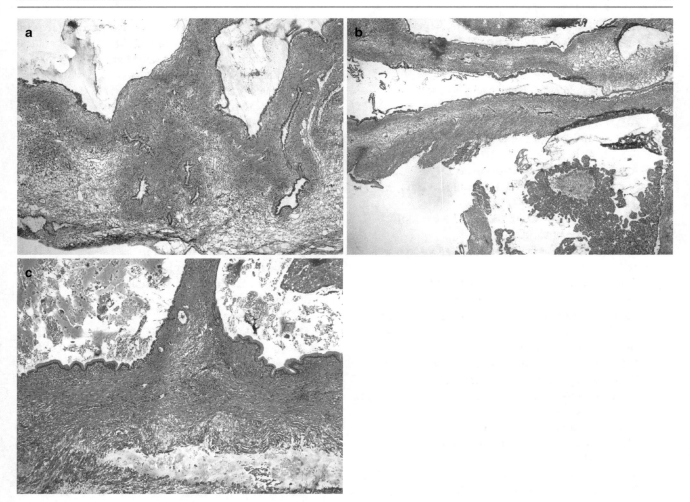

Fig. 8.20 Mucinous cystadenoma. The tumor may show invaginations of the cyst lining and have an adenofibromatous appearance (**a**). Focal epithelial proliferation comprising less than 10 % of tumor may also be seen (**b**, *right lower corner*). Acellular mucin in the ovarian stroma (pseudomyxoma ovarii) can be associated with mucinous cystadenoma (**c**, *lower portion of image*)

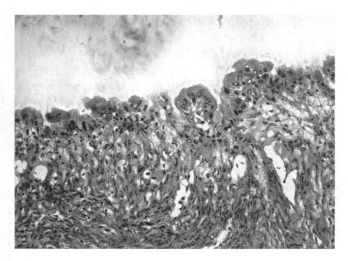

Fig. 8.21 Seromucinous cystadenoma (Mullerian-type mucinous cystadenoma). Note the admixture of serous (eosinophilic) and mucinous (endocervical-type) epithelial cells

Mucinous Borderline Tumor (MBT)/Atypical Proliferative Mucinous Tumor (APMT)

- Clinical features
  - Wide age range with a mean age in 40s.
  - Almost always unilateral (*intestinal-type* MBT/APMT).
    - *Seromucinous* MBT/APMT may be bilateral in up to 40 % of cases.
  - Almost always limited to the ovary.
  - Excellent prognosis, >99 % overall survival [6].
- Gross pathology (Fig. 8.22)
  - Size may be up to 50 cm, mean: 21.5 cm [20].
  - Smooth external surface.
  - Multiloculated, cystic cut surface and viscous mucoid cyst contents.
  - Solid component is uncommon and should raise concern for carcinoma or mural nodule.
  - Inking of ovarian surface (at least in the area where frozen sections are submitted from) is helpful in determining surface involvement.
  - Mucinous tumors often show significant morphologic heterogeneity; therefore, multiple areas—up to 3–4 tissue blocks—should be sampled to adequately assess the tumor on frozen section.
- Microscopic features (Fig. 8.23)
  - Most commonly *gastrointestinal-type* epithelium with goblet cells.
  - Epithelial proliferation (involving >10 % of epithelial lining) with stratification, tufting, intraglandular villous or filiform papillary growth and fusion of papillae.
  - Mild to moderate nuclear atypia.
    - Increased nuclear to cytoplasmic ratio, hyperchromasia, and decreased cytoplasmic mucin content.
  - Mitotic activity is variable and may be numerous.
  - Acellular mucin pools within the ovarian stroma may be seen ("pseudomyxoma ovarii").
  - Intraluminal necrotic debris may be present.
  - No stromal invasion.
  - May rarely be associated with/arising within a mature teratoma (dermoid cyst).
  - *Seromucinous-type* (endocervical- or Mullerian-type) lining is much less common (~15 % of all MBT/APMT) (Fig. 8.24).
    - Variable admixture of mucinous (endocervical-type), serous, eosinophilic, and rarely endometrioid epithelial cell proliferation.

- Architecture resembles serous borderline/atypical proliferative tumor (SBT/APST)—hierarchical branching of complex papillae and tufting.
- Mild to moderate nuclear atypia.
- Stroma often shows neutrophilic infiltration.
- Psammomatous calcifications may be present.
- May be associated with endometriosis.
- No goblet cells are seen.
  - MBT/APMT with intraepithelial carcinoma
    - Foci with marked nuclear atypia alone or in combination with architectural complexity (cribriform pattern or epithelial stratification).
    - No stromal invasion.
  - MBT/APMT with microinvasion
    - Stromal invasion of <5 mm
    - Small tumor nests, glands, or single cells, which may be "floating" in extracellular mucin
- Differential diagnosis
  - Mucinous cystadenoma
  - Mucinous cystadenoma with focal epithelial proliferation/atypia (<10 % of epithelial lining shows proliferation and atypia)
  - SBT/APST (especially for seromucinous-type MBT/APMT)
  - Primary ovarian mucinous carcinoma
  - Metastatic mucinous carcinomas
- Diagnostic pitfalls/key intraoperative consultation issues
  - Mucinous ovarian tumors are often heterogeneous, showing morphologic continuum from benign to borderline to malignant areas within the same tumor.
    - Adequate sampling is key for intraoperative frozen section diagnosis of MBT/APMT.
  - The prognosis of MBT/APMT is excellent; fertility-sparing surgery may be an option for younger patients [17, 21, 22].
  - Seromucinous borderline tumor resembles SBT/APST especially on low magnification; identification of mucinous cells may be difficult due to frozen section artifact.
    - Distinction between the two entities has no impact on surgical management at the time of frozen section.
  - MBT/APMT with intraepithelial carcinoma or microinvasion.

- Prognosis and intraoperative surgical management implications are similar to MBT/APMT [17, 21, 23, 24].
- Definitive diagnosis of *intraepithelial carcinoma or microinvasion* in MBT/APMT on the frozen sections is typically not necessary for intraoperative management; frozen section diagnosis of "mucinous borderline tumor" is adequate.
- Primary ovarian mucinous carcinoma.
  - Confluent (expansile) or infiltrative growth (>5 mm) and complex architectural patterns—cribriform or serpiginous—should raise concern for mucinous carcinoma.
  - Presence of necrosis alone is not a reliable histological feature to separate MBT/APMT from mucinous carcinoma.
  - Distinction between MBT/APMT and ovarian mucinous carcinoma with expansile-type invasion may be difficult; frozen section diagnosis of "at least mucinous borderline tumor" can be communicated.

- Metastatic mucinous carcinoma.
  - Metastatic mucinous tumors—especially from appendiceal, pancreatobiliary, and colorectal primaries—can closely mimic intestinal-type MBT/APMT.
  - Bilaterality, small size (<10 cm) and ovarian surface involvement strongly favor metastasis [18, 19].
    - Intestinal-type MBT/APMT is almost always unilateral.
  - The surgeon should be inquired about:
    - Patient's clinical history of prior malignancies.
    - Any concurrent mass lesions/imaging findings.
    - Intraoperative findings.
  - Intraoperative surgical assessment of the appendix and intestines should be recommended.
  - Additional frozen sections—from the ovarian tumor or from any additional lesions found intraoperatively—may be helpful.

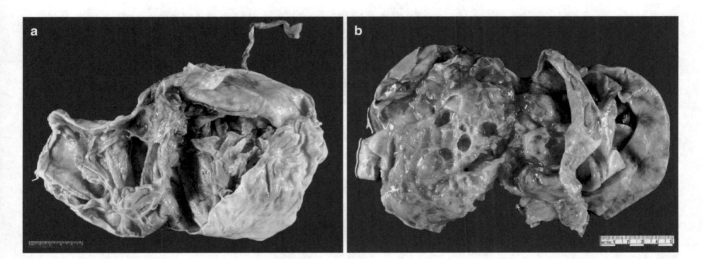

Fig. 8.22 Mucinous borderline tumor (MBT)/atypical proliferative mucinous tumor (APMT) typically shows a multiloculated cystic cut surface with viscous/mucinous cyst contents (**a**, **b**)

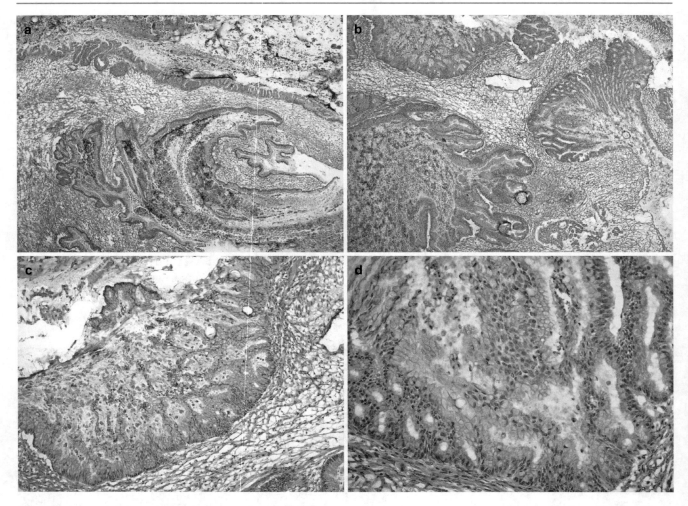

Fig. 8.23 MBT/APMT. Note the proliferation of intestinal-type epithelium in the form of complex branching glandular structures and intraglandular filiform papillae (**a**, **b**). Fusion of papillae and intralumi-nal necrotic debris are characteristic (**c**). Mild to moderate nuclear atypia with increased nuclear to cytoplasmic ratio is apparent (**d**)

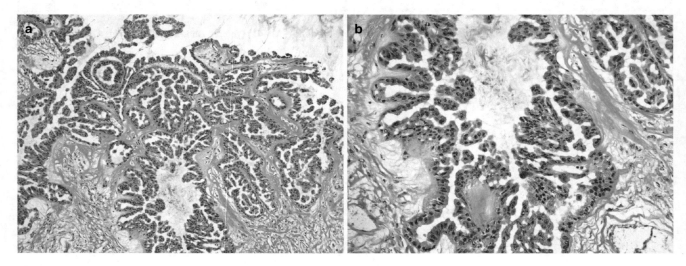

Fig. 8.24 Seromucinous (Mullerian-type) borderline tumor/atypical proliferative seromucinous tumor. Note the hierarchical branching papillae and tufting, resembling SBT/APST (**a**) and admixture of serous, eosinophilic, and mucinous cells with mild cytological atypia (**b**)

Mucinous Carcinoma

- Clinical features
  - Rare histological subtype, only 2–4 % of ovarian carcinomas.
  - Mean patient age at presentation is 45 years.
  - Most often presents with abdominal mass/pain.
  - Usually confined to the ovary at the time of presentation.
  - Most often unilateral.
- Gross pathology (Fig. 8.25)
  - Large unilateral mass, typically >10 cm (mean: 18–22 cm).
  - Complex, multicystic cut surface with solid areas.
  - Necrosis and hemorrhage may be present.
  - Inking of ovarian surface (in the area where frozen sections are submitted from) is helpful in determining surface involvement.
  - Sampling should focus on solid areas and areas near identifiable necrotic tumor.
  - Multiple tissue blocks may be necessary for adequate frozen section assessment due to morphologic heterogeneity.
- Microscopic features (Fig. 8.26)
  - Two patterns of invasion (>5 mm in size):
    - Confluent or expansile type with labyrinthine, crowded glandular growth, and lack of intervening stroma.
    - Destructive invasion is less common, showing irregular, atypical glands, nests, and single cells infiltrating the stroma.
      - Desmoplastic stromal reaction may also be seen.
    - The two invasion patterns may coexist within the same tumor.
  - Moderate to marked nuclear atypia with increased nuclear to cytoplasmic ratio.
  - Most commonly intestinal type with abundant goblet cells.
  - Abundant intraluminal necrotic debris is often present.
  - Mitotic activity is usually high.
  - Tumor heterogeneity may be significant with areas resembling MBT/APMT or mucinous cystadenoma.
  - May rarely be associated with/arising within a mature teratoma (dermoid cyst).
- Differential diagnosis
  - MBT/APMT

- Other primary ovarian carcinomas
  - Endometrioid adenocarcinoma
  - High-grade serous carcinoma
- Metastatic adenocarcinomas
  - Especially gastrointestinal (appendiceal, colorectal, and pancreatobiliary)
- Diagnostic pitfalls/key intraoperative consultation issues
  - Most important decision at the time of intraoperative frozen section is to rule out a metastatic mucinous adenocarcinoma.
    - Surgical staging is performed for ovarian primary, but not for metastatic carcinomas.
  - Tumor heterogeneity
    - Adequate sampling is key for intraoperative frozen section diagnosis of mucinous ovarian tumors.
    - Benign- or borderline-appearing foci may be present within the same tumor.
  - Bilaterality and small size (<10 cm) favor metastasis over primary ovarian mucinous carcinoma [18, 19] (Table 8.1).
  - Presence of a teratomatous component favors ovarian primary.
  - If the patient has a history of another primary, morphologic comparison with the patient's prior biopsies should be pursued.
  - The surgeon should be inquired about:
    - Patient's clinical history of prior malignancies (particularly gastrointestinal)
    - Any concurrent mass lesions/imaging findings
    - Intraoperative findings—mass lesions, pseudomyxoma peritonei, appearance of the other ovary, and the possibility of bilaterality (if only one ovary was sent for frozen section)
  - Intraoperative surgical assessment of the appendix and intestines should be recommended.
  - Distinction from other primary ovarian carcinomas:
    - Endometrioid adenocarcinoma
      - Squamous differentiation within the tumor is a characteristic feature of endometrioid histology, not seen in primary or metastatic mucinous carcinomas.
    - High-grade serous carcinoma (HGSC)
      - Papillary and slit-like glandular architecture, psammomatous calcifications, and bizarre, markedly atypical nuclei are characteristic of HGSC and not typically seen in mucinous carcinoma.
      - Rarely intracytoplasmic vacuoles and intraluminal necrosis may be seen in HGSC.

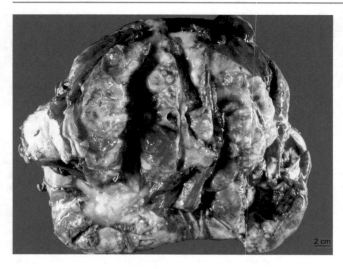

Fig. 8.25 Primary mucinous ovarian carcinoma. The tumor forms a large mass with a solid and cystic cut surface and extensive necrosis

Table 8.1 Differential diagnosis of mucinous carcinoma of the ovary

	Primary	Metastatic
Bilaterality	Rare	Common
Size >10 cm	Common	Uncommon
Surface involvement	Rare	Common
Growth pattern	Most often expansile; less commonly destructive invasion	Common destructive stromal invasion with desmoplasia
Lymphovascular invasion	Rare	Common
Ovarian hilus involvement	Rare	Common
Signet-ring cells	Rare (may be seen in teratoma-associated tumors)	May be present
Single cell infiltration	Rare	May be present
Pseudomyxoma peritonei	Rare (may be seen in teratoma-associated tumors)	May be present
Tumor morphologic heterogeneity	May be present	Common

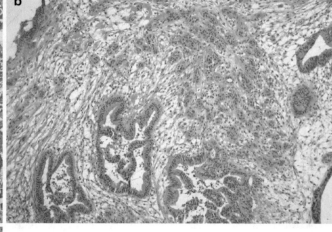

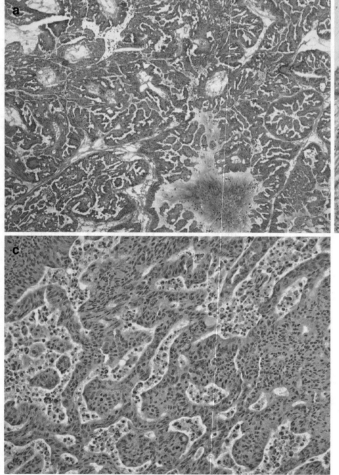

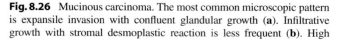

Fig. 8.26 Mucinous carcinoma. The most common microscopic pattern is expansile invasion with confluent glandular growth (**a**). Infiltrative growth with stromal desmoplastic reaction is less frequent (**b**). High magnification shows moderate to marked nuclear atypia with decreased amount of mucin-containing cytoplasm and scattered goblet cells (**c**). Also note the confluent glandular growth and intraluminal necrotic debris

Mucinous Ovarian Tumors with Mural Nodules

- Mural nodules may rarely be associated with benign, borderline/atypical proliferative, or malignant mucinous ovarian tumors
    - Reactive sarcomalike mural nodule
        - Heterogeneous cell population with multinucleated, "epulis-like" giant cells, spindle cells, and pleomorphic cells.
        - Hemorrhage, necrosis, and inflammation are common.
        - Typically occurs in younger patients and does not alter the prognosis of the associated mucinous tumor [25].
        - Does not warrant additional surgery if seen on intraoperative frozen section.

- Malignant mural nodules (Fig. 8.27)
    - Anaplastic carcinoma or sarcoma
        - Usually seen in older patients and indicates poor prognosis [26]
        - Large polygonal and spindle cells (anaplastic carcinoma) or spindle cells with a herringbone pattern (sarcoma)
        - Precise classification or designation as a mural nodule is not critical on frozen section: may be signed out as "high-grade carcinoma/sarcoma associated with mucinous ovarian tumor" or "carcinosarcoma" if associated with mucinous carcinoma, and the final classification can be deferred for permanent sections

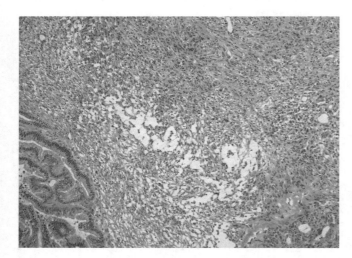

Fig. 8.27 Ovarian mucinous carcinoma with a malignant (sarcomatous) mural nodule. The mucinous carcinoma component is present in the left lower corner, with a sharp transition into the adjacent sarcoma on the right side of the image

Endometrioid Tumors

Endometrioid Adenofibroma

- Clinical features
  - Less common than serous adenofibroma.
  - Patients are usually peri- or postmenopausal.
  - Often associated with endometriosis in the same ovary or at other pelvic sites.
- Gross pathology
  - Most often unilateral.
  - Cut surface is typically solid; cystically dilated glands may be grossly visible.
- Microscopic features (Fig. 8.28)
  - Tubular or cystically dilated glands embedded in a prominent, fibrous stroma.
    - Stroma may be hypercellular.
  - Glands are lined by pseudostratified proliferative-type endometrial epithelium.
  - No significant glandular crowding, architectural complexity, or cytological atypia.

- Squamous morules may be seen.
  - Reactive stroma around squamous morules may mimic desmoplastic reaction.
- Differential diagnosis
  - Other benign ovarian tumors or conditions
    - Serous adenofibroma
    - Endometriosis
  - Endometrioid borderline tumor (atypical proliferative endometrioid tumor)
- Diagnostic pitfalls/key intraoperative consultation issues
  - Distinction from other benign entities (e.g., serous adenofibroma or endometriosis) is not crucial at the time of frozen section.
  - If the microscopic features are concerning but not definitive for a borderline/atypical proliferative endometrioid tumor, a conservative approach is recommended to avoid unnecessary staging surgery.
  - Endometrioid borderline tumors have an excellent prognosis [27].

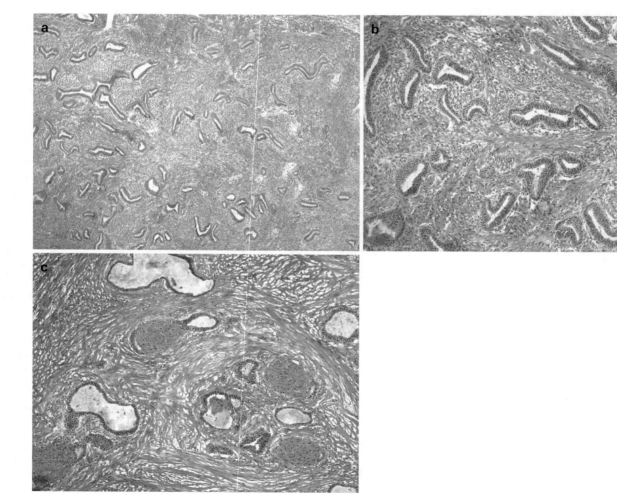

Fig. 8.28 Endometrioid adenofibroma. The histological features include endometrioid-type glands scattered in a prominent, fibrous ovarian stroma (**a**). There is no glandular crowding or architectural complexity and the pseudostratified endometrial epithelium lacks significant atypia (**b**). Squamous morule formation may be seen (**c**)

Endometrioid Borderline Tumor (EBT)/Atypical Proliferative Endometrioid Tumor (APET)

- Clinical features
  - Patients are usually peri- or postmenopausal.
- Gross pathology
  - Most often unilateral [28]
  - Predominantly solid cut surface, but may be focally cystic, or show a "spongelike" appearance (Fig. 8.29)
- Microscopic features (Fig. 8.30)
  - Glandular crowding and complex glandular architecture without confluent glandular growth pattern.
  - Glandular epithelium is pseudostratified, resembling proliferative-type endometrium.
  - Squamous metaplasia (squamous morules) is commonly seen.
  - Growth pattern may be adenofibromatous or intracystic.
  - Mild to moderate nuclear atypia.
  - Absence of stromal invasion.
  - *EBT/APET with intraepithelial carcinoma*
    - Severe cytological atypia, but no stromal invasion
  - *EBT/APET with microinvasion*
    - Confluent glandular growth or unequivocal stromal invasion of <5 mm in size (Fig. 8.31)
- Differential diagnosis
  - Endometrioid adenofibroma
  - Atypical endometriosis/endometriosis with cytological atypia or atypical hyperplasia (see Chap. 11)
  - Endometrioid adenocarcinoma
- Diagnostic pitfalls/key intraoperative consultation issues
  - Endometriosis may be associated with cytological atypia or atypical hyperplasia (especially polypoid endometriosis). Both types of "atypical endometrio-sis" are managed conservatively and are distinct from EBT/APET. However, they may be associated with more severe lesions—endometrioid or clear cell carcinoma—therefore, adequate sampling is of key importance.
  - The prognosis of EBT/APET is excellent [27, 28]; fertility-sparing surgery may be an option for younger patients.
    - Standard surgical management of EBT/APET is complete surgical staging.
  - Presence of *intraepithelial carcinoma* or *microinvasion* typically does not alter the surgical management; frozen section diagnosis of "endometrioid borderline tumor cannot rule out intraepithelial carcinoma/microinvasion" is appropriate.
    - Additional sampling on frozen section may be helpful in revealing a larger focus of unequivocal invasion.
  - *Squamous morular metaplasia* is commonly seen in both benign and borderline endometrioid tumors and should not be mistaken for solid growth pattern of an endometrioid adenocarcinoma.
    - Squamous morules in the center of irregular, branching glands of EBT/APET may result in a cribriform pattern, mimicking endometrioid adenocarcinoma.
  - Endometrioid adenocarcinoma.
    - Characterized by confluent glandular proliferation or destructive stromal invasion exceeding 5 mm in size
    - May arise in the background of EBT/APET or endometriosis—adequate sampling on frozen sections is crucial

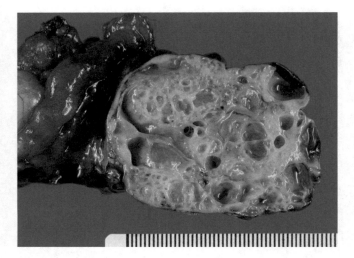

Fig. 8.29 Endometrioid borderline tumor (EBT)/atypical proliferative endometrioid tumor (APET) with a multicystic, "spongelike" cut surface

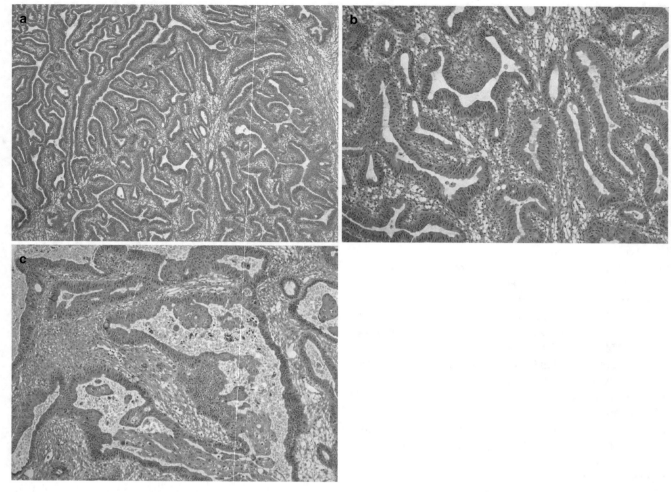

Fig. 8.30 EBT/APET on low magnification. The tumor shows crowded, complex glandular structures without confluent growth or stromal invasion (**a**). The glandular epithelium demonstrates mild to moderate nuclear atypia with some loss of polarity (**b**). Squamous metaplasia is common (**c**)

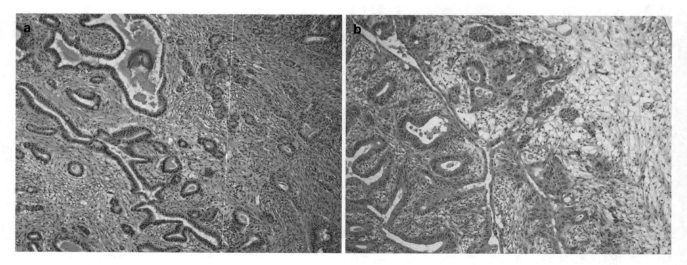

Fig. 8.31 EBT/PET with microinvasion. Note the small infiltrative component forming tubular or "sertoliform" structures (**a**) and desmoplastic stromal reaction around the invasive glands (**b**) on the right sides of the images

Endometrioid Adenocarcinoma

- Clinical features
  - Most commonly occurs during the 5th and 6th decades, and the mean patient age is 58 years [29]
  - May be asymptomatic or presents as a pelvic mass
- Gross pathology (Fig. 8.32)
  - Bilateral in up to 17 % of the cases [6].
  - Mean tumor size is 15 cm.
  - Cut surface may be solid or cystic with an intraluminal growth.
  - Hemorrhage and necrosis are common.
- Microscopic features (Figs. 8.33, 8.34, 8.35, and 8.36)
  - Two types of growth patterns:
    - Most common form is confluent, back-to-back glandular proliferation ("expansile invasion").
      - Markedly complex glandular architecture with cribriform, villoglandular, or papillary patterns, similar to endometrial endometrioid carcinomas.
      - Loss of intervening stroma.
    - Destructive stromal invasion is less common.
      - Irregular glands, cell clusters, or single cells infiltrating the stroma.
      - Stromal desmoplasia and inflammatory response may be seen.
  - Size (of either confluent growth or destructive stromal invasion) >5 mm.
    - <5 mm confluent/invasive focus within an EBT/APET is classified as microinvasion (see above).
  - Significant nuclear atypia.
  - Most tumors are well differentiated with open glandular lumens; less often show significant solid component.
  - Intraluminal necrotic debris or larger areas of necrosis may be present.
  - Tumor cells usually resemble endometrial glandular epithelium: pseudostratified, elongated nuclei and non-mucinous cytoplasm, although focal mucinous metaplasia may be seen.
  - *Squamous differentiation* is often present (in up to half of the cases) and is one of the most helpful features to confirm endometrioid histology.
  - Secretory changes are rare.
    - Cytoplasmic vacuoles, resembling early secretory phase endometrial epithelium.
    - Stromal luteinization
  - Sertoliform pattern may rarely be seen (see Fig. 8.36).
    - Small tubular glands or thin cords, resembling Sertoli cell tubules
- Differential diagnosis (Table 8.2)
  - EBT/APET
    - EBT/APET with intraepithelial carcinoma
    - EBT/APET with microinvasion (<5 mm)

- Other primary ovarian carcinomas
  - High-grade serous carcinoma
  - Mucinous carcinoma
- Sertoli cell and Sertoli-Leydig cell tumors (see Chap. 10)
- Germ cell tumors
  - Yolk sac tumor with a glandular (endometrioid-like) growth pattern
  - Struma ovarii
  - Carcinoid tumor and strumal carcinoid
- Metastatic tumors
  - Colorectal
  - Breast
  - Endocervical adenocarcinoma
  - Endometrial endometrioid adenocarcinoma
- Diagnostic pitfalls/key intraoperative consultation issues
  - EBT/APET in young patients may not require full staging; hence, adequate sampling (multiple blocks from solid and/or any necrotic areas) is important to rule out endometrioid adenocarcinoma.
    - Microinvasion (<5 mm) within an EBT/APET has not been shown to adversely affect patient outcome.
  - Precise distinction between primary ovarian serous and endometrioid adenocarcinoma is not essential for intraoperative management; however, mucinous differentiation—and the possibility of metastatic mucinous carcinoma—should be ruled out.
  - Most helpful features supporting endometrioid differentiation:
    - Squamous metaplasia/differentiation
    - Adjacent foci of EBT/APET or background endometriosis
  - Features in favor of *metastatic colorectal primary* but may also be seen in endometrioid adenocarcinoma:
    - "Garland"-type glandular pattern
    - Intraluminal "dirty" necrosis
  - Ovarian metastasis may be the first clinical presentation of clinically unsuspected endocervical adenocarcinomas [30].
    - Most often unilateral
    - Confluent glandular, villoglandular, or cribriform growth pattern
    - Scant cytoplasm, elongated nuclei, mitotic figures close to the apical portion of the cells ("jumping mitoses")
  - If the morphologic features are equivocal or raise concern for a metastatic tumor:
    - The surgeon should be inquired about the clinical history of prior malignancies and any concurrent mass lesions/imaging findings.
    - Morphology with the patient's prior biopsy—if available—should be compared.
    - Intraoperative surgical assessment of intestines should be recommended.

- Ovarian endometrioid adenocarcinomas present with *simultaneous endometrial endometrioid carcinoma* in up to 15–20 % of cases [31–33].
  - Characterization of the relationship between the endometrial and ovarian tumors (metastatic versus synchronous independent primaries) is not crucial on frozen section.
- *Struma ovarii* and *primary ovarian carcinoid tumor* (insular or trabecular type).
  - Most often have a benign clinical course and do not require staging surgery.
  - Have a follicular/glandular architecture that may resemble endometrioid adenocarcinoma.

- Lack significant cytological atypia, necrosis, or stromal desmoplasia.
- Squamous metaplasia is absent.
- Identification of adjacent other teratomatous elements (dermoid cyst) is very helpful.
- Yolk sac tumor presents at a much younger age (mean: 16–19 years) and is most often unilateral.
  - The surgeon should be inquired about the patient's serum AFP: high level is suggestive of yolk sac tumor.

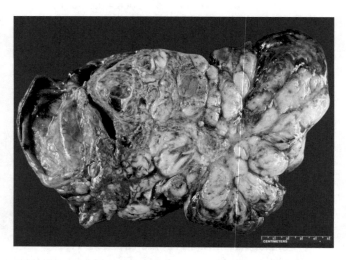

Fig. 8.32 Endometrioid adenocarcinoma of the ovary typically shows a solid or partially cystic cut surface with necrosis and hemorrhage

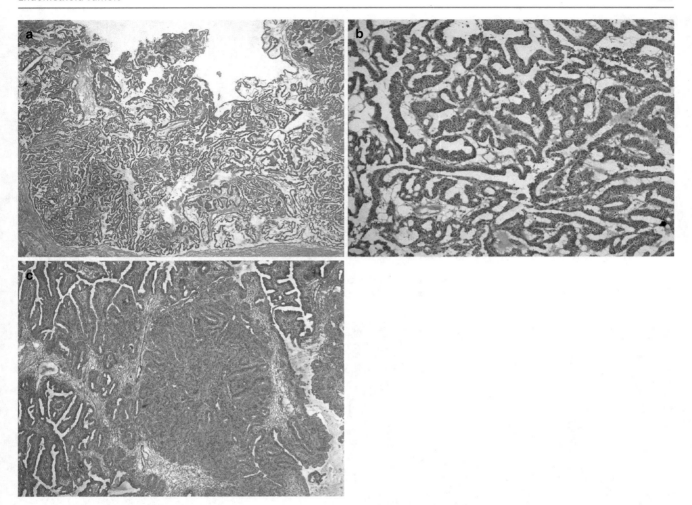

Fig. 8.33 Endometrioid adenocarcinoma of the ovary. The most common microscopic growth pattern is confluent, back-to-back glandular proliferation with loss of intervening stroma. Open glandular lumens are characteristically seen in well-differentiated tumors (**a**, **b**), while solid tumor nests are also present in moderately differentiated tumors (**c**)

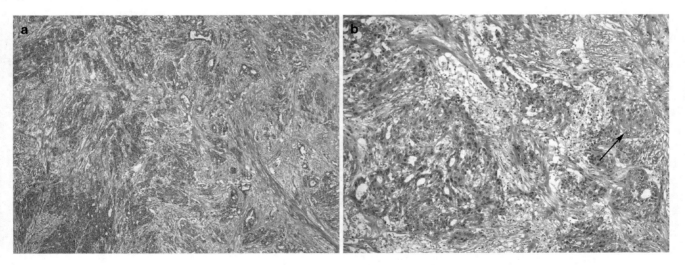

Fig. 8.34 Endometrioid adenocarcinoma of the ovary with predominantly solid tumor nests and cords with an infiltrative growth pattern and desmoplastic stroma (**a**). Presence of squamous differentiation confirms endometrioid histology (**b**, *arrow*)

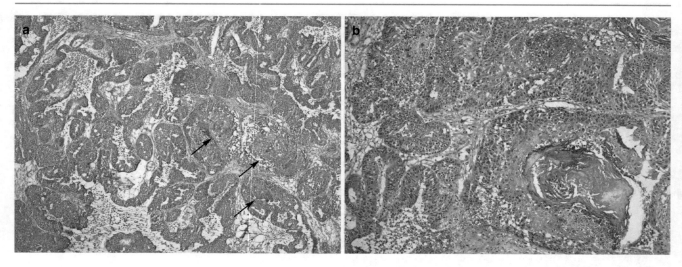

Fig. 8.35 Endometrioid adenocarcinoma of the ovary may have intraluminal necrotic debris, mimicking metastatic colorectal carcinoma (**a, b**). Squamous differentiation (**a**, *arrows*; **b**) confirms endometrioid histology

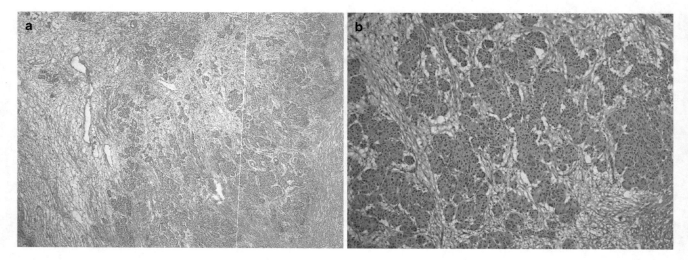

Fig. 8.36 Sertoliform endometrioid adenocarcinoma of the ovary (**a, b**). The tumor cells are arranged in small tubular glands or cords in a fibromatous stroma, resembling a Sertoli cell tumor

Table 8.2 Differential diagnosis of ovarian endometrioid adenocarcinoma

	Endometrioid adenocarcinoma	Metastatic colon adenocarcinoma	Sertoli-Leydig cell tumor	Yolk sac tumor
Age (years)	5th–6th decades (mean 58)	Over the 5th decade (median: 68)	Most common in young patients (mean: 25–30)	2nd–3rd decades (mean: 16–19)
Bilaterality	Up to 17 % of cases	Common, ~60 % of cases	Very rare	Rare
Mean tumor size	15 cm	Usually <10–12 cm	12–14 cm	15 cm
Clinical symptoms	Asymptomatic or pelvic mass/pain	Symptoms associated with colonic primary, less commonly pelvic mass/pain	Hormonal manifestations common (androgenic>estrogenic)	Pelvic mass/pain; increased serum AFP
Squamous differentiation	Common	Absent	Absent	Absent
Mucinous differentiation	Uncommon (no goblet cells)	Common (with goblet cells)	Rare (gastric- or intestinal-type heterologous elements)	Uncommon
Necrosis	Common	Common	May be seen (in poorly differentiated tumors)	Common

Clear Cell Tumors

Clear Cell Cystadenoma/Adenofibroma

- Clinical features
  - *Exceedingly rare tumors*; only few case reports [34, 35]
- Gross pathology
  - Size up to 16 cm
  - Solid cut surface, with small cysts
  - Multiple blocks should be sampled for frozen section to rule out clear cell borderline tumor or carcinoma
- Microscopic features
  - Cystic glands, lined by a single layer of cuboidal or flattened cells
  - Clear or eosinophilic cytoplasm
  - No nuclear atypia or mitotic activity
  - May be associated with endometriosis
  - Background fibromatous stroma

- Differential diagnosis
  - Clear cell borderline tumor/atypical proliferative clear cell tumor
  - Clear cell carcinoma
- Diagnostic pitfalls/key intraoperative consultation issues
  - Clear cell carcinomas may have foci with relatively mild cytological atypia, resembling a benign or borderline/atypical proliferative tumor (Fig. 8.37).
    - If a benign clear cell tumor is suspected on frozen section, multiple additional blocks should be sampled to rule out a clear cell borderline tumor or carcinoma.
    - In equivocal cases, the diagnosis may be best deferred to permanent sections.
  - Cytoplasmic clearing is often difficult to appreciate on frozen sections; eosinophilic cytoplasm is more common.

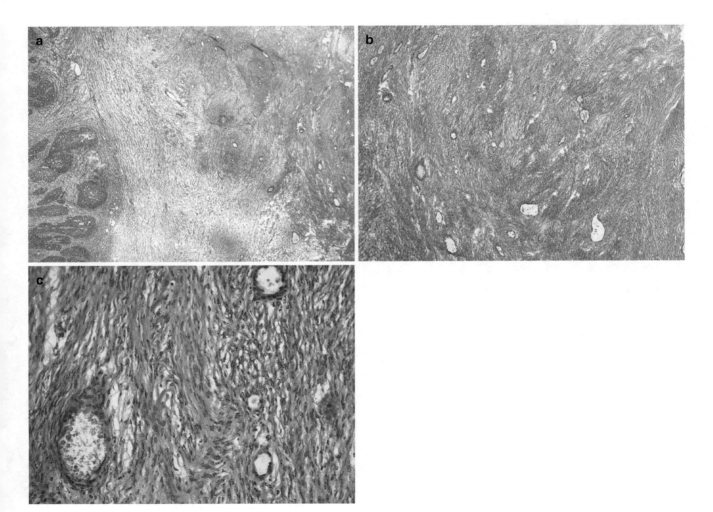

Fig. 8.37 Clear cell carcinoma of the ovary with adenofibromatous foci resembling a benign clear cell tumor. Low magnification of ovarian clear cell carcinoma (**a**, *left side*) shows an adjacent area mimicking clear cell adenofibroma (**a**, *right side*). Medium and high magnification of the adenofibromatous area demonstrates small glandular structures (**b**) with deceptively bland cytological features (**c**)

Clear Cell Borderline Tumor/Atypical Proliferative Clear Cell Tumor

- Clinical features
  - Very rare tumor
  - Less than 1 % of all borderline/atypical proliferative tumors of ovary
- Gross pathology
  - Variable size
  - Solid cut surface, may be "spongy" with small cysts [34, 35].
  - Multiple blocks should be sampled for frozen section to rule out clear cell carcinoma.
- Microscopic features (Fig. 8.38)
  - Fibromatous stroma with epithelial-lined glands and small cysts
  - Clear or eosinophilic cytoplasm
  - Mild to moderate nuclear atypia
  - Low mitotic activity
  - Absence of stromal invasion
  - May be associated with endometriosis

- Differential diagnosis
  - Clear cell carcinoma
- Diagnostic pitfalls/key intraoperative consultation issues
  - Clear cell carcinomas may have foci with relatively mild cytological atypia, resembling a benign or borderline/atypical proliferative tumor.
  - If a clear cell tumor is suspected on frozen section, multiple additional blocks should be sampled to rule out clear cell carcinoma.
  - Not all clear cell carcinomas show obvious stromal invasion.
    - Clear cell carcinomas with adenofibromatous or tubular/tubulocystic pattern may be under-interpreted as borderline/atypical proliferative clear cell tumor.
  - Potential fertility-sparing surgery has been proposed for clear cell borderline tumor/atypical proliferative tumors in young patients based on a small case series [36].

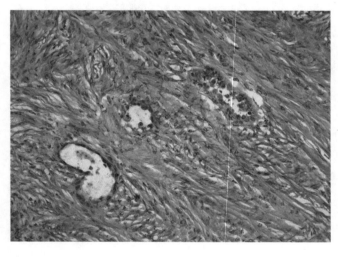

Fig. 8.38 Clear cell borderline tumor/atypical proliferative clear cell tumor showing adenofibromatous stroma with small glands, lined by atypical cells. Note hobnailing and mild to moderate nuclear atypia. The cytoplasmic clearing is often difficult to appreciate on frozen sections

Clear Cell Carcinoma

- Clinical features
  - Mean patient age is 50–55 years [37].
    - Generally tends to present at a younger age than serous carcinoma and may occur during the 3rd or 4th decades, especially if associated with endometriosis [38]
  - May be associated with thromboembolic events and hypercalcemia [39, 40].
  - Strong association with endometriosis.
- Gross pathology (Fig. 8.39)
  - Most often unilateral.
  - Mean size is 15 cm.
  - Cut surface may be solid with hemorrhage and necrosis or predominantly cystic with intraluminal growth.
- Microscopic features (Fig. 8.40)
  - Various architectural patterns often present within the same tumor:
    - Tubulocystic—variably spaced tubules and larger cystic glands
    - Solid—large sheets of tumor cells
    - Papillary—small round papillae with hyalinized fibrovascular cores
  - Polygonal cells with moderate to marked nuclear atypia. Degree of atypia may vary significantly between areas within the same tumor.
    - Foci with adenofibromatous pattern and only mild nuclear atypia may be seen, mimicking a benign or borderline/atypical proliferative tumor.
    - Tumors with a tubulocystic pattern may show flattened tumor cells with deceptively mild nuclear atypia.
  - Prominent nucleoli may be present.
  - Mitotic activity is relatively low (less than 10/10 HPF in most cases).
  - Cytoplasm is clear or eosinophilic; however, cytoplasmic clearing is not always easy to appreciate on frozen sections.
    - Cytoplasmic eosinophilic globules may also be present, resulting in a "targetoid" appearance.
  - Hobnail cells—with round, apical expansion of the cytoplasm by atypical nuclei—are often present.
  - Intraluminal mucinous or eosinophilic secretion may be seen.
  - Necrosis and hemorrhage are not uncommon.
  - Psammoma bodies may be present, but less commonly than in serous tumors.
  - Stromal desmoplastic response is not a common feature.
  - May be associated with endometriosis.
- Differential diagnosis
  - Endometriosis with cytological atypia
  - Benign and borderline/atypical proliferative clear cell tumor
  - Serous borderline tumor/atypical proliferative serous tumor (SBT/APST)
  - Other primary ovarian carcinomas
    - High-grade serous carcinoma
    - Mucinous carcinoma
    - Endometrioid adenocarcinoma
  - Other primary ovarian tumors with clear cytoplasmic features
    - Yolk sac tumor
    - Dysgerminoma
  - Struma ovarii
  - Metastatic carcinomas
    - Clear cell carcinoma from other Mullerian primaries (endometrium, cervix, and lower genital tract)
    - Breast carcinoma
    - Signet-ring cell carcinoma
    - Clear cell renal cell carcinoma
- Diagnostic pitfalls/key intraoperative consultation issues
  - Most important role of frozen section diagnosis is to identify the tumor as high-grade malignancy of Mullerian origin.
    - Distinction between other histological subtypes of primary ovarian carcinomas (high-grade serous or endometrioid) is not critical at the time of frozen section.
    - Distinction between primary ovarian and metastatic Mullerian (endometrium, cervix, lower genital tract) clear cell carcinomas may be difficult—frozen section diagnosis of "high-grade carcinoma/clear cell carcinoma consistent with Mullerian primary" is usually sufficient to cover the above possibilities.
  - Atypia may be mild, especially in tubulocystic or adenofibromatous areas—slides should be carefully evaluated for high-grade nuclear atypia in other foci.
  - Benign and borderline/atypical proliferative clear cell tumors are exceedingly rare; additional blocks should be submitted to rule out a clear cell carcinoma.
  - Clear cell carcinoma with predominantly papillary pattern may mimic SBT/APST; however, marked nuclear atypia is not a feature of SBT/APST
  - Endometriosis may show focal cytological atypia—additional blocks may be submitted for frozen section, especially if there is an intracystic solid mass on gross examination.

– Yolk sac tumor and dysgerminoma also commonly have clear cytoplasmic features, however, they typically occur at a younger age group (2nd and 3rd decades) than clear cell carcinoma (Table 8.3)
  • Fertility-preserving surgery is an option for young patients with malignant germ cell tumors.
  • Role of fertility-sparing surgery in clear cell carcinoma is not uniformly agreed upon, although small case series of stage I tumors showed comparable outcome to patients treated with radical surgery [41, 42].
– Struma ovarii may mimic the tubulocystic pattern of clear cell carcinoma but lacks significant nuclear atypia.
  • Identification of adjacent other teratomatous elements (dermoid cyst) is very helpful.

– Metastasis from renal clear cell carcinoma and adeno-carcinomas with signet ring—or clear cytoplasmic features (breast, gastrointestinal)—may also mimic primary clear cell carcinoma of the ovary.
  • The morphology of the patient's prior biopsy should be compared.
  • The surgeon should be inquired about clinical history of prior malignancies, any concurrent mass lesions/imaging findings, and intraoperative findings.

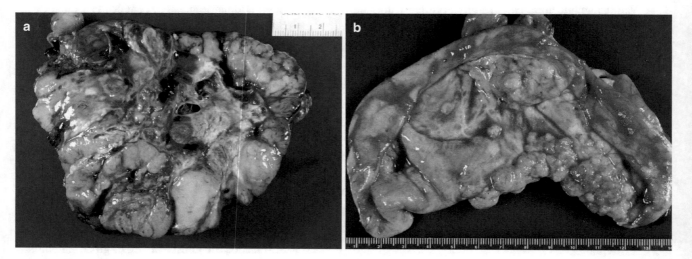

Fig. 8.39 Clear cell carcinoma of ovary. The tumor may have a solid cut surface with apparent necrosis (**a**) or may show a predominantly cystic appearance with intraluminal papillary or solid growth (**b**)

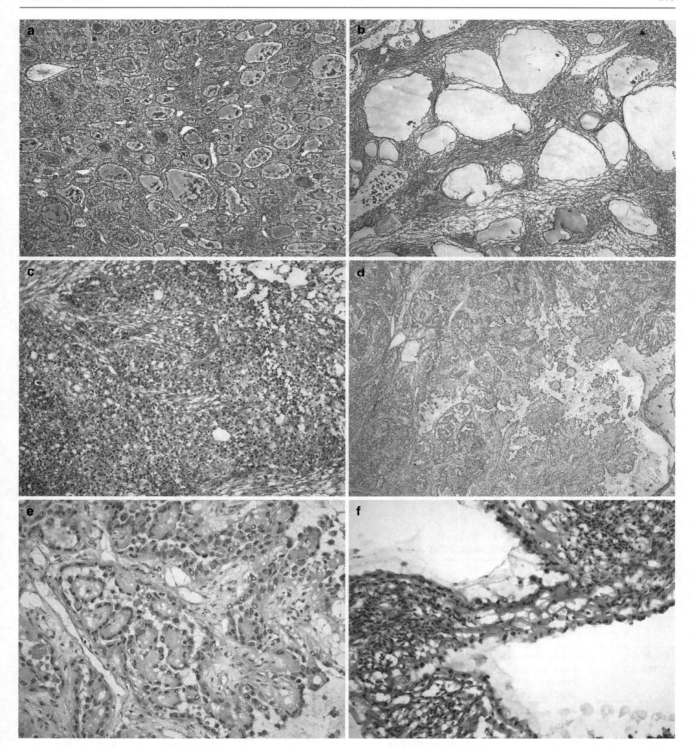

Fig. 8.40 Clear cell carcinoma of ovary. The tumor shows various architectural patterns: tubulocystic (**a, b**), solid (**c**), and papillary with characteristic small round papillae and hyalinized fibrovascular cores (**d, e**). The degree of cytological atypia often ranges from mild (**f, g**) to severe (**h, i**), even within the same tumor. Hobnail cells (**e, g**) and intra-luminal eosinophilic or basophilic secretion (**g–i**) are often seen. Cytoplasmic clearing may not be prominent on frozen sections, but rare cases may demonstrate abundant clear cytoplasm (**j**) mimicking signet-ring cell carcinoma

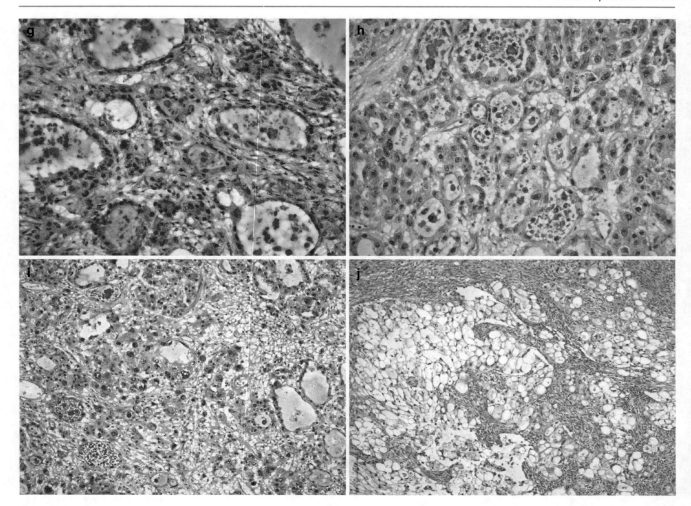

Fig. 8.40   (continued)

Table 8.3   Differential diagnosis of ovarian clear cell carcinoma

	Clear cell carcinoma	SBT/APST	Yolk sac tumor	Dysgerminoma	Struma ovarii	Metastatic adenocarcinoma
Age (years)	3rd–7th decades (mean: 50–55)	Mean age: 42 years	2nd–3rd decades (mean: 16–19)	2nd–3rd decades (mean: 22)	Reproductive years	Usually over 5th decade
Bilaterality	Rare	Common	Rare	10–20 %	Other ovary may show dermoid cyst	Common
Clinical symptoms	Pelvic mass/pain, thromboembolic events, hypercalcemia	Pelvic mass/pain	Pelvic mass/pain; Increased serum AFP	Pelvic mass/pain; increased serum LDH	Rarely hyperthyroidism	Variable, depending on the primary tumor
Helpful features in background ovary	Endometriosis	–	–	Rarely gonadal dysgenesis or gonadoblastoma	Other teratomatous elements (dermoid)	–
Architectural pattern	Variable: papillary, tubulocystic, solid	Papillary	Variable: reticular, solid, alveolar-glandular	Solid	Glandular, may be cystic	Variable: glandular or single cell infiltration
Nuclear atypia	Variable; at least focally high grade	Mild	Moderate to marked with prominent nucleoli	Uniform nuclear enlargement with prominent nucleoli	Minimal to none	Variable, depending on primary tumor
Necrosis	Common	Absent	Common	Common	Absent	Common

SBT/APST serous borderline tumor/atypical proliferative serous tumor

Brenner Tumors

Benign Brenner Tumor

- Clinical features
  - Most common in the 5th–7th decades but can occur at any age [43, 44].
  - Most often incidental; rarely presents with pelvic mass/pain.
  - Endocrine symptoms due to stromal hormone production may rarely occur [45].
- Gross pathology (Fig. 8.41)
  - Most often less than 2 cm in size [44].
  - Most often unilateral [43].
  - Cut surface is usually solid, firm, tan-yellow, or white.
  - Cystic component may be present (most often represents an associated mucinous neoplasm) [46].
- Microscopic features (Fig. 8.42)
  - Abundant, dense fibromatous stroma with round or irregularly shaped and variably sized transitional-type epithelial nests.
    - Tumor nests may have central lumens lined by transitional or mucinous epithelium and filled with mucinous or eosinophilic material.
    - Squamous metaplasia may rarely be seen.
  - Oval nuclei with longitudinal grooves and small nucleoli.
  - No nuclear atypia or significant mitotic activity.
  - Pale eosinophilic or clear cytoplasm.
  - Prominent cell membranes.
  - Stromal hyalinization and calcification are common.
  - May be associated with other tumor types, most commonly mucinous tumors, less often dermoid cyst, struma ovarii, or serous cystadenoma.

- Differential diagnosis
  - Borderline/atypical proliferative Brenner tumor
  - Adult granulosa cell tumor
- Diagnostic pitfalls/key intraoperative consultation issues
  - Fibromatous stroma with irregular glands may mimic an infiltrative process.
    - Lack of desmoplastic stromal response or nuclear atypia
  - Focal mucinous lumen/cyst formation may mimic a glandular or microfollicular pattern.
    - Typically, it is very focal; other areas of tumor show characteristic transitional cell nests with oval nuclei and nuclear grooves.
  - Gross appearance, nuclear grooves, and focal small lumen formation may raise suspicion for adult granulosa cell tumor.
    - Unlike adult granulosa cell tumor, Brenner tumor has abundant pale eosinophilic cytoplasm and well-defined cell membranes.
    - The nuclear membrane contours are typically smooth in Brenner tumor, whereas adult granulosa cell tumors have irregular nuclear membranes in addition to longitudinal grooves.
  - Unlike borderline/atypical proliferative Brenner tumors, benign Brenner tumors:
    - Do not have intracystic papillary or undulating transitional epithelial proliferation
    - Have no significant nuclear atypia
  - Associated mucinous tumor is most often a benign mucinous cystadenoma, but may rarely show borderline/atypical proliferative histology.
    - Adequate sampling of the cystic component (if present) is important (see *Mucinous Tumors*).

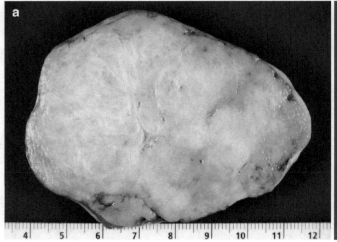
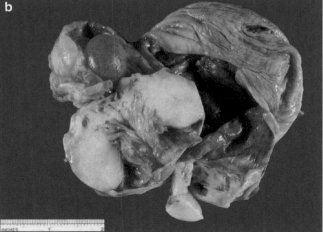

Fig. 8.41 Benign Brenner tumor with a solid firm, tan-yellow cut surface (**a**). Less often the tumor may be partially cystic due to an associated mucinous neoplasm (**b**)

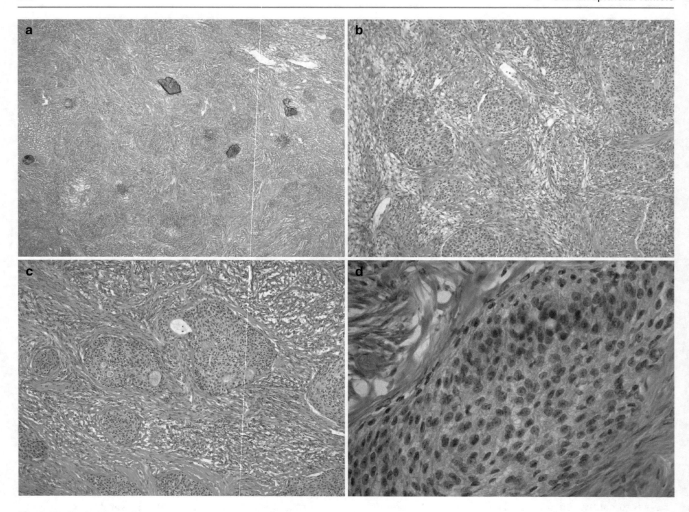

Fig. 8.42 Benign Brenner tumor. The tumor shows dense, fibromatous stroma with irregularly shaped nests composed of transitional-type epithelium (**a**, **b**). Stromal calcifications (**a**) and mucinous change with lumen formation are common (**c**). The nuclei are round or oval with longitudinal nuclear grooves, smooth nuclear membranes and small nucleoli. Nuclear atypia is absent (**d**)

Borderline Brenner Tumor/Atypical Proliferative Brenner Tumor

- Clinical features
  - Rare tumor [47–51].
  - Mean patient age is 59 years [6].
  - May present with pelvic pain/mass.
- Gross pathology (Fig. 8.43)
  - Unilateral.
  - Larger than benign Brenner tumor (size range 10–28 cm).
  - Cut surface is usually cystic with intraluminal polypoid projections and variable solid component.
- Microscopic features (Fig. 8.44)
  - Intracystic component resembles low-grade papillary urothelial tumors or shows undulating, tortuous transitional-type epithelial lining.
  - Crowded nests of transitional-type epithelium.
  - Mild to moderate nuclear atypia.
  - Mitotic figures may be present.
  - Absence of stromal invasion.
  - Adjacent areas of benign Brenner tumor are often present.
  - Often shows mucinous metaplasia or may be associated with a mucinous tumor.

- Differential diagnosis
  - Benign Brenner tumor
  - Malignant Brenner tumor
- Diagnostic pitfalls/key intraoperative consultation issues
  - Rare local recurrence has been reported, but majority of borderline/atypical proliferative Brenner tumors have a benign clinical course [47–51].
    - Similar to other histological subtypes of borderline/atypical proliferative tumors, staging surgery is typically performed.
  - If high-grade nuclear atypia is present without stromal invasion, the term *borderline/atypical proliferative Brenner tumor with intraepithelial carcinoma* should be used.
  - Malignant Brenner tumors are usually associated with benign or borderline/atypical proliferative Brenner tumors but show marked nuclear atypia, high mitotic activity, and stromal invasion
    - If stromal invasion cannot be ruled out on frozen section, intraoperative diagnosis of "at least borderline/atypical proliferative Brenner tumor" can be communicated.

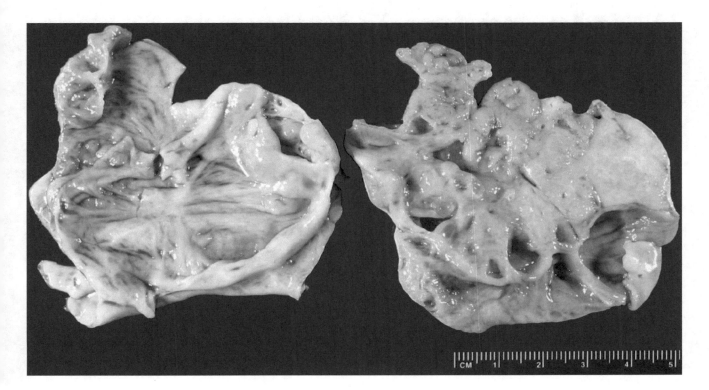

Fig. 8.43 Borderline Brenner tumor/atypical proliferative Brenner tumor typically shows a cystic cut surface with intraluminal tan-yellow polypoid or solid growth

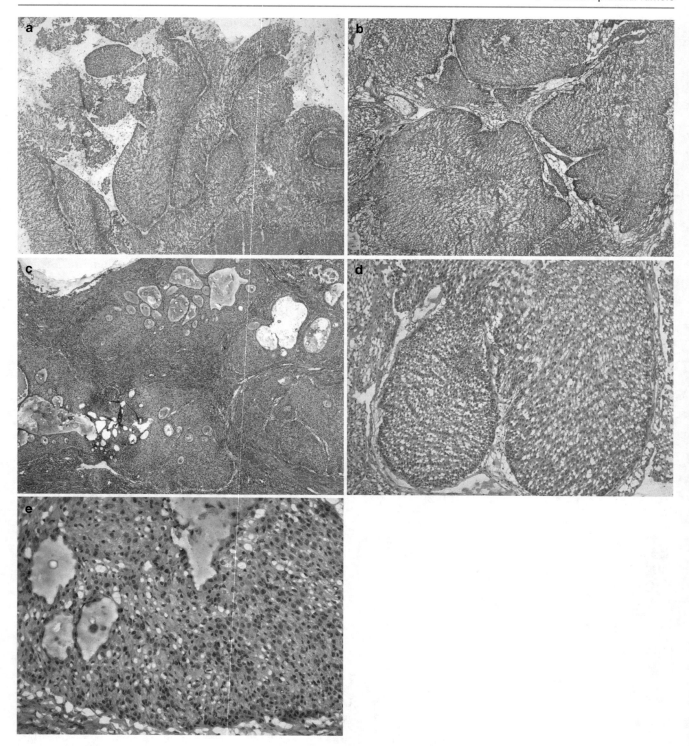

Fig. 8.44 Borderline Brenner tumor/atypical proliferative Brenner tumor. Intracystic papillary or undulating epithelial proliferation is seen on low magnification, resembling low-grade urothelial tumors (**a**, **b**). Mucinous epithelial change and intraluminal mucin are often present (**c**). Nuclear atypia is typically mild. Mitotic figures and stromal invasion are absent (**d**, **e**)

Malignant Brenner Tumor

- Clinical features
  - Rare tumor
  - Usually occurs in patients over 50 years of age
  - Presents with pelvic pain/mass
- Gross pathology
  - Typically large, may be up to 40 cm in size.
  - Cut surface usually shows both solid and cystic components.
  - Necrosis may be grossly apparent.
  - Up to 12 % of tumors are bilateral [52].
  - Sampling multiple blocks for frozen section may be necessary to demonstrate malignant component.
    - Inadequate sampling may only show the benign or borderline/atypical proliferative Brenner tumor component.
- Microscopic features (Fig. 8.45)
  - Irregular nests of transitional-type epithelial cells, resembling high-grade urothelial carcinoma.
  - Stromal invasion
    - Irregular small nests or single cells.
    - Desmoplastic stromal response may be seen.
  - Moderate to marked nuclear atypia.
  - Mitotic figures are usually easily found.
  - Associated or contiguous with benign or borderline/atypical proliferative Brenner tumor.
  - Squamous and mucinous differentiation may be present.
  - Necrosis may be seen.
- Differential diagnosis
  - Borderline/atypical proliferative Brenner tumor

- Other primary ovarian carcinomas
  - High-grade serous carcinoma
  - Endometrioid adenocarcinoma
  - Mucinous carcinoma
  - Squamous cell carcinoma—arising in a mature teratoma
- Metastatic transitional cell carcinoma
- Diagnostic pitfalls/key intraoperative consultation issues
  - High-grade serous and endometrioid carcinomas may show transitional cell features.
    - Should not be classified as malignant Brenner tumor without background benign or borderline/atypical proliferative Brenner tumor component
    - Distinction between various histological subtypes of primary ovarian carcinomas (malignant Brenner tumor, high-grade serous or endometrioid adenocarcinoma) is not critical at the time of frozen section as it does not alter the intraoperative management.
  - Presence of unequivocal stromal invasion may be difficult to identify on frozen section—intraoperative diagnosis of "at least borderline/atypical proliferative Brenner tumor" can be communicated.
  - Metastatic transitional cell carcinoma can be ruled out by identifying associated benign or borderline/atypical proliferative Brenner tumor components.
    - If the patient has history of a known malignancy, morphologic comparison should be made.
    - The surgeon should be inquired about any concurrent mass lesions, imaging and intraoperative findings.

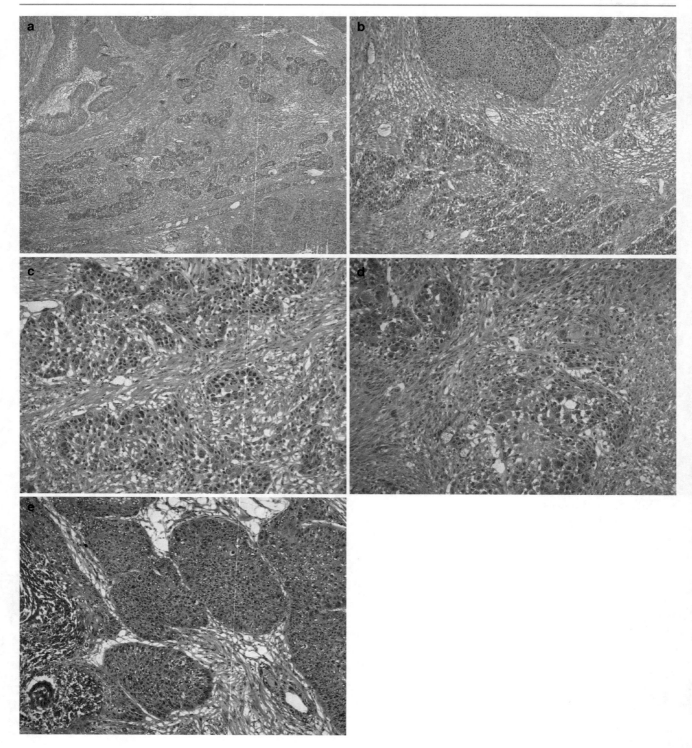

Fig. 8.45 Malignant Brenner tumor. Note the stromal invasion by irregular nests of transitional epithelial cells, arising in the background of borderline/atypical proliferative Brenner tumor (**a**; associated bor-derline Brenner tumor is seen in the left upper corner of image). The tumor cells are markedly atypical and mitotic figures are frequent (**b–e**). Squamous differentiation may be present (**d, e**)

Mixed Epithelial-Mesenchymal Tumors

Carcinosarcoma (Malignant Mixed Mullerian Tumor, MMMT)

- Clinical features
  - Most often occurs during the 6th or 7th decade [53]
  - Presents with pelvic pain/mass
  - Usually advanced stage at presentation
- Gross pathology (Fig. 8.46)
  - Mean tumor size is 14 cm [54].
  - Solid and cystic cut surface often with necrosis and hemorrhage.
  - Up to one-third with bilateral ovarian involvement.
- Microscopic features (Fig. 8.47)
  - High-grade epithelial component—most often high-grade serous carcinoma, but endometrioid, clear cell and undifferentiated carcinoma components or a mixed carcinomatous component may also be seen.
  - Mesenchymal (sarcomatous) component may be homologous—high-grade, nonspecific spindle cell sarcoma—or heterologous: rhabdomyosarcoma, chondrosarcoma, or rarely osteosarcoma or liposarcoma.
  - Marked nuclear atypia in both components.
  - High mitotic activity.
  - Necrosis and hemorrhage are common.
- Differential diagnosis
  - High-grade primary ovarian carcinomas
  - Metastatic carcinomas
  - Metastatic carcinosarcoma from other Mullerian primaries (fallopian tube, endometrium)
  - Immature teratoma
  - Sertoli-Leydig cell tumor, poorly differentiated

- Diagnostic pitfalls/key intraoperative consultation issues
  - Sarcomatous component may be very focal and may not be sampled on the frozen sections.
    - Identification of a sarcomatous component and distinction between primary high-grade ovarian carcinoma and carcinosarcoma is not critical at the time of frozen section, as it does not change intraoperative management.
  - Identification of a sarcomatous component is helpful in ruling out metastatic non-Mullerian carcinomas.
  - Distinction between primary ovarian and metastatic Mullerian (endometrial and fallopian tube) carcinosarcomas is not critical on frozen section, as it does not change the intraoperative management.
  - Carcinosarcoma—especially if containing chondrosarcomatous elements—may mimic immature teratoma.
    - Immature teratoma typically occurs in a much younger patient population (during the first 3 decades) and almost never seen after the menopause.
    - Degree of nuclear atypia in carcinosarcoma is much more severe in both components than in the immature neuroectodermal and mesenchymal elements of immature teratoma.
  - Sertoli-Leydig cell tumors (SLCT)
    - Typically occur in young patients (<30 years of age).
    - Show lesser degree of nuclear atypia.
    - Well-differentiated areas are often present focally, even in poorly differentiated SLCT.
    - May rarely contain cartilagenous heterologous elements.

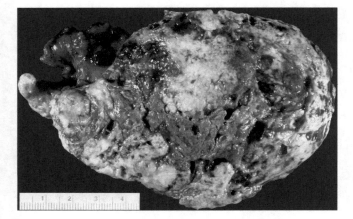

Fig. 8.46 Carcinosarcoma (malignant mixed Mullerian tumor) typically forms a large mass with a solid and cystic cut surface and areas of necrosis and hemorrhage

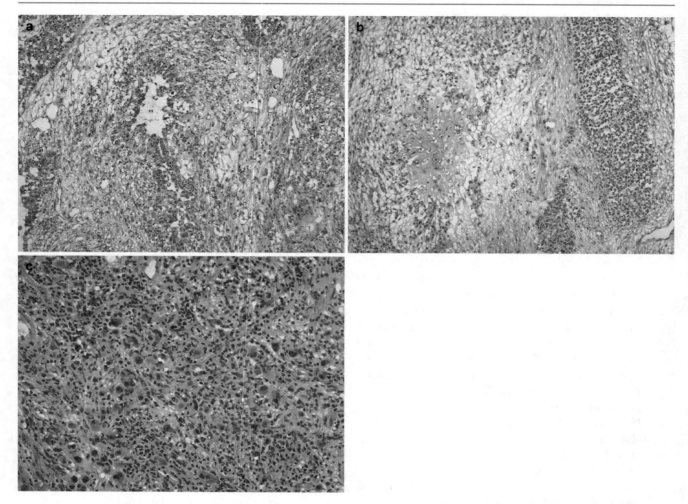

Fig. 8.47 Carcinosarcoma (malignant mixed Mullerian tumor). The high-grade epithelial component may form glandular structures (**a**, *center*) or irregular solid nests (**b**, *right side of image*). The sarcomatous component may be homologous or nonspecific spindle cell sarcoma (**a**, surrounding the malignant glands) or heterologous chondrosarcoma (**b**, *left side of image*) or rhabdomyosarcoma with characteristic dense eosinophilic cytoplasm and eccentrically located atypical nuclei (**c**)

References

1. Lim-Tan SK, Cajigas HE, Scully RE. Ovarian cystectomy for serous borderline tumors: a follow-up study of 35 cases. Obstet Gynecol. 1988;72:775–81.
2. Bostwick DG, Tazelaar HD, Ballon SC, Hendrickson MR, Kempson RL. Ovarian epithelial tumors of borderline malignancy. A clinical and pathologic study of 109 cases. Cancer. 1986;58:2052–65.
3. Lim FK, Yeoh CL, Chong SM, Arulkumaran S. Pre and intraoperative diagnosis of ovarian tumours: how accurate are we? Aust N Z J Obstet Gynaecol. 1997;37:223–7.
4. Allison KH, Swisher EM, Kerkering KM, Garcia RL. Defining an appropriate threshold for the diagnosis of serous borderline tumor of the ovary: when is a full staging procedure unnecessary? Int J Gynecol Pathol. 2008;27:10–7.
5. Seidman JD, Soslow RA, Vang R, GErman JJ, Stoler MH, Sherman ME, et al. Borderline ovarian tumors: diverse contemporary viewpoints on terminology and diagnostic criteria with illustrative images. Hum Pathol. 2004;35:918–33.
6. Kurman RJ, Carcanglu ML, Herrington CS, Young RH. WHO classification of tumours of female reproductive organs. 4th ed. Lyon: International Agency for Research on Cancer (IARC); 2014.
7. Longacre TA, McKenney JK, Tazelaar HD, Kempson RL, Hendrickson MR. Ovarian serous tumors of low malignant potential (borderline tumors): outcome-based study of 276 patients with long-term (> or =5-year) follow-up. Am J Surg Pathol. 2005;29:707–23.
8. McKenney JK, Balzer BL, Longacre TA. Patterns of stromal invasion in ovarian serous tumors of low malignant potential (borderline tumors): a reevaluation of the concept of stromal microinvasion. Am J Surg Pathol. 2006;30:1209–21.
9. Bell DA. Low-grade serous tumors of ovary. Int J Gynecol Pathol. 2014;33:348–56.
10. Hannibal CG, Vang R, Junge J, Frederiksen K, Kjaerbye-Thygesen A, Andersen KK, et al. A nationwide study of serous "borderline" ovarian tumors in Denmark 1978–2002: centralized pathology review and overall survival compared with the general population. Gynecol Oncol. 2014;134(2):267–73.
11. Seidman JD, Kurman RJ. Subclassification of serous borderline tumors of the ovary into benign and malignant types. A clinicopathologic study of 65 advanced stage cases. Am J Surg Pathol. 1996;20:1331–45.
12. Eichhorn JH, Bell DA, Young RH, et al. Ovarian serous borderline tumors with micropapillary and cribriform patterns: a study of 40 cases and comparison with 44 cases without these patterns. Am J Surg Pathol. 1999;23:397–409.
13. Prat J, De Nictolis M. Serous borderline tumors of the ovary: a long-term follow-up study of 137 cases, including 18 with a micropapillary pattern and 20 with microinvasion. Am J Surg Pathol. 2002;26:1111–28.
14. Malpica A, Deavers MT, Lu K, Bodurka DC, Atkinson EN, Gershenson DM, Silva EG. Grading ovarian serous carcinoma using a two-tier system. Am J Surg Pathol. 2004;28:496–504.
15. Gershenson DM, Sun CC, Bodurka D, Coleman RL, Lu KH, Sood AK, et al. Recurrent low-grade ovarian carcinoma is relatively chemoresistant. Gynecol Oncol. 2009;114:48–52.
16. Seidman JD, Yemelyanova A, Cosin JA, Smith A, Kurrman RJ. Survival rates for international federation of gynecology and obstetrics stage III ovarian carcinoma by cell type: a study of 262 unselected patients with uniform pathologic review. Int J Gynecol Cancer. 2012;22:367–71.
17. Ronnett BM, Kajdacsy-Balla A, Gilks CB, Merino MJ, Silva E, Werness BA, Young RH. Mucinous borderline ovarian tumors: points of general agreement and persistent controversies regarding nomenclature, diagnostic criteria, and behavior. Hum Pathol. 2004;35:949–60.
18. Lee KR, Young RH. The distinction between primary and metastatic mucinous carcinomas of the ovary: gross and histologic findings in 50 cases. Am J Surg Pathol. 2003;27:281–92.
19. Seidman JD, Kurman RJ, Ronnett BM. Primary and metastatic mucinous adenocarcinomas in the ovaries: incidence in routine practice with a new approach to improve intraoperative diagnosis. Am J Surg Pathol. 2003;27:985–93.
20. Yemelyanova AV, Vang R, Judson K, Wu LS, Ronnett BM. Distinction of primary and metastatic mucinous tumors involving the ovary: analysis of size and laterality data by primary site with reevaluation of an algorithm for tumor classification. Am J Surg Pathol. 2008;32:128–38.
21. Riopel MA, Ronnett BM, Kurman RJ. Evaluation of diagnostic criteria and behavior of ovarian intestinal-type mucinous tumors: atypical proliferative (borderline) tumors and intraepithelial, microinvasive, invasive, and metastatic carcinomas. Am J Surg Pathol. 1999;23:617–35.
22. Rodriguez IM, Prat J. Mucinous tumors of the ovary: a clinicopathologic analysis of 75 borderline tumors (of intestinal type) and carcinomas. Am J Surg Pathol. 2002;26:139–52.
23. Lee KR, Scully RE. Mucinous tumors of the ovary: a clinicopathologic study of 196 borderline tumors (of intestinal type) and carcinomas, including an evaluation of 11 cases with 'pseudomyxoma peritonei'. Am J Surg Pathol. 2000;24:1447–64.
24. Kim KR, Lee HI, Lee SK, Ro JY, Robboy SJ. Is stromal microinvasion in primary mucinous ovarian tumors with "mucin granuloma" true invasion? Am J Surg Pathol. 2007;31:546–54.
25. Bague S, Rodriguez IM, Prat J. Sarcoma-like mural nodules in mucinous cystic tumors of the ovary revisited: a clinicopathologic analysis of 10 additional cases. Am J Surg Pathol. 2002;26:1467–76.
26. Provenza C, Young RH, Prat J. Anaplastic carcinoma in mucinous ovarian tumors: a clinicopathologic study of 34 cases emphasizing the crucial impact of stage on prognosis, their histological spectrum, and overlap with sarcomalike mural nodules. Am J Surg Pathol. 2008;32:383–9.
27. Bell KA, Kurman RJ. A clinicopathologic analysis of atypical proliferative (borderline) tumors and well-differentiated endometrioid adenocarcinomas of the ovary. Am J Surg Pathol. 2000;24:1465–79.
28. Roth LM, Emerson RE, Ulbright TM. Ovarian endometrioid tumors of low malignant potential: a clinicopathologic study of 30 cases with comparison to well-differentiated endometrioid adenocarcinoma. Am J Surg Pathol. 2003;27:1253–9.
29. Storey DJ, Rush R, Stewart M, Rye T, Al-Nafussi A, Williams AR, et al. Endometrioid epithelial ovarian cancer : 20 years of prospectively collected data from a single center. Cancer. 2008;112:2211–20.
30. Ronnett BM, Yemelyanova AV, Vang R, Gilks CB, Miller D, Gravitt PE, Kurman RJ. Endocervical adenocarcinomas with ovarian metastases: analysis of 29 cases with emphasis on minimally invasive cervical tumors and the ability of the metastases to simulate primary ovarian neoplasms. Am J Surg Pathol. 2008;32:1835–53.
31. Sheu BC, Lin HH, Chen CK, Chao KH, SHun CT, Huang SC. Synchronous primary carcinomas of the endometrium and ovary. Int J Gynaecol Obstet. 1995;51:141–6.
32. Kline RC, Wharton JT, Atkinson EN, Burke TW, Gershenson DM, Edwards CL. Endometrioid carcinoma of the ovary: retrospective review of 145 cases. Gynecol Oncol. 1990;39:337–46.
33. Zaino R, Whitney C, Brady MF, DeGeest K, Burger RA, Buller RE. Simultaneously detected endometrial and ovarian carcinomas–a prospective clinicopathologic study of 74 cases: a gynecologic oncology group study. Gynecol Oncol. 2001;83:355–62.
34. Bell DA, Scully RE. Benign and borderline clear cell adenofibromas of the ovary. Cancer. 1985;56:2922–31.

35. Roth LM, Langley FA, Fox H, Wheeler JE, Czernobilsky B. Ovarian clear cell adenofibromatous tumors. Benign, of low malignant potential, and associated with invasive clear cell carcinoma. Cancer. 1984;53:1156–63.

36. Uzan C, Dufeu-Lefebvre M, Fauvet R, Gouy S, Duvillard P, Darai E, Morice P. Management and prognosis of clear cell borderline ovarian tumor. Int J Gynecol Cancer. 2012;22:993–9.

37. Chan JK, Teoh D, Hu JM, Shin JY, Osann K, Kapp DS. Do clear cell ovarian carcinomas have poorer prognosis compared to other epithelial cell types? A study of 1411 clear cell ovarian cancers. Gynecol Oncol. 2008;109:370–6.

38. Scarfone G, Bergamini A, Noli S, Villa A, Cipriani S, Taccagni G, et al. Characteristics of clear cell ovarian cancer arising from endometriosis: a two center cohort study. Gynecol Oncol. 2014;133:480–4.

39. Matsuura Y, Robertson G, Marsden DE, Kim SN, Gebski V, Hacker NF. Thromboembolic complications in patients with clear cell carcinoma of the ovary. Gynecol Oncol. 2007;104:406–10.

40. Savvari P, Peitsidis P, Alevizaki M, Dimopoulos MA, Antsaklis A, Papadimitriou CA. Paraneoplastic humorally mediated hypercalcemia induced by parathyroid hormone-related protein in gynecologic malignancies: a systematic review. Onkologie. 2009;32:517–23.

41. Kajiyama H, Shibata K, Mizuno M, Hosono S, Kawai M, Nagasaka T, Kikkawa F. Fertility-sparing surgery in patients with clear-cell carcinoma of the ovary: is it possible? Hum Reprod. 2011;26:3297–302.

42. Kajiyama H, Shibata K, Suzuki S, Ino K, Yamamoto E, Mizuno K, et al. Is there any possibility of fertility-sparing surgery in patients with clear-cell carcinoma of the ovary? Gynecol Oncol. 2008;111:523–6.

43. Kondi-Pafiti A, Kairi-Vassilatou E, Iavazzo C, Vouza E, Mavrigiannaki P, Kleanthis C, et al. Clinicopathological features and immunoprofile of 30 cases of Brenner ovarian tumors. Arch Gynecol Obstet. 2012;285:1699–702.

44. Fox H, Agrawal K, Langley FA. The Brenner tumour of the ovary. A clinicopathological study of 54 cases. J Obstet Gynaecol Br Commonw. 1972;79:661–5.

45. de Lima GR, de Lima OA, Baracat EC, Vasserman J, Burnier Jr M. Virilizing Brenner tumor of the ovary: case report. Obstet Gynecol. 1989;73:895–8.

46. Seidman JD, Khedmati F. Exploring the histogenesis of ovarian mucinous and transitional cell (Brenner) neoplasms and their relationship with Walthard cell nests: a study of 120 tumors. Arch Pathol Lab Med. 2008;132:1753–60.

47. Miles PA, Norris HJ. Proliferative and malignant brenner tumors of the ovary. Cancer. 1972;30:174–86.

48. Roth LM, Dallenbach-Hellweg G, Czernobilsky B. Ovarian Brenner tumors. I. Metaplastic, proliferating, and of low malignant potential. Cancer. 1985;56:582–91.

49. Roth LM, Sternberg WH. Proliferating Brenner tumors. Cancer. 1971;27:687–93.

50. Woodruff JD, Dietrich D, Genadry R, Parmley TH. Proliferative and malignant Brenner tumors. Review of 47 cases. Am J Obstet Gynecol. 1981;141:118–25.

51. Uzan C, Dufeu-Lefebvre M, Fauvet R, Gouy S, Duvillard P, Darai E, Morice P. Management and prognosis of borderline ovarian Brenner tumors. Int J Gynecol Cancer. 2012;22:1332–6.

52. Austin RM, Norris HJ. Malignant Brenner tumor and transitional cell carcinoma of the ovary: a comparison. Int J Gynecol Pathol. 1987;6:29–39.

53. George EM, Herzog TJ, Neugut AI, Lu YS, Burke WM, Lewin SN, et al. Carcinosarcoma of the ovary: natural history, patterns of treatment, and outcome. Gynecol Oncol. 2013;131:42–5.

54. Kunkel J, Peng Y, Tao Y, Krigman H, Cao D. Presence of a sarcomatous component outside the ovary is an adverse prognostic factor for primary ovarian malignant mixed mesodermal/mullerian tumors: a clinicopathologic study of 47 cases. Am J Surg Pathol. 2012;36:831–7.

Ovarian Germ Cell Tumors

9

Introduction

Germ cell tumors account for approximately 30 % of primary ovarian neoplasms, comprising the second most common tumor type after epithelial tumors. However, vast majority of them are benign and the group represents only 2–3 % of ovarian malignancies. While the intraoperative diagnosis of the most common mature cystic teratoma (dermoid cyst) is usually straightforward, frozen section evaluation of malignant germ cell tumors is often challenging given their rarity and the clinical implications of the diagnosis. Most malignant germ cell tumors occur in young patients—children and young adults less than 30 years of age, hence preservation of fertility is of great importance. Thanks to recent advances in adjuvant chemotherapy, fertility-sparing surgery—intact removal of tumor, pelvic washings, surgical examination, and removal/biopsy of any suspicious areas from omentum and regional lymph nodes—now became the standard of care for this group of tumors [1–4]. The frozen section pathologist has a crucial role in recognizing these neoplasms and distinguishing them from their mimics—most importantly the more aggressive epithelial ovarian cancers—to guide appropriate surgical management.

The importance of the clinical presentation and laboratory findings as an aid in the frozen section diagnosis cannot be overemphasized in ovarian pathology in general, but this is especially true for germ cell tumors. The patient's age, hormonal manifestations (e.g., precocious puberty), and serum tumor markers can provide important diagnostic clues and significantly narrow down the differential diagnosis during intraoperative consultation.

© Springer International Publishing Switzerland 2015
P. Hui, N. Buza, *Atlas of Intraoperative Frozen Section Diagnosis in Gynecologic Pathology*,
DOI 10.1007/978-3-319-21807-6_9

Dysgerminoma

- Clinical features
  - Most common malignant germ cell tumor (approximately 50 % of all malignant germ cell tumors).
  - Occurs most often during the 2nd and 3rd decades with a mean patient age of 22 years.
  - Rapidly growing tumor; frequently presents with abdominal mass and pain.
  - May be an incidental finding, e.g., during pregnancy.
  - Serum LDH is often elevated.
  - Rarely may be associated with paraneoplastic hypercalcemia [5].
  - May arise in dysgenetic gonads with gonadoblastoma.
    - Patients in this setting may have an abnormal (46XY or 45X/46XY) karyotype [6, 7].
- Gross pathology (Fig. 9.1)
  - Bilateral in 10–20 % of cases
  - Large, usually more than 10 cm in diameter [8]
  - Cut surface is solid, fleshy, and tan-yellow
    - Small foci of necrosis, hemorrhage, and cystic degeneration may be seen.
- Microscopic features (Fig. 9.2)
  - Solid nests, sheets, or cords of relatively uniform polygonal cells.
  - Abundant clear or eosinophilic cytoplasm with well-defined cell membranes.
  - Prominent nucleoli.
  - High mitotic activity.
  - Intersecting fibrous septae, infiltrated by small lymphocytes.
    - Ratio between tumor cells and fibrous stroma may vary, in some tumors hyalinized stroma may predominate
  - Sarcoid-like granulomas with multinucleated giant cells may be seen in up to 20 % of cases.
  - Syncytiotrophoblastic giant cells may rarely be seen.
    - May be associated with elevated serum beta human chorionic gonadotropin (hCG)
  - Focal necrosis and hemorrhage are not uncommon.
  - Calcifications may be present.

- Differential diagnosis
  - Diffuse large B-cell lymphoma
  - Clear cell carcinoma
  - Yolk sac tumor
  - Embryonal carcinoma
  - Gonadoblastoma
- Diagnostic pitfalls/key intraoperative consultation issues
  - Contralateral ovarian biopsy should be performed to rule out bilateral involvement by dysgerminoma or underlying gonadal dysgenesis and/or gonadoblastoma.
    - Bilateral oophorectomy is indicated for gonadal dysgenesis and gonadoblastoma.
    - Abundant calcifications should raise suspicion for gonadoblastoma.
  - Fertility-preserving surgery—unilateral salpingo-oophorectomy with peritoneal biopsies and lymph node sampling—is the standard first-line treatment [1, 9].
    - Other malignant germ cell tumors in the differential diagnosis—yolk sac tumor and embryonal carcinoma—have essentially the same surgical management.
  - Entities in the differential with the most significant impact on intraoperative management:
    - Diffuse large B-cell lymphoma
      - Primarily nonsurgical treatment.
      - Fresh tissue sample should be submitted for hematopathology—flow cytometry and molecular studies—workup.
      - Lymphoma cells are more polymorphous and have less cytoplasm than dysgerminoma.
    - Epithelial malignancies (e.g., clear cell carcinoma and small cell carcinoma)
      - More aggressive tumors, typically requiring more extensive staging—tumor debulking—surgery

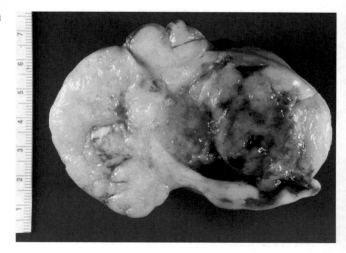

Fig. 9.1 Dysgerminoma. Note the solid, tan-yellow, fleshy cut surface with foci of hemorrhage and necrosis

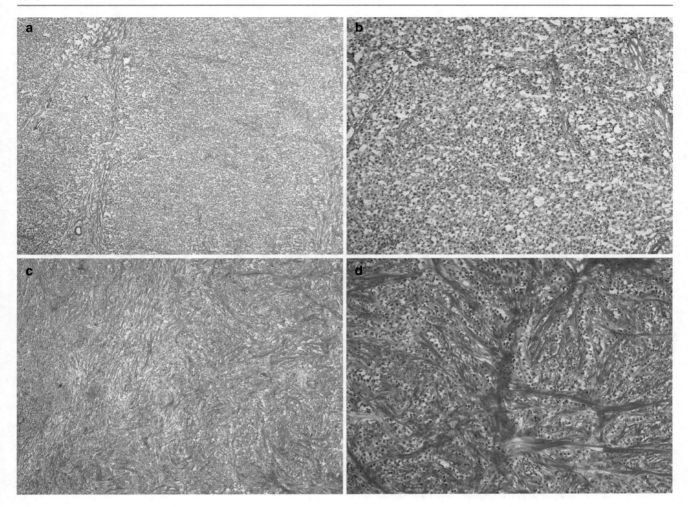

Fig. 9.2 Dysgerminoma, microscopic features. The tumor cells form solid sheets or nests, divided by fibrous septa with lymphocytic infiltrate (**a**, **b**). Marked stromal fibrosis and hyalinization may be seen (**c**, **d**). The tumor cells are relatively uniform, polygonal with prominent nucleoli and abundant eosinophilic or clear cytoplasm (**e**). Granulomatous reaction with multinucleated giant cells is present in some cases (**f**, **g**)

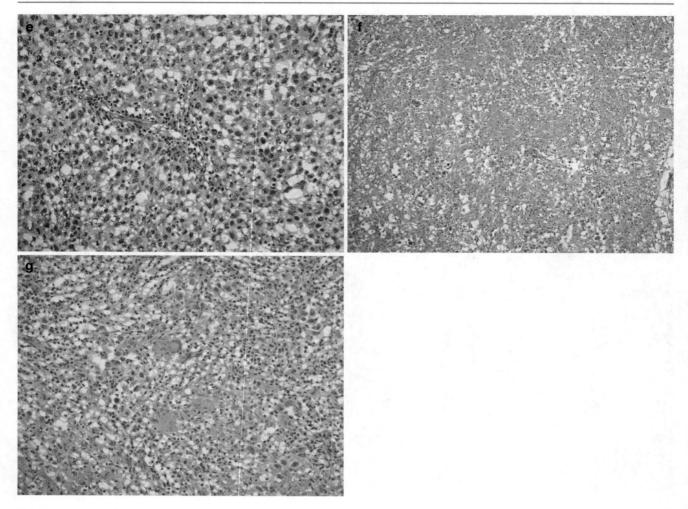

Fig. 9.2 (continued)

Yolk Sac Tumor (YST)

- Clinical features
  - Accounts for approximately 20 % of malignant germ cell tumors
  - Occurs during the 2nd and 3rd decades with a mean patient age of 16–19 years
  - Rapidly growing pelvic mass
  - Abdominal pain, may be due to torsion
  - Elevated serum alfa-fetoprotein (AFP)
- Gross pathology (Fig. 9.3)
  - Nearly always unilateral [10, 11].
  - Large tumors, usually more than 10 cm in diameter [11].
  - Cut surface is predominantly solid and tan-yellow, with areas of necrosis, hemorrhage, and cyst formation.
- Microscopic features (Fig. 9.4)
  - Various different microscopic growth patterns, often within the same tumor:
    - Reticular pattern: most common, composed of microcysts and anastomosing network of irregular luminal structures
    - Endodermal sinus pattern with characteristic peri-vascular Schiller-Duval bodies, only seen in approximately 20 % of cases
    - Solid pattern
    - Alveolar-glandular pattern
    - Other rare patterns: polyvesicular vitelline, hepatoid, papillary, and myxomatous
  - Cytoplasm may be clear or pale eosinophilic.
  - Eosinophilic cytoplasmic or extracellular hyaline globules are often present.
  - Intestinal differentiation may be seen with goblet cells and mucin production.
  - Moderate to marked nuclear pleomorphism with prominent nucleoli and frequent mitotic figures.
  - Loose, myxoid stroma is often prominent in areas with alveolar-glandular pattern.
  - Necrosis and hemorrhage are common.
- Differential diagnosis
  - Primary ovarian carcinomas
    - Endometrioid adenocarcinoma
    - Clear cell carcinoma
  - Other malignant germ cell tumors
    - Dysgerminoma
    - Embryonal carcinoma
    - Immature teratoma
  - Sertoli-Leydig cell tumor, especially retiform variant

- Diagnostic pitfalls/key intraoperative consultation issues
  - For intraoperative surgical management, the most important entities in the differential are primary ovarian—endometrioid and clear cell—carcinomas:
    - Typically require more extensive staging—tumor debulking—surgery.
    - Endometrioid and clear cell ovarian carcinomas usually affect older patients, but there is some overlap in patient age with YST.
    - Both endometrioid and clear cell carcinomas are more uniform architecturally and may be associated with endometriosis.
  - Examination of multiple tissue blocks is useful in identifying the various different growth patterns, characteristic of YST.
  - Hyaline globules are nonspecific and may be also seen in other entities in the differential, e.g., clear cell carcinoma.
  - Distinction between YST and other malignant germ cell tumors on frozen section is not critical for intraoperative management.
    - Other malignant germ cell tumors in the differential have essentially the same intraoperative management: fertility-preserving surgery (unilateral salpingo-oophorectomy with peritoneal biopsies and lymph node sampling) [1].
    - Dysgerminomas are more uniform than YST, both at the architectural and cytological level.

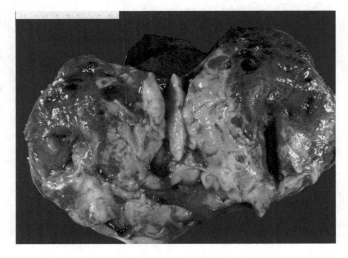

Fig. 9.3 Yolk sac tumor with a solid and cystic, tan-yellow cut surface

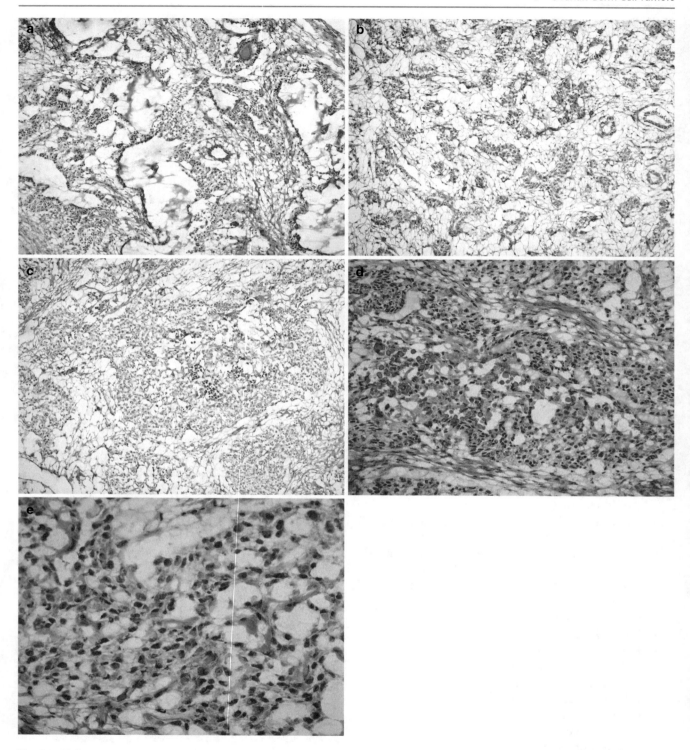

Fig. 9.4 Yolk sac tumor, microscopic features. The tumor shows various growth patterns, including reticular (**a**), alveolar-glandular (**b**), and solid architecture (**c**). The tumor cells have pleomorphic nuclei with prominent nucleoli and clear or pale eosinophilic cytoplasm containing hyaline globules (**d**, **e**)

Choriocarcinoma (Non-gestational)

- Clinical features
  - Rare tumor, less than 1 % of malignant germ cell tumors
  - Usually occurs in children and young adults
    - Rare case reports in postmenopausal patients [12, 13]
  - Symptoms may include:
    - Abdominal mass/pain, rarely hemoperitoneum
    - Isosexual pseudoprecocity
    - Vaginal bleeding
  - Elevated serum beta-hCG with positive pregnancy test
  - May mimic ectopic pregnancy clinically
- Gross pathology
  - Typically unilateral
  - Large tumor with solid and cystic cut surface, often with hemorrhage and necrosis
- Microscopic features
  - Bi- or triphasic appearance with sheets of mononuclear cytotrophoblast, intermediate-type trophoblast, and multinucleated syncytiotrophoblast.
  - Marked nuclear pleomorphism and frequent mitotic figures.
  - May be mixed with other malignant germ cell tumor components.
  - Necrosis and hemorrhage are often present.
- Differential diagnosis
  - Gestational choriocarcinoma
  - Other malignant germ cell tumors (e.g., dysgerminoma, embryonal carcinoma, YST) with isolated syncytiotrophoblastic giant cells
  - Poorly differentiated ovarian carcinomas (somatic, non-germ cell origin) with trophoblastic differentiation
- Diagnostic pitfalls/key intraoperative consultation issues
  - Distinction between choriocarcinoma and other malignant germ cell tumors on frozen section is not critical for intraoperative management.
  - Ovarian carcinomas of somatic origin with trophoblastic differentiation typically present in older patients, often postmenopausal, in contrast to choriocarcinoma.
    - Unlike choriocarcinoma, somatic (non-germ cell) ovarian carcinomas require aggressive surgery.
    - In postmenopausal patients—if the histological features are equivocal—additional tissue blocks may be sampled to help identifying the morphologically more typical somatic carcinoma component (e.g., poorly differentiated endometrioid adenocarcinoma), and a frozen section diagnosis of "carcinoma with probable trophoblastic differentiation" can be communicated.
  - Non-gestational (germ cell origin) and gestational choriocarcinomas are morphologically identical.
    - Gestational origin can be ruled out in preadolescent patients.
  - Distinction between the two pathogenetic entities is typically not crucial for intraoperative management.

Embryonal Carcinoma

- Clinical features
  - Very rare tumor
  - Occurs in young patients (<30 years of age), with a mean age of 15 years [14]
  - Clinical presentation may include:
    - Abdominal mass/pain
    - Isosexual pseudoprecocity
    - Vaginal bleeding
    - Elevated serum AFP and beta-hCG (positive pregnancy test)
- Gross pathology
  - Unilateral.
  - Mean tumor size is 15 cm.
  - Cut surface is solid tan-grey, often with foci of hemorrhage and necrosis.
- Microscopic features
  - Sheets of large, polygonal cells.
  - Pleomorphic, hyperchromatic nuclei with prominent nucleoli.
  - High mitotic activity and numerous apoptotic bodies.
  - Abundant, amphophilic cytoplasm.
  - Syncytiotrophoblastic giant cells are often present.
  - Necrosis and hemorrhage are common.
  - May be mixed with other malignant germ cell tumor components.
- Differential diagnosis
  - Other malignant germ cell tumors (e.g., dysgerminoma, choriocarcinoma, and YST)
  - Poorly differentiated ovarian carcinomas (somatic, non-germ cell origin)
- Diagnostic pitfalls/key intraoperative consultation issues
  - Distinction between embryonal carcinoma and other malignant germ cell tumors on frozen section is not critical for intraoperative management.
    - The tumor cells in dysgerminoma are more uniform, and characteristic fibrovascular septae with lymphocytic infiltrate are present.
    - YST typically shows various growth patterns, compared to the relatively homogeneous morphology of embryonal carcinoma.
  - Poorly differentiated ovarian carcinomas of somatic (non-germ cell) origin typically present in older patients—often postmenopausal—in contrast to embryonal carcinoma and require extensive staging surgery.

Mixed Germ Cell Tumor

- Occurs in children and young adults.
- Admixture of two or more types of malignant germ cell tumors.
  - Most common combination is dysgerminoma and yolk sac tumor, but any combination of tumor types may occur.
- Precise identification of different histological components of a mixed germ cell tumor is most important for adjuvant therapy and prognostication; however, it is not critical for intraoperative management, and a frozen section diagnosis of "malignant germ cell tumor, favor/probable mixed components" is usually sufficient.

Teratomas

Mature Teratoma/Mature Cystic Teratoma/Dermoid Cyst

- Clinical features
  - Very common, accounting for up to 44 % of all ovarian tumors [15, 16] and over 95 % of ovarian teratomas
  - May occur at any age, but most commonly during the reproductive years
  - May be asymptomatic or presents with pelvic mass/pain
  - May undergo torsion
  - Often an incidental finding—on imaging studies or during unrelated surgery
  - Rarely may be associated with autoimmune hemolytic anemia or encephalitis (anti-N-methyl-D-aspartate (NMDA) receptor encephalitis)
- Gross pathology (Fig. 9.5)
  - Bilateral in 10–15 % of cases.
  - Almost always cystic—usually unilocular cyst filled with sebaceous material (typically still liquid at the time of frozen section) and hair.
    - Solid nodule (Rokitansky protuberance) is also commonly present.
    - Rare tumors may be entirely solid—*mature solid teratoma.*
  - Average tumor size is between 5 and 10 cm.
  - Approximately one-third of cases show well-formed teeth, usually arising from the Rokitansky protuberance [17].
    - Rare cases with a fetus-like structure have also been described (fetiform teratoma, homunculus) [18, 19].

- Sampling for frozen section should focus on solid areas, including the Rokitansky protuberance.
  - One block is usually sufficient for frozen section, unless unusual gross features are noted.
- Microscopic features (Fig. 9.6)
  - Admixture of tissues from all three germ cell layers, usually with ectodermal predominance.
  - Ectoderm:
    - Cyst lining is keratinizing squamous epithelium with abundant adnexal structures—sebaceous and eccrine glands and hair follicles.
    - Brain/neural tissues—glial tissue, ganglia, cerebellar, retinal and/or ependymal tissue, and choroid plexus.
  - Mesoderm:
    - Adipose tissue—may have associated histiocytic (lipogranulomatous) reaction
    - Cartilage, bone, and smooth muscle
  - Endoderm:
    - Gastrointestinal and respiratory-type epithelium
    - Salivary gland tissue
    - Thyroid tissue
  - Foreign body giant cell reaction may be seen in adjacent ovarian tissue or within the tumor as a reaction to the tumor contents, i.e., keratin and hair shaft.
  - May rarely be associated with a mucinous neoplasm—benign cystadenoma, borderline/atypical proliferative mucinous tumor, and mucinous carcinoma.
- Differential diagnosis
  - Immature teratoma
  - Monodermal teratomas (struma ovarii, carcinoid tumor)
  - Secondary, somatic-type malignancy arising in a mature teratoma
- Diagnostic pitfalls/key intraoperative consultation issues
  - Some neural elements, especially cerebellar, retinal, or ependymal tissue, in a mature teratoma may mimic the primitive/immature neuroepithelial tissue of immature teratomas.
  - Foci of choroid plexus may mimic a papillary neoplasm.
  - In cases with paraneoplastic encephalitis (anti-NMDA receptor encephalitis), the surgeon may request margin evaluation if a partial oophorectomy/cystectomy is performed in a young patient.
  - Adequate sampling of solid areas—particularly in large tumors—is important to rule out an immature teratoma or a secondary malignancy arising in a mature teratoma.

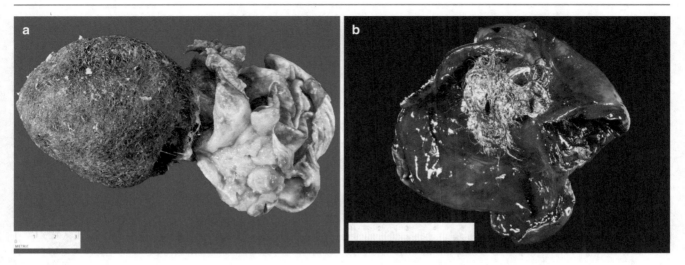

Fig. 9.5 Mature cystic teratoma (dermoid cyst). The cut surface typically shows a unilocular cyst filled with hair and sebaceous material. Solid areas may also be present (**a**, *right side of image*). Hemorrhagic infarction may be seen as a result of torsion (**b**)

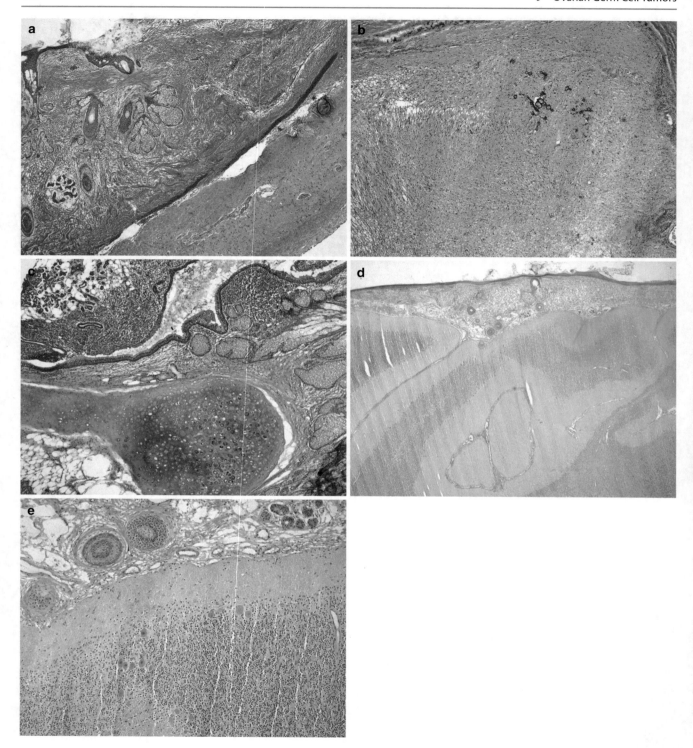

Fig. 9.6 Mature cystic teratoma (dermoid cyst). The tumor shows admixture of tissues from all three germ cell layers: the cyst lining is keratinizing squamous epithelium with abundant sebaceous glands and other skin adnexal structures (**a**, *upper left side of image*). Mature glial tissue is often present (**a**, *lower right side of image*; **b**) and may contain calcifications (**b**). Respiratory-type epithelium and cartilage are also common (**c**). Mature cerebellar tissue with numerous small and large neuronal cells (**d**, **e**) may mimic immature neuroepithelial tissue

Immature Teratoma

- Clinical features
  - Rare tumor representing 1–3 % of all teratomas and approximately 20–30 % of malignant germ cell tumors [20, 21]
  - Occurs in children and young adults, most commonly during the first two decades of life
  - Presents with pelvic mass/pain, which may be related to torsion
  - Elevated serum AFP—lower level than YST
- Gross pathology (Fig. 9.7)
  - Usually unilateral, but the contralateral ovary may have mature teratoma in 10–15 % of cases.
  - Mean tumor size is 18 cm [22].
  - Cut surface is solid and cystic.
    - Cystic areas often contain hair and sebaceous material, similar to dermoid cysts.
    - Solid areas are tan-yellow and fleshy, usually corresponding to immature neural tissue.
  - Hemorrhage and necrosis may be grossly apparent.
- Microscopic features (Fig. 9.8)
  - Immature—embryonal-appearing—tissues of neuroepithelial/neuroectodermal type, composed of small uniform blue cells forming primitive rosettes and tubules.
    - Numerous apoptotic bodies and frequent mitotic figures
  - Immature epithelial and mesenchymal elements (e.g., cartilage and skeletal muscle) are also common.
  - Mature tissues are commonly admixed with the immature elements.
  - Implants/metastases from immature teratoma may consist entirely of mature glial tissues.

- Immature teratoma is also a frequent component of mixed germ cell tumors (see above).
  - Necrosis may be seen.
- Differential diagnosis
  - Mature teratoma (cystic or solid)
  - Yolk sac tumor with hepatoid or glandular differentiation
  - Carcinosarcoma (malignant mixed Mullerian tumor)
- Diagnostic pitfalls/key intraoperative consultation issues
  - Some neural elements of mature teratomas, especially cerebellar, retinal, or ependymal tissue, may mimic the primitive/immature neuroepithelial tissue of immature teratomas.
  - Immature mesenchymal and endodermal elements are more difficult to distinguish from their mature forms, especially on frozen section.
    - Diagnosis of immature teratoma should always rely on identification of immature neuroectodermal/neuroepithelial tissues.
  - Distinction between YST and immature teratoma is not critical on frozen section, as their intraoperative surgical management is similar.
  - Carcinosarcomas usually present in an older age group—most often postmenopausal—while immature teratomas virtually never occur after the menopause.
    - Immature teratomas have a much greater heterogeneity in terms of tissue types from all three germ cell layers and degree of maturation.
    - Carcinosarcomas usually have predominance of carcinomatous component with marked nuclear pleomorphism, which is not a typical feature of immature teratomas.

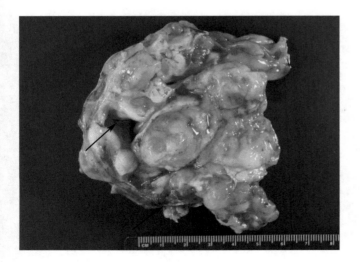

Fig. 9.7 Immature teratoma with a cystic and solid, tan fleshy cut surface. Note the presence of hair in the cystic areas (*arrows*)

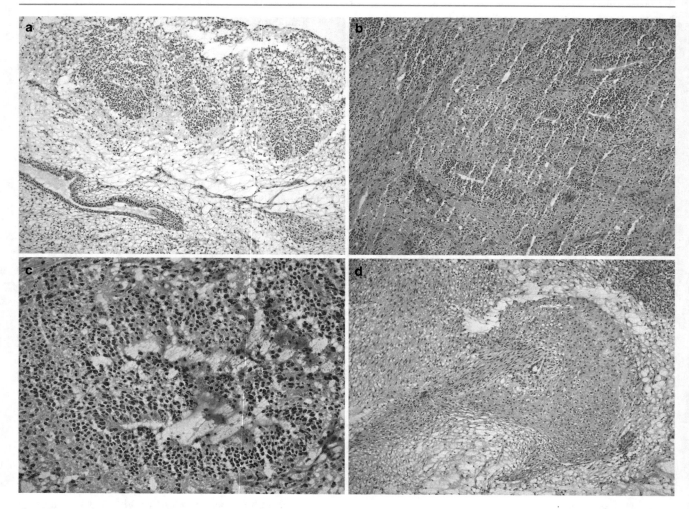

Fig. 9.8 Immature teratoma. The tumor characteristically contains immature neuroepithelium forming primitive tubules and rosettes (**a**, **b**), composed of small blue cells with scant cytoplasm and numerous mitotic figures and apoptotic bodies (**c**). Immature mesenchymal elements, including cartilage, are also common (**d**)

Monodermal Teratomas

Struma Ovarii

- Clinical features
  - Most common type of monodermal teratoma, representing approximately 3 % of ovarian teratomas [23].
  - Patients present at a wide age range, though most commonly during the reproductive years [15, 23].
  - May present with abdominal pain or as a mass lesion.
  - Ascites may be associated, but it does not indicate malignant behavior [24].
  - Hyperfunction of the thyroid tissue may occur.
- Gross pathology (Fig. 9.9)
  - Usually unilateral.
  - Tumor size is typically less than 10 cm.
  - Cut surface may show admixture of solid and cystic areas or may entirely be solid or cystic.
  - Solid areas are tan-brown or reddish-brown, glistening, similar to eutopic thyroid tissue.
- Microscopic features (Fig. 9.10)
  - Tumor is composed predominantly or entirely of thyroid tissue.
    - Up to 20 % of mature ovarian teratomas (dermoid cysts) contain thyroid tissue.
  - Variably sized thyroid follicles filled with thick eosinophilic colloid.
    - Architectural pattern may be macrofollicular, microfollicular, tubular ("sertoliform"), or cystic.
    - Calcium-oxalate crystals may be seen within the colloid.
    - Colloid material is prone to frozen artifacts—folding and "bubbles."
  - Uniform cells with round nuclei and large eosinophilic—or rarely clear—cytoplasm.
  - No significant nuclear atypia or mitotic activity.
  - May be admixed with carcinoid tumor: strumal carcinoid.
- Differential diagnosis
  - Serous cystadenoma
  - Primary ovarian carcinomas—endometrioid and clear cell

- Sertoli-Leydig cell tumor
- Carcinoid tumor
- Adult granulosa cell tumor
- Metastatic thyroid carcinoma
- Diagnostic pitfalls/key intraoperative consultation issues
  - Most struma ovarii are benign and removal of the affected ovary is sufficient.
    - Rare cases may show aggressive behavior with extraovarian spread [25].
      - A subset of them are histologically *papillary thyroid carcinoma*—arising in struma ovarii—with the same characteristic morphologic features as papillary thyroid carcinoma of the thyroid gland and should be reported on the frozen section as such.
      - Other cases may resemble follicular adenomas or normal thyroid tissue; however, the histological features cannot reliably predict malignant behavior [26].
  - Follicles of struma ovarii may resemble the glandular proliferation of endometrioid adenocarcinoma.
    - Endometrioid adenocarcinomas often show at least moderate nuclear atypia, increased mitotic activity, and squamous metaplasia.
    - Identification of adjacent other teratomatous elements (dermoid cyst) is helpful to confirm struma ovarii.
  - Carcinoid tumors lack colloid material and typically have less cytoplasm than thyroid epithelial cells.
    - Distinction between struma ovarii and carcinoid tumor is generally not crucial on frozen section, as almost all insular, trabecular, and strumal carcinoid tumors are clinically benign.
  - Metastasis from a primary thyroid carcinoma to the ovary is extremely rare, and the most helpful hints at the time of frozen section are:
    - Clinical history of known thyroid cancer
      - Slides from the known thyroid primary should be reviewed and the histological features should be compared.
    - Identification of adjacent other teratomatous elements (dermoid cyst)

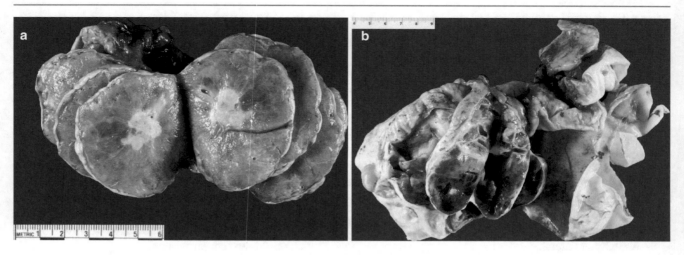

Fig. 9.9 Struma ovarii may have a solid (**a**) or predominantly cystic (**b**), tan-brown or red, glistening gross appearance

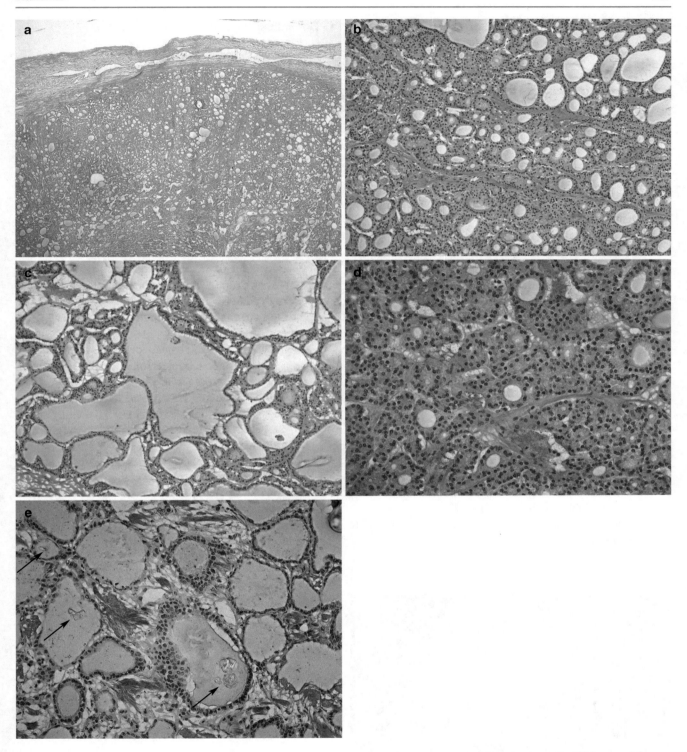

Fig. 9.10 Struma ovarii. Note the characteristic micro- and macrofollicular pattern, composed of variably sized thyroid follicles with dense eosinophilic intraluminal colloid (**a–c**). The cells have uniform, round nuclei and abundant eosinophilic cytoplasm (**d**). Calcium-oxalate crystals may be seen within the colloid (**e**, *arrows*)

Carcinoid Tumor

- Clinical features
  - Patients' age at presentation ranges from 14 to 79 years with a mean age of 53 years [8].
  - Often an incidental finding.
  - Approximately one-third of patients have clinical carcinoid syndrome [27, 28].
- Gross pathology (Fig. 9.11)
  - Unilateral.
  - Size may be from microscopic to over 20 cm [28–30].
  - Cut surface is solid, tan-yellow, or may be cystic if associated with a dermoid cyst or a mucinous cystic neoplasm.
- Microscopic features (Fig. 9.12)
  - Three histological subtypes
    - Insular:
      - Most common type, composed of solid nests or small, round acini.
      - Uniform, small, round nuclei with finely stippled chromatin.
      - Mitotic activity is typically low.
      - Moderate amount of eosinophilic cytoplasm.
      - Fibrous stroma, which is often dense and hyalinized.
    - Trabecular:
      - Tumor cells form ribbons and thin trabeculae, separated by fibrous stroma.
    - Mucinous (goblet cell):
      - Tumor cells are arranged in small glands, sometimes "floating" in extracellular mucin.
      - Variable number of goblet cells.
  - May be associated with dermoid cyst or mucinous neoplasm.

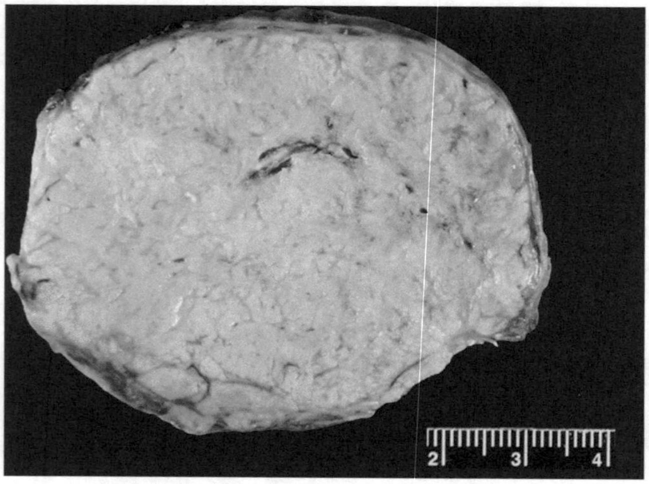

- Differential diagnosis
  - Metastatic carcinoid tumor
  - Adult granulosa cell tumor
  - Sertoli-Leydig cell tumor
  - Endometrioid adenocarcinoma
  - Struma ovarii
  - Metastatic signet-ring cell carcinoma
- Diagnostic pitfalls/key intraoperative consultation issues
  - Features in favor of metastatic carcinoid tumor include bilaterality, multinodular involvement of the ovary, extraovarian disease, and clinical history of known carcinoid tumor (usually in the gastrointestinal tract).
    - Comparison with the histological features of prior known carcinoid tumor may be helpful.
  - Identification of associated dermoid cyst, mucinous tumor, or struma ovarii supports the diagnosis of primary ovarian carcinoid tumor.
    - Cystic areas should be included for frozen section sampling.
  - Acini within the solid nests of an insular carcinoid tumor may mimic the microfollicular pattern of adult granulosa cell tumor (AGCT).
    - Carcinoid tumors have round nuclei with smooth nuclear membranes, in contrast to the elongated or oval-shaped, irregular nuclei with longitudinal grooves in AGCT.
  - Endometrioid adenocarcinomas have more significant nuclear pleomorphism, glandular growth with larger luminal spaces, and often squamous differentiation.
  - Mucinous (goblet cell) carcinoid may mimic metastatic signet-ring cell carcinoma.

Fig. 9.11 Carcinoid tumor has a characteristic solid, yellow cut surface

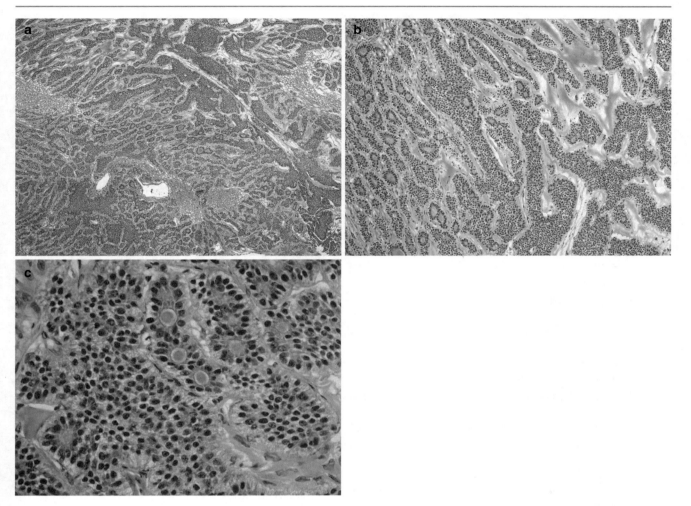

Fig. 9.12 Carcinoid tumor with insular pattern. The tumor cells are arranged in solid nests and small acini in the background of hyalinized stroma (**a**, **b**) and show characteristic uniform, round nuclei with finely stippled chromatin pattern (**c**)

Somatic Malignancy Arising in Mature Teratoma

- Clinical features
  - Malignant transformation of mature teratoma is rare, occurring in 1–2 % of cases [15, 31, 32].
  - Most common in postmenopausal patients.
  - May present as a rapidly growing mass or may be an incidental finding.
- Gross pathology (Fig. 9.13)
  - Usually large, mean tumor size is 7 cm [32].
  - Cut surface is typically cystic and solid, with the solid area representing the malignant component often with necrosis and hemorrhage.
    - Hair and sebaceous material are often seen in the cystic component and are helpful in identifying the associated teratoma.
    - Malignant melanoma arising in a dermoid cyst usually shows characteristic pigmentation.
- Microscopic features (Figs. 9.14, 9.15, and 9.16)
  - Most common histological type is squamous cell carcinoma, accounting for approximately 80 % of cases [31, 33].
  - Less commonly mucinous adenocarcinoma, malignant melanoma, and rarely sarcomas (e.g., leiomyosarcoma, chondrosarcoma) may also arise in a dermoid cyst [8].
  - Morphologic features of tumors are similar to those of presenting at other sites.
- Differential diagnosis
  - Metastatic tumors
  - Primary ovarian carcinomas (not associated with a teratoma)
    - Endometrioid, clear cell, and mucinous carcinoma
- Diagnostic pitfalls/key intraoperative consultation issues
  - Associated teratoma component and lack of other known primary strongly favor malignancy arising in a teratoma.
    - Unlike metastatic tumors, teratomas with malignant transformation require full surgical staging [34].

- Carcinomas and melanoma arising in association with a teratoma may also mimic other primary ovarian carcinomas, i.e., endometrioid, clear cell, and mucinous carcinoma, especially if the underlying teratoma is not recognized grossly and microscopically.
- No significant impact on the immediate surgical management, staging procedure is typically performed in both scenarios.

Mixed Germ Cell and Sex-Cord Stromal Tumors

Gonadoblastoma

- Clinical features
  - Very rare tumor in young patients under 30 years of age, almost always occurs in dysgenetic gonads.
  - Most patients with gonadoblastoma are phenotypic females but almost always have an abnormal (46XY or 45X/46XY) karyotype [6, 7].
- Gross pathology
  - Usually small, measuring less than 8 cm [35, 36]
- Microscopic features
  - Admixture of germ cells and sex-cord type cells, resembling immature Sertoli or granulosa cells.
  - Small, round acini, filled with eosinophilic material.
  - Mitotic activity may be noticeable.
  - Calcification is common.
- Differential diagnosis
  - Dysgerminoma
  - Sex-cord tumor with annular tubules
- Diagnostic pitfalls/key intraoperative consultation issues
  - Pure gonadoblastoma is benign; however, it may give rise to dysgerminoma in approximately 50 % of cases [35, 36].
    - Bilateral oophorectomy is typically performed, due to associated gonadal dysgenesis and risk of malignancy.

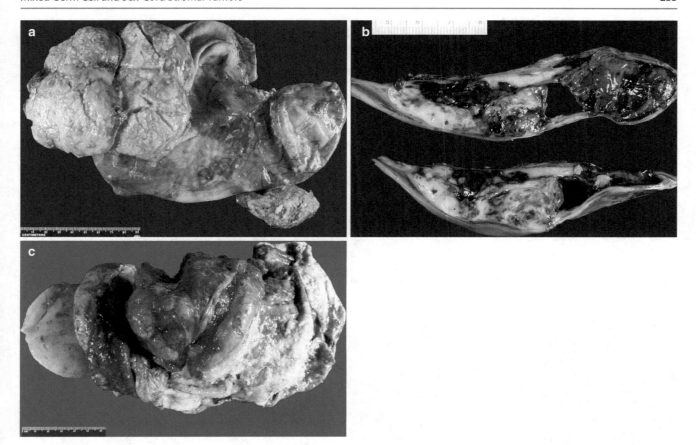

Fig. 9.13 Somatic malignancies arising in mature teratoma. Squamous cell carcinoma presents as an intracystic solid nodule with a tan-pink, gritty cut surface (**a**, *left upper corner of image*). Note the cyst contents—hair and sebaceous material (**a**, right lower corner of image). Melanoma arising in mature teratoma shows dark brown-black pigmentation (**b**). Mucinous carcinoma associated with mature teratoma shows a solid, glistening cut surface with rare hair and sebaceous material (**c**, *right side of image*)

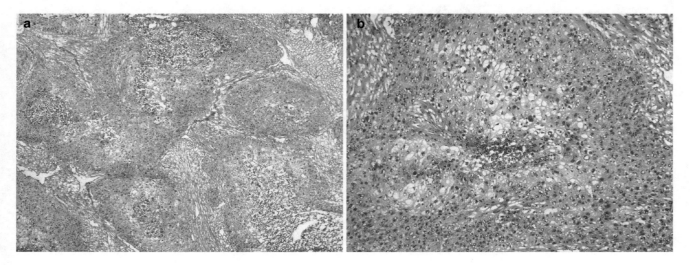

Fig. 9.14 Squamous cell carcinoma arising in mature teratoma (**a, b**). Note the large solid nests of pleomorphic tumor cells with abundant eosinophilic or clear cytoplasm and central necrosis

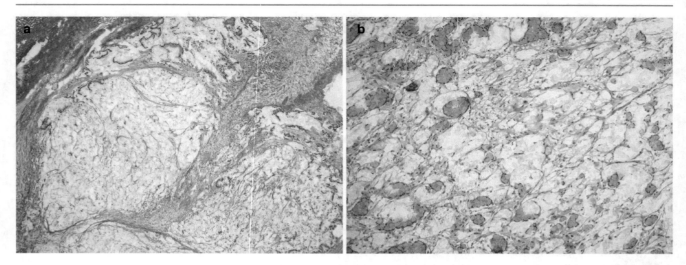

Fig. 9.15 Mucinous adenocarcinoma arising in mature teratoma (**a**, **b**). Note the presence of goblet cells and abundant extracellular mucin dissecting the ovarian stroma

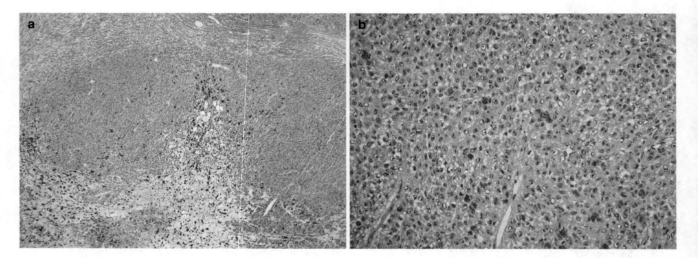

Fig. 9.16 Melanoma arising in mature teratoma. The tumor shows solid nests of epithelioid tumor cells with necrosis (**a**). The nuclei are markedly atypical with prominent eosinophilic nucleoli, and the cytoplasm is abundant, containing brown melanin pigment (**b**)

References

1. Eskander RN, Randall LM, Berman ML, Tewari KS, Disala PJ, Bristwo RE. Fertility preserving options in patients with gynecologic malignancies. Am J Obstet Gynecol. 2011;205:103–10.

2. Liu Q, Ding X, Yang J, Cao D, Shen K, Lang J, et al. The significance of comprehensive staging surgery in malignant ovarian germ cell tumors. Gynecol Oncol. 2013;131:551–4.

3. Gershenson DM. Fertility-sparing surgery for malignancies in women. J Natl Cancer Inst Monogr. 2005;34:43–7

4. Schwartz PE. Surgery of germ cell tumours of the ovary. Forum (Genova). 2000;10:355–65.

5. Evans KN, Taylor H, Zehnder D, Kilby MD, Bulmer JN, Shah F, et al. Increased expression of 25-hydroxyvitamin D-1alpha-hydroxylase in dysgerminomas: a novel form of humoral hypercalcemia of malignancy. Am J Pathol. 2004;165:807–13.

6. Joki-Erkkila MM, Karikoski R, Rantala I, Lenko HL, Visakorpi T, Heinonen PK. Gonadoblastoma and dysgerminoma associated with XY gonadal dysgenesis in an adolescent with chronic renal failure: a case of Frasier syndrome. J Pediatr Adolesc Gynecol. 2002;15:145–9.

7. Hanlon AJ, Kimble RM. Incidental gonadal tumors at the time of gonadectomy in women with Swyer Syndrome: a case series. J Pediatr Adolesc Gynecol. 2015;28:e27–9.

8. Kurman RJ, Carcanglu ML, Herrington CS, Young RH. WHO classification of tumours of female reproductive organs. 4th ed. Lyon: International Agency for Research on Cancer (IARC); 2014.

9. Billmire DF. Malignant germ cell tumors in childhood. Semin Pediatr Surg. 2006;15:30–6.

10. Gershenson DM, Del Junco G, Herson J, Rutledge FN. Endodermal sinus tumor of the ovary: the M. D. Anderson experience. Obstet Gynecol. 1983;61:194–202.

11. Kurman RJ, Norris HJ. Endodermal sinus tumor of the ovary: a clinical and pathologic analysis of 71 cases. Cancer. 1976;38:2404–19.

12. Park SH, Park A, Kim JY, Kwon JH, Koh SB. A case of non-gestational choriocarcinoma arising in the ovary of a postmenopausal woman. J Gynecol Oncol. 2009;20:192–4.

13. Hirabayashi K, Yasuda M, Osamura RY, Hirasawa T, Murakami M. Ovarian nongestational choriocarcinoma mixed with various epithelial malignancies in association with endometriosis. Gynecol Oncol. 2006;102:111–7.

14. Kurman RJ, Norris HJ. Embryonal carcinoma of the ovary: a clinicopathologic entity distinct from endodermal sinus tumor resembling embryonal carcinoma of the adult testis. Cancer. 1976;38:2420–33.

15. Roth LM, Talerman A. Recent advances in the pathology and classification of ovarian germ cell tumors. Int J Gynecol Pathol. 2006;25:305–20.

16. Koonings PP, Campbell K, Mishell Jr DR, Grimes DA. Relative frequency of primary ovarian neoplasms: a 10-year review. Obstet Gynecol. 1989;74:921–6.

17. Blackwell WJ, Dockerty MB, et al. Dermoid cysts of the ovary: their clinical and pathologic significance. Am J Obstet Gynecol. 1946;51:151–72.

18. Abbott TM, Hermann Jr WJ, Scully RE. Ovarian fetiform teratoma (homunculus) in a 9-year-old girl. Int J Gynecol Pathol. 1984;2:392–402.

19. Weldon-Linne CM, Rushovich AM. Benign ovarian cystic teratomas with homunculi. Obstet Gynecol. 1983;61:88S–94.

20. Gershenson DM, del Junco G, Silva EG, Copeland LJ, Wharton JT, Rutledge FN. Immature teratoma of the ovary. Obstet Gynecol. 1986;68:624–9.

21. Smith HO, Berwick M, Verschraegen CF, Wiggins C, Lansing L, Muller CY, Qualls CR. Incidence and survival rates for female malignant germ cell tumors. Obstet Gynecol. 2006;107:1075–85.

22. Norris HJ, Zirkin HJ, Benson WL. Immature (malignant) teratoma of the ovary: a clinical and pathologic study of 58 cases. Cancer. 1976;37:2359–72.

23. Woodruff JD, Rauh JT, Markley RL. Ovarian struma. Obstet Gynecol. 1966;27:194–201.

24. Smith FC. Pathology and physiology of struma ovarii. Arch Surg. 1946;53:603–26.

25. Robboy SJ, Shaco-Levy R, Peng RY, Snyder MJ, Donahue J, Bentley RC, et al. Malignant struma ovarii: an analysis of 88 cases, including 27 with extraovarian spread. Int J Gynecol Pathol. 2009;28:405–22.

26. Shaco-Levy R, Peng RY, Snyder MJ, Osmond GW, Veras E, Bean SM, et al. Malignant struma ovarii: a blinded study of 86 cases assessing which histologic features correlate with aggressive clinical behavior. Arch Pathol Lab Med. 2012;136:172–8.

27. Davis KP, Hartmann LK, Keeney GL, Shapiro H. Primary ovarian carcinoid tumors. Gynecol Oncol. 1996;61:259–65.

28. Robboy SJ, Norris HJ, Scully RE. Insular carcinoid primary in the ovary. A clinicopathologic analysis of 48 cases. Cancer. 1975;36:404–18.

29. Soga J, Osaka M, Yakuwa Y. Carcinoids of the ovary: an analysis of 329 reported cases. J Exp Clin Cancer Res. 2000;19:271–80.

30. Talerman A, Evans MI. Primary trabecular carcinoid tumor of the ovary. Cancer. 1982;50:1403–7.

31. Stamp GW, McConnell EM. Malignancy arising in cystic ovarian teratomas. A report of 24 cases. Br J Obstet Gynaecol. 1983;90:671–5.

32. Ayhan A, Bukulmez O, Genc C, Karamursel BS, Ayhan A. Mature cystic teratomas of the ovary: case series from one institution over 34 years. Eur J Obstet Gynecol Reprod Biol. 2000;88:153–7.

33. Hirakawa T, Tsuneyoshi M, Enjoji M. Squamous cell carcinoma arising in mature cystic teratoma of the ovary. Clinicopathologic and topographic analysis. Am J Surg Pathol. 1989;13:397–405.

34. Choi EJ, Koo YJ, Jeon JH, Kim TJ, Lee KH, Lim KT. Clinical experience in ovarian squamous cell carcinoma arising from mature cystic teratoma: a rare entity. Obstet Gynecol Sci. 2014;57:274–80.

35. Scully RE. Gonadoblastoma. A review of 74 cases. Cancer. 1970;25:1340–56.

36. Talerman A, Roth LM. Recent advances in the pathology and classification of gonadal neoplasms composed of germ cells and sex cord derivatives. Int J Gynecol Pathol. 2007;26:313–21.

Ovarian Sex Cord-Stromal Tumors

10

Introduction

Sex cord-stromal tumors represent the third group of ovarian tumors in decreasing order of frequency, with approximately 5–10 % of cases falling within this category. The most common entity among these tumors—ovarian fibroma—is readily recognized on frozen sections by a general surgical pathologist; however, other sex cord-stromal tumors may present a significant challenge due to their diverse morphology. In addition, unlike in other tumor types, the biological behavior of sex cord-stromal tumors is usually not directly linked to their microscopic degree of pleomorphism or cytological atypia. As an example, most adult granulosa cell tumors have uniform nuclei and relatively low mitotic activity, despite their locally aggressive behavior and overall 20–30 % recurrence rate. Similarly, the nuclear atypia may not be obvious in juvenile granulosa cell tumors and in biologically aggressive forms of Sertoli-Leydig cell tumors. While histological subtyping of primary ovarian epithelial malignancies on frozen section is typically not necessary and may be deferred for permanent sections, mere identification of an ovarian tumor as sex cord-stromal in origin, without recognition of the specific entity, is not sufficient for predicting outcome and guiding intraoperative management.

Endocrine/hormonal manifestations—estrogenic or androgenic—are relatively frequent in these tumors compared with other groups of ovarian neoplasms and may be helpful in the differential diagnosis at the time of frozen section.

© Springer International Publishing Switzerland 2015
P. Hui, N. Buza, *Atlas of Intraoperative Frozen Section Diagnosis in Gynecologic Pathology*,
DOI 10.1007/978-3-319-21807-6_10

Fibroma

- Clinical features
  - Most common pure ovarian stromal tumor.
  - Most often occurs in middle-aged patients (mean 48 years).
  - May be associated with ascites, or rarely both ascites and pleural effusion—Meigs syndrome—in approximately 1 % of cases [1, 2].
    - Ascites is more common in tumors >10 cm.
  - May occur in patients with Gorlin syndrome (nevoid basal cell carcinoma syndrome) [3].
  - May present with acute abdominal pain due to torsion [4].
- Gross pathology (Fig. 10.1)
  - Mean tumor size is 6.8 cm [5].
  - Up to 8 % of cases are bilateral, mostly those that are associated with Gorlin syndrome.
  - Smooth ovarian surface.
  - Cut surface is solid, firm, white, or tan.
  - Hemorrhage and necrosis may be present, due to torsion.
- Microscopic features (Fig. 10.2)
  - Intersecting bundles/fascicles of spindle cells.
  - Storiform pattern, hyalinization, collagen bands, or plaques are often present.
  - Cellularity is variable.
    - Approximately 10 % of cases show dense cellularity and are designated as *cellular fibroma* [6, 7].
  - Edema, hemorrhage, and hemorrhagic infarction may be seen due to torsion.
  - Nuclear atypia is absent or mild.
  - Low mitotic activity (≤3/10 high power field (HPF)).
    - Cellular tumors with mitotic activity of ≥4/10 HPF and no more than mild atypia have been termed *mitotically active cellular fibroma* [7].
  - No atypical mitotic figures.
  - Minor sex cord elements—granulosa cells or sertoliform tubules—may be present (<10 % of tumor on any slide) [8].

- Differential diagnosis
  - Metastatic signet-ring cell tumors (Krukenberg tumor)
  - Adult granulosa cell tumor
  - Fibrosarcoma
  - Thecoma
  - Stromal hyperplasia/stromal hyperthecosis
- Diagnostic pitfalls/key intraoperative consultation issues
  - The most clinically relevant differential diagnoses are adult granulosa cell tumor and metastatic carcinomas with reactive ovarian stromal proliferation.
  - Presence of minor sex cord elements (<10 % of tumor) has not been reported to have clinical significance in an otherwise typical fibroma.
    - Thorough sampling with additional blocks for frozen section is recommended to rule out an adult granulosa cell tumor or Sertoli-Leydig cell tumor.
  - Adult granulosa cell tumors may show a spindle-cell, "sarcomatoid" morphology, mimicking a fibroma/cellular fibroma.
    - Characteristic nuclear features of adult granulosa cell tumors—irregular nuclear membranes with nuclear grooves—may be difficult to appreciate due to frozen section artifact.
    - Identification of other morphologic patterns of adult granulosa cell tumor (i.e., insular, trabecular, or microfollicular) can be helpful—additional blocks may be sampled for frozen section.
  - Krukenberg tumor must be ruled out by careful microscopic examination.
    - Bilaterality should raise suspicion for metastasis, although up to 8 % of fibromas may be bilateral.
    - Scattered individual metastatic tumor cells with signet-ring or breast lobular carcinoma morphology may be missed on low magnification in a reactive/hyperplastic ovarian stroma.
  - Ovarian fibrosarcoma shows at least moderate nuclear atypia and increased mitotic activity (≥4/10 HPF), often with atypical mitotic figures.
  - Distinction between fibroma and other benign entities—thecoma, stromal hyperplasia/stromal hyperthecosis is not crucial at the time of frozen section.

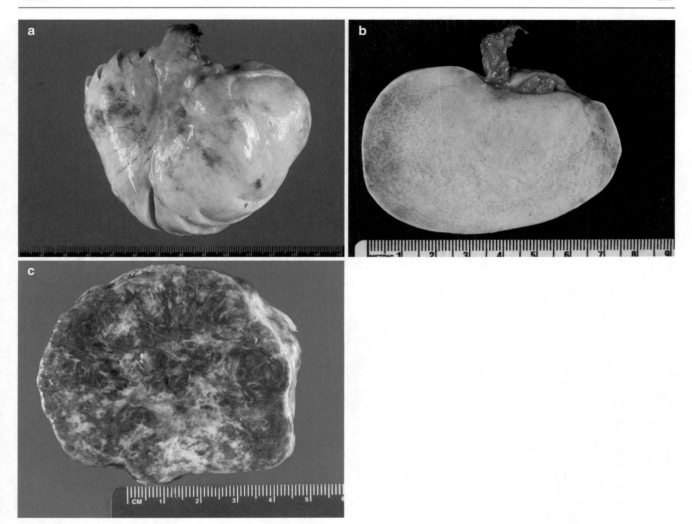

Fig. 10.1 Fibroma. The ovarian surface is smooth and glistening (**a**). The cut surface is solid, firm, tan white (**b**) and may also be hemorrhagic due to torsion (**c**)

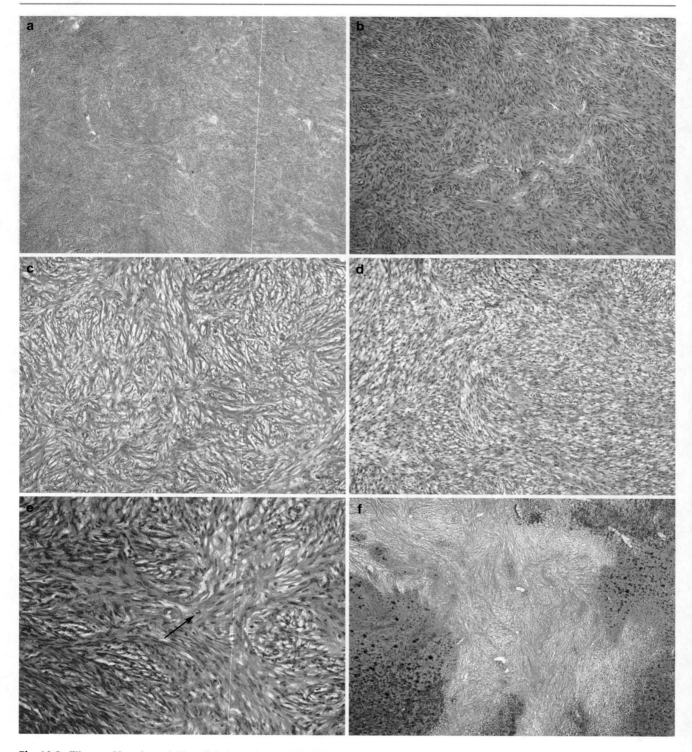

Fig. 10.2 Fibroma. Note the variable cellularity and stromal hyalinization (**a**, **b**). The spindled tumor cells are arranged in a storiform pattern (**c**) or form intersecting fascicles (**d**). Mitotic figures may be seen (**e**, *arrow*). Hemorrhagic infarction of fibroma due to torsion (**f**) is not uncommon

Thecoma

- Clinical features
  - Uncommon ovarian tumor.
  - Typically occurs in postmenopausal women.
  - May show symptoms associated with hormone production (most often estrogenic).
  - *Luteinized thecomas* tend to occur in younger (premenopausal) patients and may produce androgens [9].
- Gross pathology
  - Most often unilateral.
  - Average size is 5–10 cm.
  - Cut surface is solid, yellow, but may contain white areas.
- Microscopic features (Fig. 10.3)
  - Sheets composed of oval or round cells.
  - Moderate to abundant amount of pale eosinophilic cytoplasm.
  - Atypia is absent or minimal.
  - Mitoses are rare.
  - Hyalin plaques and focal calcifications may be seen.
  - May contain clusters of luteinized cells with pink or clear cytoplasm.
  - Areas resembling a fibroma are not uncommon; these tumors can be designated as *fibrothecoma*.
- Differential diagnosis
  - Adult granulosa cell tumor
  - Sertoli-Leydig cell tumor
  - Fibroma
  - Steroid cell tumor
  - Leydig cell tumor
  - Stromal-Leydig cell tumor
  - Stromal hyperplasia/stromal hyperthecosis
- Diagnostic pitfalls/key intraoperative consultation issues
  - The most clinically relevant differential diagnosis is adult granulosa cell tumor, which typically requires complete surgical staging.
    - Adult granulosa cell tumors may show luteinization, closely resembling thecomas/luteinized thecomas, and on frozen sections—without the help of ancillary studies—the distinction between the two entities may be very difficult.
    - In such cases, the frozen section slide could be interpreted as "sex cord-stromal tumor with luteinization," and the diagnosis could be deferred for permanent sections to avoid overdiagnosis.
  - Luteinized cells in thecomas may raise the possibility of a Leydig cell or Sertoli-Leydig cell tumor. While distinction between a Leydig cell tumor and a luteinized thecoma is not critical at the time of frozen section, identification of a Sertoli cell component is important, as a surgical staging procedure is typically performed for Sertoli-Leydig cell tumors [10]
    - Presence of intracytoplasmic Reinke crystals—which may be better preserved on frozen sections than on permanent sections after formalin fixation—confirms Leydig cells
  - Distinction between fibroma and other benign entities—thecoma, stromal hyperplasia/stromal hyperthecosis is not crucial at the time of frozen section.
    - Tumors with fibromatous areas and foci of luteinization or features of thecoma may be designated as *fibrothecoma*.

Luteinized Thecoma with Sclerosing Peritonitis

- Rare, distinctive clinicopathologic entity
- Typically occurs in young women (median 27 years) and presents with abdominal distension due to ascites and occasionally bowel adhesions [11].
- Most often bilateral with tan to red-brown cut surface.
- Hypercellular with spindled tumor cells and rare round, luteinized cells.
- Edema, microcyst formation, and increased mitotic activity are not uncommon.

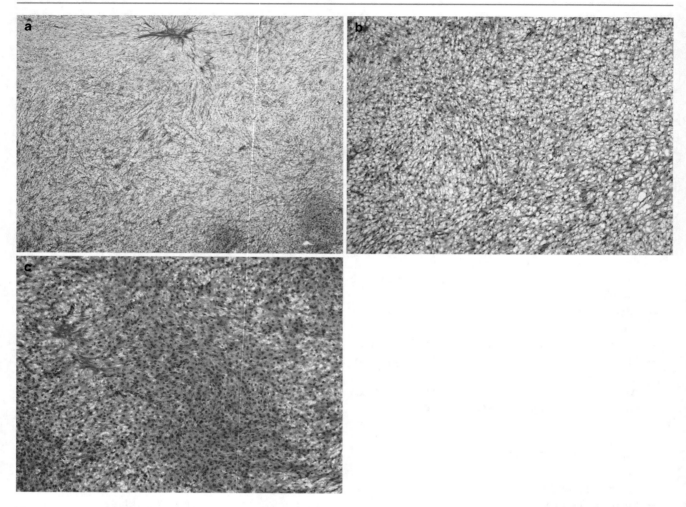

Fig. 10.3 Thecoma. Note the sheets of round to oval, uniform cells with abundant eosinophilic or clear cytoplasm (**a–c**). Hyaline plaques may be seen (**a, c**)

Adult Granulosa Cell Tumor (AGCT)

- Clinical features
  - May occur at any age, but most often in postmenopausal patients—the peak incidence is between 50 and 55 years of age [12–14].
  - May present with pelvic mass/pain.
  - Endocrine—most often estrogenic—manifestations are common and include abnormal bleeding: postmenopausal bleeding, menorrhagia, metrorrhagia, or amenorrhea.
    - Concurrent endometrial hyperplasia or well-differentiated endometrioid endometrial adenocarcinoma may be seen in approximately 25 % and 5 % of cases, respectively [15].
  - Progesterone and androgen production are much less frequent [16, 17].
  - Approximately 10 % of patients present with acute abdomen, due to tumor rupture, hemoperitoneum, or torsion [13].
- Gross pathology (Fig. 10.4)
  - Most often unilateral (>95 % of cases).
  - Size may vary from microscopic up to 40 cm; average 10–12 cm [12].
  - Cut surface is typically solid and cystic, tan-yellow, or white.
    - Less often it may be entirely solid or entirely cystic (uni- or multilocular).
  - Foci of hemorrhage are common.
  - Consistency may be firm or soft, friable, depending on the amount of fibrous stroma.
- Microscopic features (Figs. 10.5, 10.6, and 10.7)
  - Various morphologic patterns, often admixed within the same tumor.
    - *Common patterns*
      - Diffuse: most common pattern with nonspecific arrangement of tumor cells in large sheets
      - Insular: well-defined nests of tumor cells surrounded by fibromatous stroma
      - Trabecular: trabecular or cordlike arrangement
    - *Less common/uncommon patterns*
      - Microfollicular: tumor cells surrounding small round spaces filled with eosinophilic material (Call-Exner bodies)—only seen in minority of granulosa cell tumors
      - Macrofollicular: larger cystic spaces lined by tumor cells
      - "Watered silk" and gyriform patterns: undulating files or rows of tumor cells
      - Pseudopapillary: central vascular core lined by tumor cells—may be a degenerative phenomenon
      - Sarcomatoid: spindled cells, resembling cellular fibroma

  - Tumor cells are relatively uniform with scant pale cytoplasm and round to oval nuclei.
  - The chromatin pattern is pale and the nuclear membrane is characteristically irregular with folds resulting in nuclear grooves.
    - Nuclear grooves may be difficult to appreciate on frozen sections due to freezing artifact.
  - Luteinized AGCTs have a more abundant pink cytoplasm and most often lack nuclear grooves.
  - Mitotic activity is variable, but usually <3/10 HPF in most tumors.
    - Atypical mitotic figures are usually absent.
  - Rare tumors may show marked cytological atypia with bizarre nuclei [18].
  - Hemorrhage and necrosis may be seen, the latter usually secondary to torsion.
- Differential diagnosis (Table 10.1)
  - Primary ovarian carcinomas—endometrioid adenocarcinoma, clear cell carcinoma, and small cell carcinoma
  - Metastatic carcinomas—breast, pancreatic, and small cell carcinoma
  - Carcinoid tumor—primary or metastatic
  - Sex cord-stromal tumors—Sertoli-Leydig cell tumor, juvenile granulosa cell tumor, thecoma, and fibroma
  - Germ cell tumors—dysgerminoma
  - Lymphoma
  - Follicle cyst versus unilocular AGCT
- Diagnostic pitfalls/key intraoperative consultation issues
  - In postmenopausal patients with AGCT, the surgical treatment includes total hysterectomy, bilateral salpingo-oophorectomy as part of the complete surgical staging [19].
    - Fertility-sparing surgery may be performed in younger patients with tumors confined to one ovary (without surface involvement) and includes unilateral salpingo-oophorectomy, staging procedure (with or without lymphadenectomy), and intraoperative assessment of the contralateral ovary [19, 20].
    - Ovarian surface involvement should be reported if identified grossly or microscopically on frozen section, as it may preclude fertility-sparing surgery.
  - Clinically the most important distinction at the time of frozen section is between AGCT and its benign mimics among sex cord-stromal tumors and carcinomas metastatic to the ovary, as no surgical staging would be required for the latter two categories of lesions.
    - Bilaterality, marked nuclear atypia and high mitotic activity with abnormal mitotic figures are not typical features of AGCT and should raise suspicion for carcinoma—primary or metastatic.

- Clinical history of prior malignancy and morphologic comparison with prior biopsies—if available—is very helpful.
- Carcinomas typically have more abundant cytoplasm than AGCT.
- Characteristic nuclear features of AGCT—uniform, oval nuclei with irregular, folded nuclear membranes and grooves—are distinct from those of carcinomas.
- Distinction between primary ovarian carcinoma and AGCT is less critical on frozen section, as the surgical management is the same in most cases.
  - In young patients, fertility-sparing surgery may be performed for AGCT, but its role in epithelial malignancies is more controversial.
- AGCT with microfollicular pattern can mimic carcinoid tumors—primary or metastatic.
  - Carcinoid tumors characteristically have round nuclei with smooth nuclear membranes, stippled chromatin pattern in contrast to the oval nuclei and grooves of AGCT.
- AGCT with a diffuse morphologic pattern may mimic a fibroma or cellular fibroma.
  - Identification of other morphologic patterns of AGCT—insular, trabecular or microfollicular—is most helpful, and it may require careful microscopic examination or sampling of additional tissue blocks.

- AGCT with luteinization can pose a significant diagnostic challenge on frozen section evaluation, closely mimicking a thecoma/fibrothecoma.
  - Luteinized AGCT usually has more abundant pink cytoplasm and lacks nuclear grooves.
  - Distinct tumor nodules are more in favor of AGCT, while a diffuse pattern is more common in thecomas.
  - In difficult cases, the frozen section slide could be interpreted as "sex cord-stromal tumor with luteinization," and the diagnosis could be deferred for permanent sections.
- Distinction between adult and juvenile granulosa cell tumors on frozen section is typically not critical for intraoperative management.
- Frozen section artifacts often hamper the morphologic interpretation:
  - Artifactual cytoplasmic clearing may raise the possibility of clear cell carcinoma or dysgerminoma.
  - Artifactual clearing of nuclei may obscure the characteristic nuclear features.
- Evaluation of endometrium: If the diagnosis of AGCT is made on frozen section, evaluation of the endometrium is also recommended—at least grossly or both grossly and microscopically—if a hysterectomy specimen is available
  - If the uterus will be spared, an endometrial curettage during the same procedure is recommended to rule out endometrial hyperplasia or carcinoma.

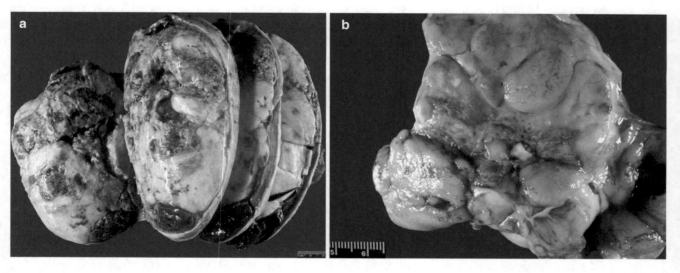

Fig. 10.4 Adult granulosa cell tumor (AGCT). The cut surface of the tumor is solid, tan-yellow (**a**) or tan-pink (**b**). Hemorrhage and cystic changes are commonly present (**a**)

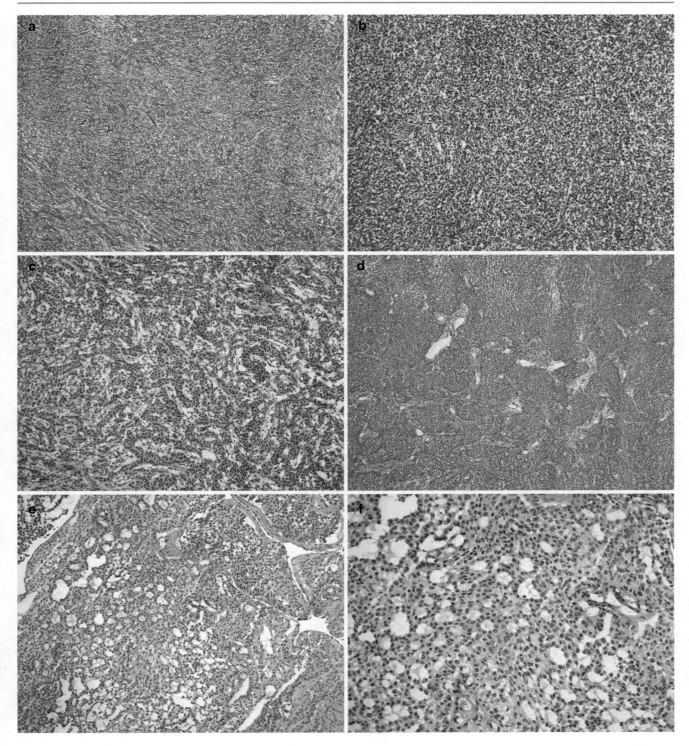

Fig. 10.5 Histological features of adult granulosa cell tumor (AGCT). Note the various morphologic patterns: diffuse (**a**, **b**), trabecular (**c**), insular (**d**), microfollicular (**e**, **f**), macrofollicular (**g**), pseudopapillary (**h**), and sarcomatoid (**i**, **j**). Hemorrhage is not uncommon (**k**)

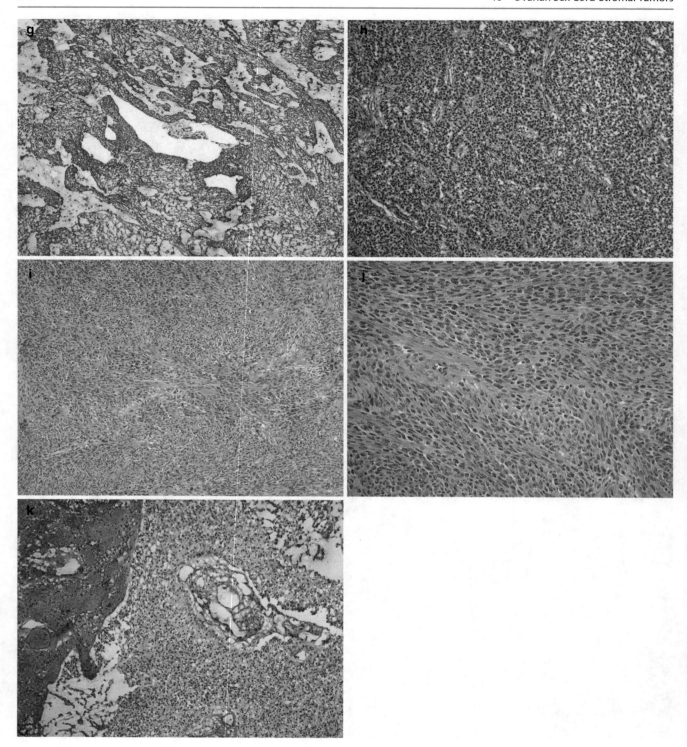

Fig. 10.5 (continued)

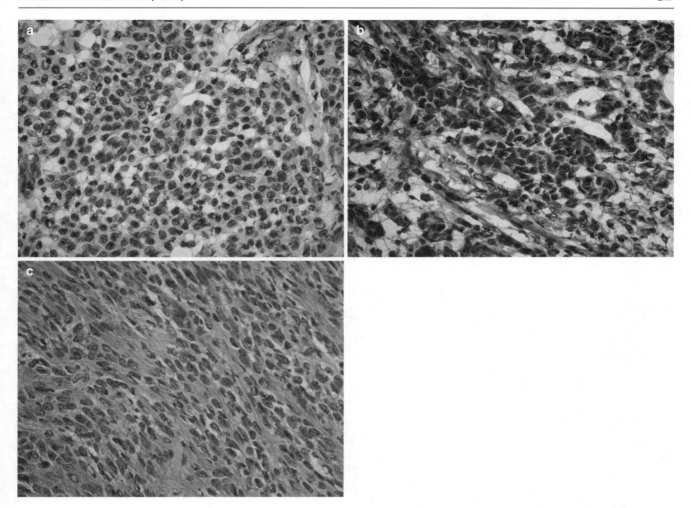

Fig. 10.6 Cytological features of adult granulosa cell tumor (AGCT). The tumor cells have round to oval nuclei with irregular nuclear membranes and longitudinal grooves, pale chromatin, small nucleoli, and scant eosinophilic cytoplasm (**a–c**). Note the vague trabecular arrangement of tumor cells (**b**) in a tumor with a predominant diffuse growth pattern

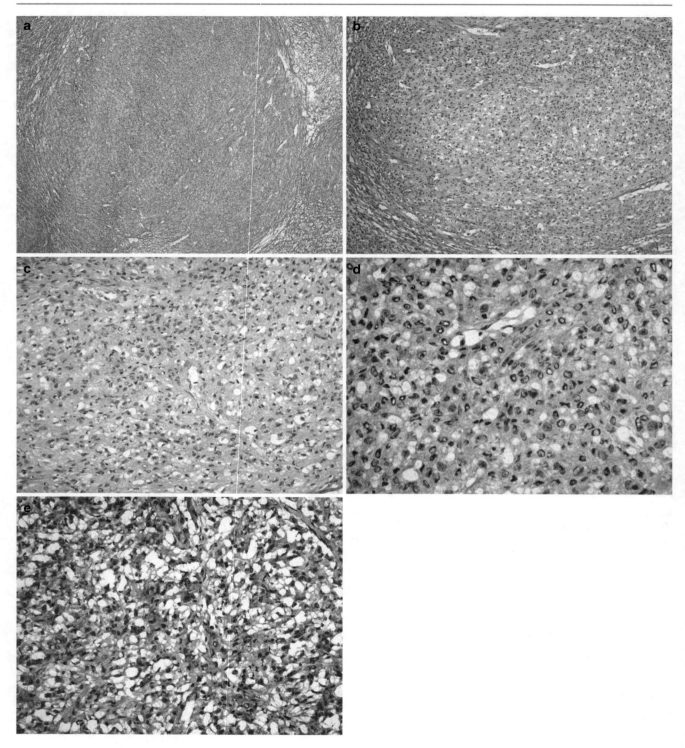

Fig. 10.7 Luteinized adult granulosa cell tumor (AGCT). Note the diffuse growth pattern (**a, b**) and characteristic abundant eosinophilic cytoplasm and round nuclei lacking grooves (**c, d**). Frozen section artifact may result in cytoplasmic clearing, mimicking signet-ring cells (**e**)

Table 10.1 Differential diagnosis of adult granulosa cell tumor (AGCT)

	AGCT	Endometrioid adenocarcinoma	Sertoli-Leydig cell tumor	Carcinoid tumor (primary)	Dysgerminoma
Age (years)	Most often postmenopausal (mean 50–55)	5th–6th decades (mean 58)	Most common in young patients (mean: 25–30)	14–79 years (mean 53)	2nd–3rd decades (mean: 22)
Bilaterality	Very rare	Up to 17 %	Very rare	Very rare (suspect metastasis if bilateral)	10–20 %
Size (mean)	10–12 cm	15 cm	12–14 cm	Variable	Most often >10 cm
Clinical symptoms	Pelvic mass/pain; hormonal (estrogenic > androgenic) manifestations	Asymptomatic or pelvic mass/pain	Hormonal manifestations common (androgenic > estrogenic)	May be incidental; one-third of patients have carcinoid syndrome	Pelvic mass/pain; increased serum LDH
Cytoplasmic features	Little cytoplasm, cell membrane not well defined, except luteinized AGCT	Moderate to abundant; may show squamous and mucinous differentiation	Leydig cells with abundant eosinophilic cytoplasm containing lipofuscin pigment and Reinke crystals	Moderate amount, may show mucinous differentiation (goblet cell carcinoid)	Abundant clear or pale eosinophilic cytoplasm; well-defined cell borders
Nuclear features	Most often uniform, pale nuclei with membrane folds and grooves	Variable nuclear atypia; no grooves	Grade dependent; nuclear membrane folds and grooves may be seen in Sertoli cells	Uniform, small, round nuclei with finely stippled chromatin	Uniform nuclear enlargement with prominent nucleoli
Necrosis	May be seen	Common	May be seen (in poorly differentiated tumors)	Absent	Common

Juvenile Granulosa Cell Tumor (JGCT)

- Clinical features
  - Much less common than AGCT, representing approximately 5 % of granulosa cell tumors.
  - Usually occurs within the first three decades, although rarely may also occur in older women [21].
  - May present with pelvic pain and/or estrogenic endocrine manifestations: isosexual precocity and abnormal vaginal bleeding.
  - Ascites may be present.
  - May undergo rupture or torsion resulting in acute abdomen.
- Gross pathology (Fig. 10.8)
  - Usually unilateral [21].
  - Mean size is 12.5 cm (range 3–32 cm) [21].
  - Cut surface is solid and cystic but may be uniformly solid or cystic only.
  - Hemorrhagic areas may be present.
- Microscopic features (Figs. 10.9 and 10.10)
  - Solid sheets of cells with variably sized follicles and cystic spaces, filled with basophilic secretions.
  - Pseudopapillary pattern may occur.
  - Stromal fibrosis may rarely be prominent.
  - Tumor cells have abundant eosinophilic, amphophilic, or clear cytoplasm.
  - Round nuclei with pale chromatin pattern and absence of grooves.
  - Mild to moderate nuclear atypia.
    - Marked, focal atypia in 10–15 % of tumors
  - Frequent mitotic figures.
  - Necrosis and hemorrhage may be seen.
- Differential diagnosis
  - Cystic follicles/follicular cyst
  - Adult granulosa cell tumor
  - Malignant germ cell tumors (e.g., dysgerminoma, yolk sac tumor)
  - Clear cell carcinoma

- Diagnostic pitfalls/key intraoperative consultation issues
  - Fertility-sparing surgery with unilateral salpingo-oophorectomy and staging procedure may be sufficient in young patients with JGCT limited to one ovary without surface involvement [19, 20].
    - Ovarian surface involvement should be reported if identified grossly or microscopically on frozen section, as it may preclude fertility-sparing surgery.
  - Most important differential diagnoses during frozen section are benign cysts (follicle cyst/cystic follicles).
    - Small follicle formation within the granulosa cell layers is a feature of cystic JCGT and is absent in follicle cyst.
    - Benign lesions, e.g., follicle cysts or cystic follicles may be treated by cystectomy only.
  - JGCT may mimic dysgerminoma and other malignant germ cell tumors due to similar clinical characteristics (patient age) and morphologic overlap.
    - Clinical presentation and tumor markers may be helpful:
      - Estrogenic manifestations are common in JGCT.
      - Patients with malignant germ cell tumors may have increased serum tumor markers: dysgerminoma—LDH, yolk sac tumor—AFP.
    - Dysgerminoma has characteristic stromal lymphocytic infiltrate, which is not a feature of JGCT.
    - Variably sized follicles are seen in JGCT and not in dysgerminoma.
    - Intraoperative management of malignant germ cell tumors and JGCT is usually similar.
  - The histological features between adult and juvenile granulosa cell tumors may show overlap or admixture of the two tumor types.
  - Distinction between adult and juvenile granulosa cell tumor on frozen section is not critical for intraoperative management.
    - Frozen section diagnosis of "granulosa cell tumor, favor juvenile/or adult type" is sufficient in difficult cases.

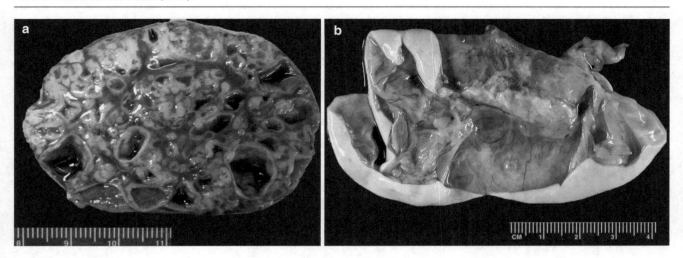

Fig. 10.8 Juvenile granulosa cell tumor (JGCT) with a predominantly solid (**a**) and oligolocular, cystic (**b**), gross appearance

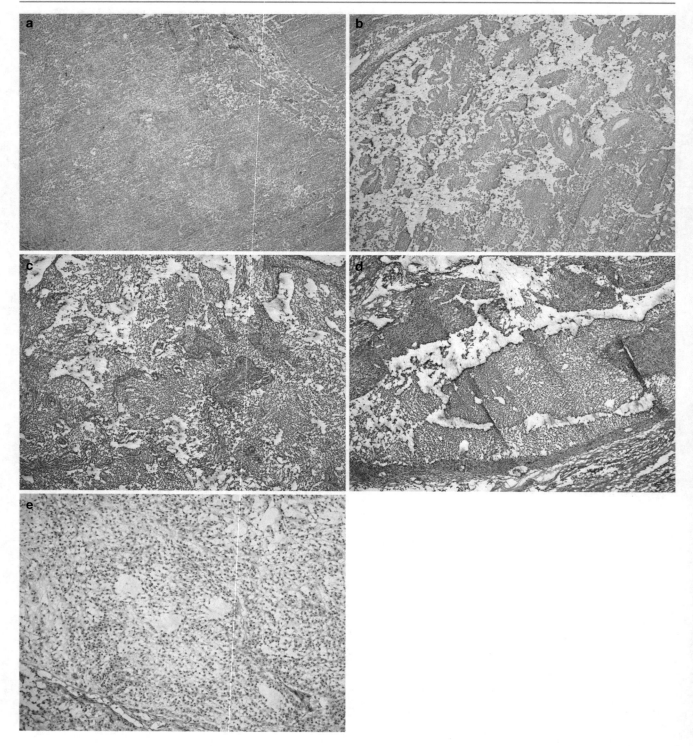

Fig. 10.9 Histological features of juvenile granulosa cell tumor (JGCT). The growth pattern may be solid (**a**), pseudopapillary (**b**) or may show cystic spaces (**c**) and follicles (**d**, **e**). Note the follicle forma-tion within the multilayered granulosa cell cyst lining (**d**) characteristic of JGCT. The cystic spaces contain basophilic secretion (**e**)

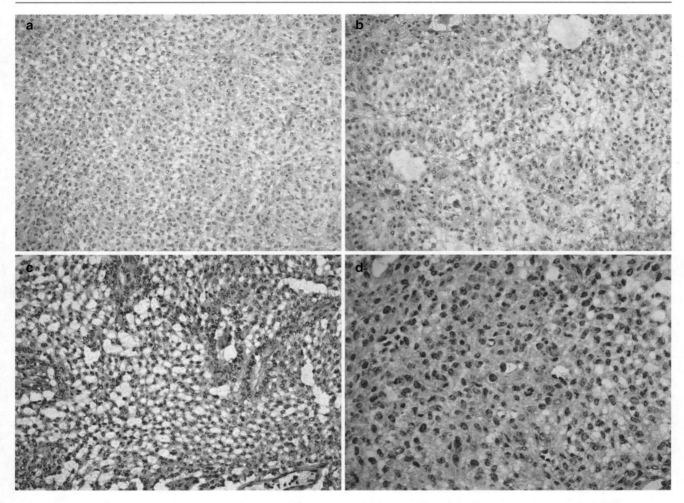

Fig. 10.10 Cytological features of juvenile granulosa cell tumor (JGCT). The tumor cells have round, moderately to markedly atypical nuclei without grooves, and abundant eosinophilic, amphophilic, or clear cytoplasm (**a–d**). Mitotic figures are easily found (**d**)

Sertoli-Leydig Cell Tumor (SLCT)

- Clinical features
  - Rare tumors accounting for less than 0.5 % of all ovarian neoplasms.
  - Most common in young patients <30 years of age—mean age is 25 years [22].
    - Less commonly, it may also occur in postmenopausal patients.
  - Patients may present with pelvic mass/pain.
  - Over 50 % of patients have androgenic hormonal manifestations: hirsutism, clitoromegaly, and amenorrhea
    - Estrogenic symptoms are rare.
  - Ascites and tumor rupture may rarely be seen.
- Gross pathology (Fig. 10.11)
  - Most often (>98 %) unilateral [22].
  - Tumor size ranges from <1 cm to 35 cm (mean 12–14 cm).
  - The cut surface is most often solid and tan-yellow or may be partially cystic.
    - Cystic component is more common in retiform SLCT and tumors with heterologous (mucinous epithelial) elements.
  - Necrosis and hemorrhage are not uncommon in poorly differentiated tumors.
- Microscopic features
  - *Well-differentiated SLCT* (Fig. 10.12)
    - Sertoli cells forming easily recognizable open or solid/compressed tubules.
    - Leydig cells are present in the intervening stroma singly or in small clusters.
    - Sertoli cells have oval or round nuclei; may have small nucleoli and nuclear grooves
    - Leydig cells have round nuclei and characteristic abundant eosinophilic cytoplasm with lipofuscin pigment.
      - Intracytoplasmic Reinke crystals may be seen and may actually be better preserved on frozen sections than on permanent sections after formalin fixation.
    - No significant nuclear pleomorphism or mitotic activity in either components.
  - *Intermediate-grade SLCT* (Fig. 10.13)
    - Diffuse or lobulated pattern on low magnification with alternating cellular areas and hypocellular edematous background stroma.
    - Sertoli cells form diffuse sheets or thin cords and solid, compressed tubules, admixed with dispersed Leydig cell component.
      - Leydig cells are usually fewer than in a well-differentiated SLCT.
    - Sertoli cell nuclei are hyperchromatic, oval, or spindled, with mild to moderate pleomorphism.
    - Mitotic figures may be present.
    - Rare cases show foci of bizarre, degenerative-type atypia.

- *Poorly differentiated SLCT* (Fig. 10.14)
  - Diffuse sheets of immature Sertoli cells with sarcomatoid or primitive gonadal stromal appearance.
  - Compressed tubule or cord formation is only focal and vague, usually difficult to identify.
  - Leydig cells are rare, typically located at the periphery of tumor nodules.
  - Sertoli cells show moderate to marked nuclear pleomorphism.
  - Mitotic activity may be up to 20/10 HPF.
- *SLCT with heterologous elements* (Fig. 10.15)
  - Approximately 20 % of SLCTs have heterologous elements, most often mucinous (intestinal or gastric type) epithelium.
    - Mucinous epithelium associated with SLCT may be benign, borderline, or malignant.
  - Heterologous mesenchymal tissues—cartilage or skeletal muscle—are less common.
  - Heterologous elements occur only in moderately or poorly differentiated SLCT and retiform SLCT.
- *Retiform SLCT*
  - Rare, approximately 15 % of SLCTs show focal or diffuse retiform pattern.
  - Anastomosing irregular, slit-like spaces resembling rete testis.
  - Papillary or multicystic architecture may also be seen.
- Differential diagnosis (Table 10.2)
  - Endometrioid adenocarcinoma of ovary
  - AGCT
  - Mucinous tumors—primary ovarian and metastatic (versus SLCT with heterologous elements)
  - Tubular Krukenberg tumor
  - Teratoma (versus SLCT with heterologous elements)
  - Carcinosarcoma (versus SLCT with heterologous elements)
  - Yolk sac tumor (versus retiform SLCT)
  - Serous borderline tumor or carcinoma (versus retiform SLCT)
  - Sarcomas (versus poorly differentiated SLCT)
  - Fibroma
  - Sertoli cell tumor
- Diagnostic pitfalls/key intraoperative consultation issues
  - Biological behavior of SLCT correlates with histological grade, subtype, and stage.
    - Well-differentiated SLCTs show a benign clinical course [22].
    - Intermediate-grade SLCTs had malignant behavior in 11 % of cases in the largest series [22].
    - Up to 59 % of poorly differentiated SLCTs are clinically malignant (rate of malignancy ranging between 13 and 59 % in various series) [10, 22–24].
    - Retiform pattern and presence of heterologous elements are also adverse prognostic factors.

– Conservative fertility-sparing surgery—unilateral salpingo-oophorectomy and staging procedure (with or without lymphadenectomy) is usually performed in young patients with stage I tumors [10, 23, 24].

– Bilateral salpingo-oophorectomy, total hysterectomy, and complete surgical staging (with or without lymphadenectomy) are typically performed for patients who do not wish to preserve fertility.

– Intraoperative management of AGCT and SLCT (especially moderately or poorly differentiated tumors) is usually similar; frozen section diagnosis of "sex cord-stromal tumor, differential includes AGCT and SLCT" is usually sufficient in cases showing overlapping morphologic features.

– Distinction from malignant epithelial ovarian tumors is critical on frozen sections, especially in young patients.

  • Role of fertility-preserving surgery in epithelial ovarian cancer is less established.

  • Surgical staging procedure is more extensive in ovarian epithelial malignancy, compared with SLCT.

  • Endometrioid adenocarcinoma of the ovary may have a sertoliform growth pattern mimicking a well-differentiated SLCT. Helpful clues in favor of SLCT:

    – Unilateral tumor
    – Younger patient age
    – Absence of squamous differentiation

    – Presence of Leydig cells in the stroma, although luteinized stromal cells in endometrioid adenocarcinomas may mimic Leydig cells
    – Lack of significant nuclear atypia and mitotic activity (well-differentiated SLCT)

Sertoli Cell Tumor

• Rare tumor composed purely of Sertoli cells.
• May occur at any age (mean 30 years).
• Hormonal manifestations (estrogenic > androgenic) may be seen [25].
• Rare cases have been associated with Peutz-Jeghers syndrome.
• Unilateral, tumor size ranging between 0.8 and 30 cm [26].
• Majority of tumors have a benign clinical course; rare malignant cases have also been reported [25, 26].
• Solid or hollow tubules composed of Sertoli cells, arranged in a lobular pattern with intervening stroma.

  – Less common patterns include diffuse, pseudopapillary, retiform, spindled, and nested [26].
  – Most tumors lack nuclear atypia and have low mitotic activity.
  – Moderate to severe nuclear atypia, >5 mitoses/10 HPF, and necrosis have been found in rare, clinically malignant tumors [26].

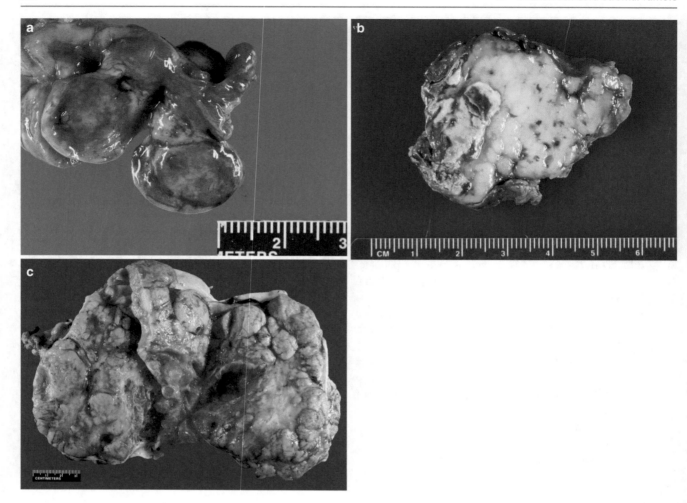

Fig. 10.11 Sertoli-Leydig cell tumor (SLCT). A small, incidental well-differentiated SLCT shows a solid, tan-yellow cut surface (**a**). Poorly differentiated SLCT has a solid, tan-yellow, fleshy gross appear- ance with areas of necrosis (**b**). Note the solid and cystic cut surface in a poorly differentiated SLCT with heterologous mucinous epithelial elements (**c**)

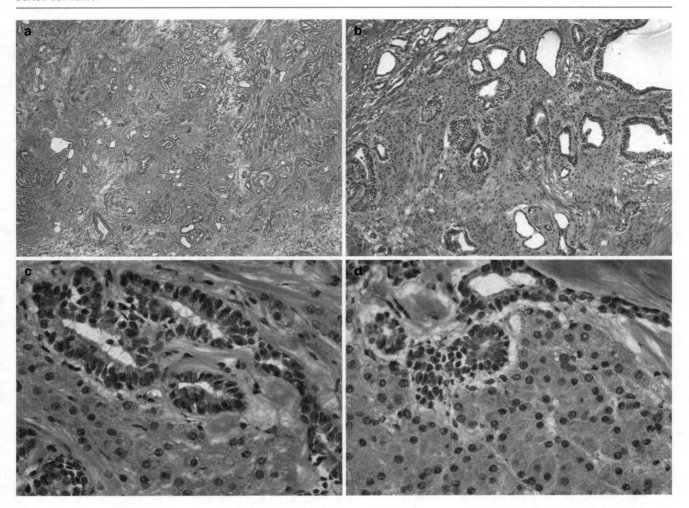

Fig. 10.12 Well-differentiated Sertoli-Leydig cell tumor (SLCT). The Sertoli cells form easily recognizable, irregular, branching tubules (**a**). Abundant Leydig cells are present in the intervening stroma (**b**). The nuclei of Sertoli cells are round to oval and hyperchromatic and may show longitudinal grooves (**c**, **d**). The Leydig cells have round nuclei with small nucleoli and abundant eosinophilic cytoplasm containing Reinke crystals (**c**, *lower portion of image*) and lipofuscin pigment (**d**)

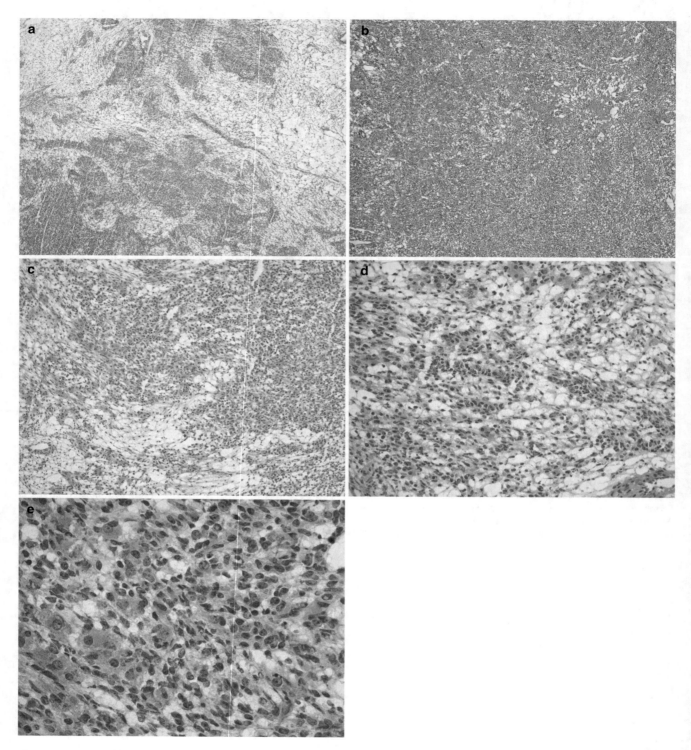

Fig. 10.13 Intermediate-grade Sertoli-Leydig cell tumor (SLCT). Low magnification shows lobulated (**a**) or diffuse (**b**) growth pattern. The hyperchromatic, oval, or spindled Sertoli cells form compressed tubules and cords and are admixed with round, eosinophilic Leydig cells (**c, d**). The Sertoli cell nuclei display moderate nuclear atypia with conspicuous nucleoli (**e**)

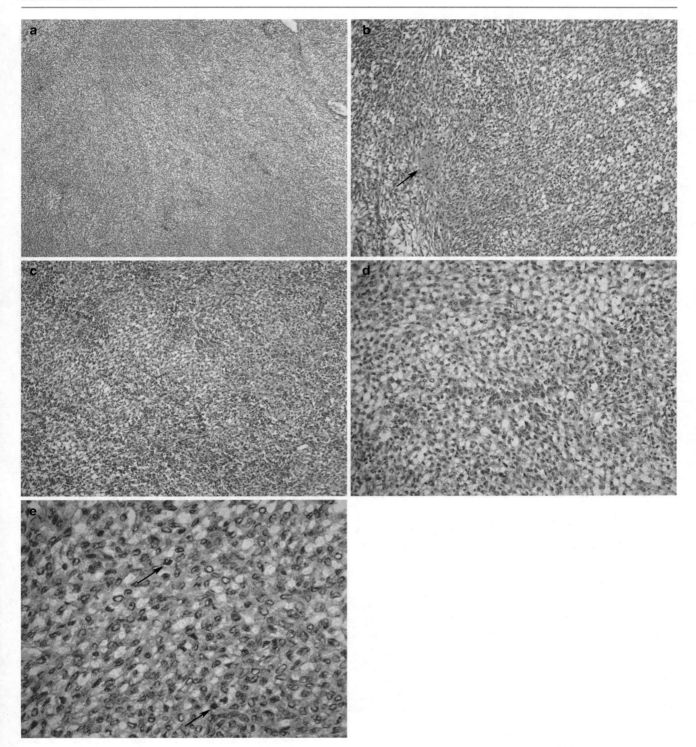

Fig. 10.14 Poorly differentiated Sertoli-Leydig cell tumor (SLCT). Note the diffuse sheets of immature Sertoli cells (**a**) with rare Leydig cells that are usually located at the periphery of tumor (**b**, *arrow*). Focal, vague corded arrangement of Sertoli cells is an important diagnostic clue (**c**, **d**). Moderate to marked nuclear pleomorphism and frequent mitotic figures (**e**, *arrows*) are also characteristic

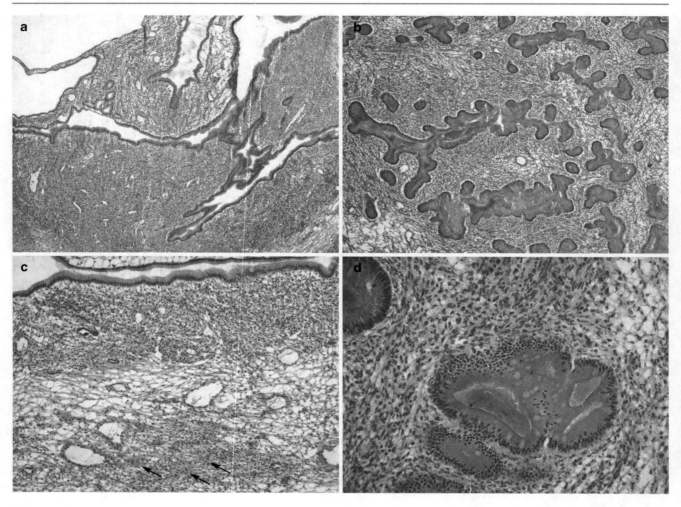

Fig. 10.15 Sertoli-Leydig cell tumor (SLCT) with heterologous elements. Gastric foveolar- and intestinal-type epithelium is surrounded by immature Sertoli cell proliferation (**a**, **b**). Leydig cells may be diffi-cult to identify but often provide an important diagnostic clue (**c**, *arrows*). Note the primitive, sarcomatoid appearance of Sertoli cells surrounding an intestinal-type gland with goblet cells (**d**)

Table 10.2 Differential diagnosis of Sertoli-Leydig cell tumor

	Sertoli/Sertoli-Leydig cell tumor	Endometrioid adenocarcinoma	Adult granulosa cell tumor	Ovarian mucinous tumors (primary)
Age (years)	Most common in young patients (mean: 25–30)	5th–6th decades (mean 58)	Most often postmenopausal (mean 50–55)	Mean age: 45 years
Bilaterality	Very rare	Up to 17 %	Very rare	Uncommon
Size (mean)	12–14 cm	15 cm	10–12 cm	>10 cm (mean: 18–22 cm)
Clinical symptoms	Hormonal manifestations common (androgenic > estrogenic)	Asymptomatic or Pelvic mass/pain	Pelvic mass/pain; hormonal (estrogenic > androgenic) manifestations	Pelvic mass/pain
Squamous differentiation	Absent	Common	Absent	Absent
Mucinous differentiation	Rare (gastric- or intestinal-type heterologous elements)	Uncommon (no goblet cells)	Absent	Yes, abundant goblet cells
Nuclear features	Grade dependent; nuclear grooves may be seen in Sertoli cells	Variable nuclear atypia; no grooves	Most often uniform, pale nuclei with membrane folds and grooves	Moderate to marked nuclear atypia
Necrosis	May be seen (in poorly differentiated tumors)	Common	May be seen	Common

Leydig Cell Tumor

- Clinical features
  - Rare tumor, approximately 20 % of steroid cell tumors of ovary.
  - Mean patient age is 58 years.
  - Androgenic manifestations are common.
- Gross pathology (Fig. 10.16)
  - Usually unilateral, mean size is 2.4 cm [27, 28].
  - Solid, red-brown, or yellow cut surface.
- Microscopic features (Fig. 10.17)
  - May be located in the ovarian hilum ("hilar type") or within the ovarian stroma ("nonhilar type").
  - Sheets of Leydig cells with abundant eosinophilic or pale cytoplasm containing lipofuscin pigment and characteristic Reinke crystals
  - Uniform, round nuclei with small nucleoli.
  - Nuclear pleomorphism and significant mitotic activity are rare.

- Tumors with admixture of ovarian stromal and Leydig cell proliferation have been termed *stromal-Leydig cell tumor* (Fig. 10.18) [29].
- Differential diagnosis
  - Steroid cell tumor, not otherwise specified (NOS)
  - Sertoli-Leydig cell tumor
  - Luteinized thecoma
  - Nonneoplastic lesions of ovary, e.g., hilus cell hyperplasia, corpus luteum
- Diagnostic pitfalls/key intraoperative consultation issues
  - Leydig cell tumors are benign; therefore, the most important distinction for intraoperative management is to distinguish it from other entities with potentially malignant clinical behavior: steroid cell tumor, NOS, and Sertoli-Leydig cell tumor.
    - Reinke crystals are absent in steroid cell tumor, NOS.

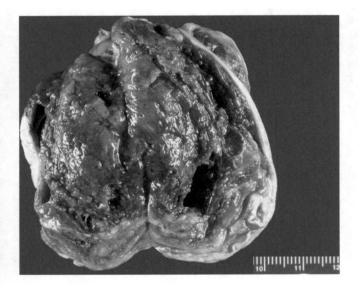

Fig. 10.16 Leydig cell tumor. Note the characteristic solid, red-brown cut surface (with focal cystic changes also seen in this case)

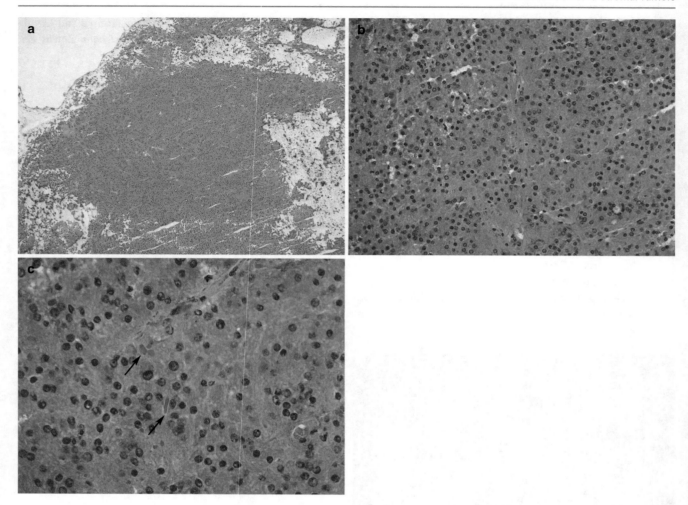

Fig. 10.17 Leydig cell tumor histological features. Note the diffuse sheets of uniform Leydig cells (**a**) with round nuclei and abundant eosinophilic cytoplasm (**b**) containing Reinke crystals (**c**, *arrows*)

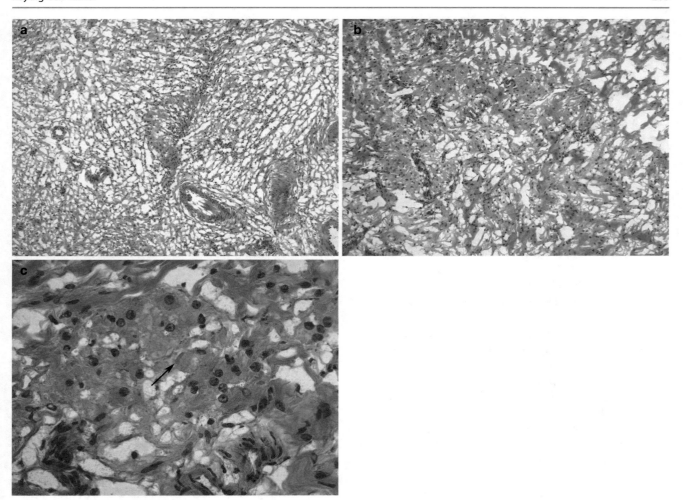

Fig. 10.18 Stromal-Leydig cell tumor is characterized by an admixture of ovarian stromal cells and Leydig cells (**a**, **b**). The Leydig cells have uniform round nuclei with conspicuous nucleoli and abundant eosinophilic cytoplasm containing Reinke crystals (**c**, *arrow*)

Steroid Cell Tumor, Not Otherwise Specified (NOS)

- Clinical features
  - Accounts for approximately 0.1 % of all ovarian tumors and 80 % of steroid cell tumors
  - Patient age is usually younger than those with Leydig cell tumors; the mean age is 43 years (range: 2–80 years) [30]
  - Hormonal manifestations are common, most often androgenic
- Gross pathology (Fig. 10.19)
  - Usually unilateral—approximately 5 % of tumors are bilateral.
  - Mean tumor size is 8.4 cm [30].
  - Solid yellow, brown, red, or black cut surface.
  - Hemorrhage and necrosis may be seen.
- Microscopic features (Fig. 10.20)
  - Diffuse or nested arrangement of round or polygonal tumor cells.
  - Abundant eosinophilic, pale, or clear foamy cytoplasm, which may contain lipochrome pigment.
    - Reinke crystals are absent.
  - Round nuclei with prominent nucleoli.
  - Nuclear atypia is usually mild, and the mitotic activity is <2/10 HPF.
  - Less commonly moderate to severe atypia and increased mitotic activity (>2/10 HPF) may be seen and has been shown to be associated with a malignant clinical course [30].
  - Tumor size larger than 7 cm and hemorrhage and necrosis are also adverse prognostic factors [30].
  - Stromal changes may include hyalinization, edema, myxoid change, and calcifications
  - Vascular network surrounding the tumor cells may be prominent.

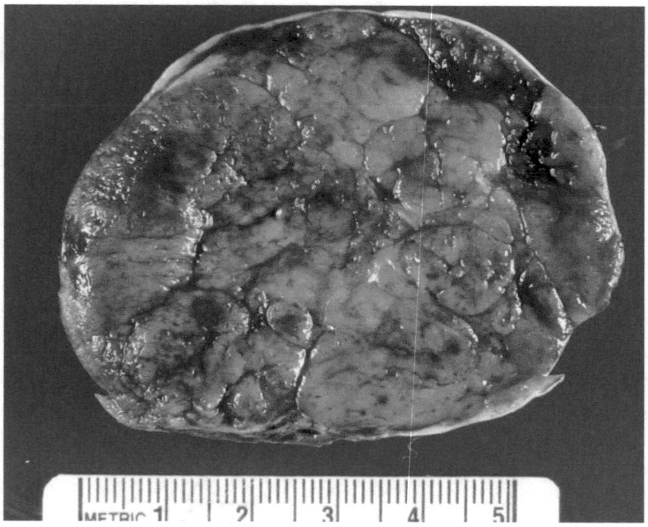

- Differential diagnosis
  - Leydig cell tumor
  - Clear cell carcinoma of ovary
  - Metastatic tumors: melanoma, hepatocellular carcinoma, clear cell renal cell carcinoma, and neuroendocrine carcinoma
  - Nonneoplastic lesions of ovary, e.g., hilus cell hyperplasia, corpus luteum
- Diagnostic pitfalls/key intraoperative consultation issues
  - Leydig cell tumors are benign, whereas large (>7 cm) steroid cell tumors with moderate to severe atypia, increased mitotic activity, hemorrhage, and necrosis may have a malignant clinical course.
    - Presence of Reinke crystals is diagnostic of Leydig cell tumor.
  - Steroid cell tumor, NOS, may mimic metastatic tumors to the ovary.
    - Clinical history of prior malignancy, especially melanoma, hepatocellular carcinoma, clear cell renal cell carcinoma, and neuroendocrine carcinoma should raise suspicion for metastasis.
    - Morphologic comparison with the patient's prior specimens—if available—is helpful.
    - Bilaterality is more common in metastatic lesions; only about 5 % of steroid cell tumors are bilateral.
  - Clear cell carcinoma of the ovary typically has a variety of morphologic patterns, including tubulocystic and papillary, which are not characteristic of steroid cell tumor.
    - Additional sampling may be helpful to identify various patterns within the tumor.

Fig. 10.19 Steroid cell tumor, NOS, showing a solid, yellow-brown cut surface

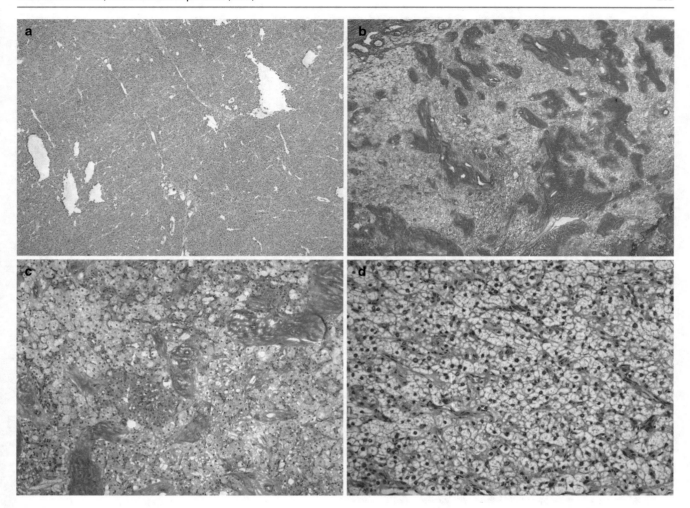

Fig. 10.20 Steroid cell tumor, NOS, microscopic features. Note the diffuse (**a**) or nested arrangement of tumor cells, often with stromal hyalinization (**b**, **c**). The tumor cells are characterized by abundant eosinophilic (**c**) or clear, foamy cytoplasm (**d**, **e**) and round, uniform nuclei. Moderate to severe nuclear atypia (**f**) and necrosis (**g**, *right side of image*) are less common

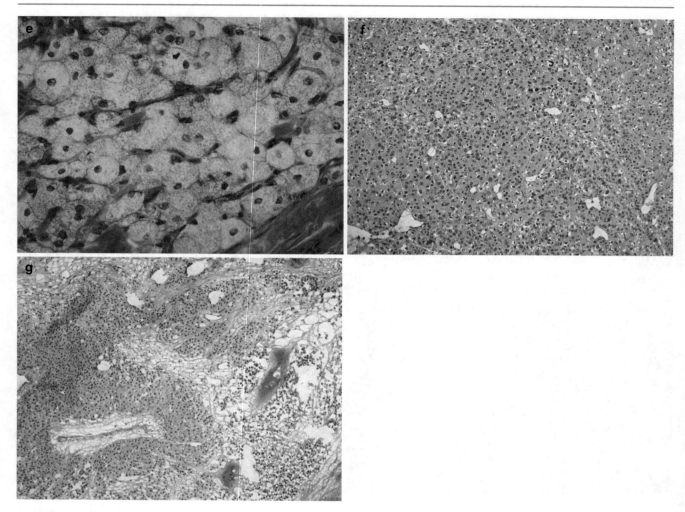

Fig. 10.20   (continued)

Sclerosing Stromal Tumor

- Clinical features
  - Rare benign stromal tumor
  - Most often occurs during the first three decades—mean age is 27 years [31, 32]
  - Presents with pelvic mass/pain and rarely hormonal manifestations (androgenic or estrogenic) [33, 34]
- Gross pathology (Fig. 10.21)
  - Usually unilateral.
  - Size ranges between 1.5 and 17 cm (mean 10 cm) [31].
  - Cut surface is solid white to yellow.
- Microscopic features (Fig. 10.22)
  - Pseudo-lobular architecture of alternating hypo- and hypercellular areas.
  - Cellular nodules are composed of oval or spindled cells in a disorganized or storiform pattern.
  - Characteristic thin-walled, branching, "hemangiopericytoma-like" vasculature.
  - Nuclei are small, relatively uniform with small nucleoli.
  - No significant nuclear atypia or mitotic activity.
  - Luteinized cells may be seen.
  - Cytoplasm may show vacuolization, resembling signet-ring cells.
- Differential diagnosis
  - Fibroma
  - Thecoma
  - Stromal hyperplasia/hyperthecosis
  - Metastatic signet-ring cell carcinoma
- Diagnostic pitfalls/key intraoperative consultation issues
  - Distinction between sclerosing stromal tumor and other benign entities (i.e., fibroma, thecoma, stromal hyperthecosis/hyperplasia) is not crucial at the time of frozen section.
    - Frozen section interpretation of "benign stromal tumor favor sclerosing stromal tumor" or "benign stromal tumor, classification deferred for permanent sections" is usually sufficient.
  - Clinical history of prior gastrointestinal tract or breast carcinoma and bilaterality should raise suspicion for possible metastatic carcinoma with reactive stromal proliferation.
  - Cytoplasm is nondistinct and the cell borders are ill defined in sclerosing stromal tumor in contrast with metastatic signet-ring cell carcinomas.

Signet-Ring Stromal Tumor

- Very rare benign ovarian stromal tumor.
- Occurs in adults, ranging between 21 and 83 years of age [35–37].
- Unilateral, with a mean tumor size of 8.4 cm.
- Solid or partially cystic, white-pink cut surface.
- Sheets or individual signet-ring cells in a background of cellular fibromatous or edematous stroma:
  - Bland, eccentric nuclei and absent or low mitotic activity
  - Clear cytoplasmic vacuoles, sometimes containing eosinophilic globules
- Main differential diagnosis is metastatic signet-ring cell carcinoma (Krukenberg tumor).
  - Clinical history of prior gastrointestinal tract or breast carcinoma and bilaterality should raise suspicion for metastatic carcinoma.
  - In either case (benign stromal tumor or metastatic carcinoma), no surgical staging procedure is performed.

Microcystic Stromal Tumor

- Very rare benign ovarian stromal tumor.
- Occurs in adults (mean age 45 years) [38].
- Unilateral with a mean tumor size of 8.7 cm [38].
- Cut surface is tan white, solid, cystic, or a combination of both.
- Solid sheets of tumor cells with round to oval microcysts.
  - Smaller intracytoplasmic vacuoles are also present.
- No significant nuclear atypia or mitotic activity.

Fibrosarcoma

- Rare malignant stromal tumor.
- Most patients are postmenopausal and present with a pelvic mass.
- Large, usually unilateral tumors, often with necrosis and hemorrhage [6].
- Microscopically hypercellular fascicles composed of moderately to markedly atypical spindle cells.
  - Mitotic activity ≥4/10 HPF.
  - Atypical mitoses may also be seen.
- Differential diagnosis includes benign tumors—fibroma, cellular fibroma, and sarcomas, e.g., endometrial stromal sarcoma.

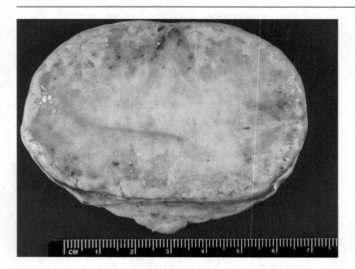

Fig. 10.21 Sclerosing stromal tumor showing a solid, tan-yellow cut surface

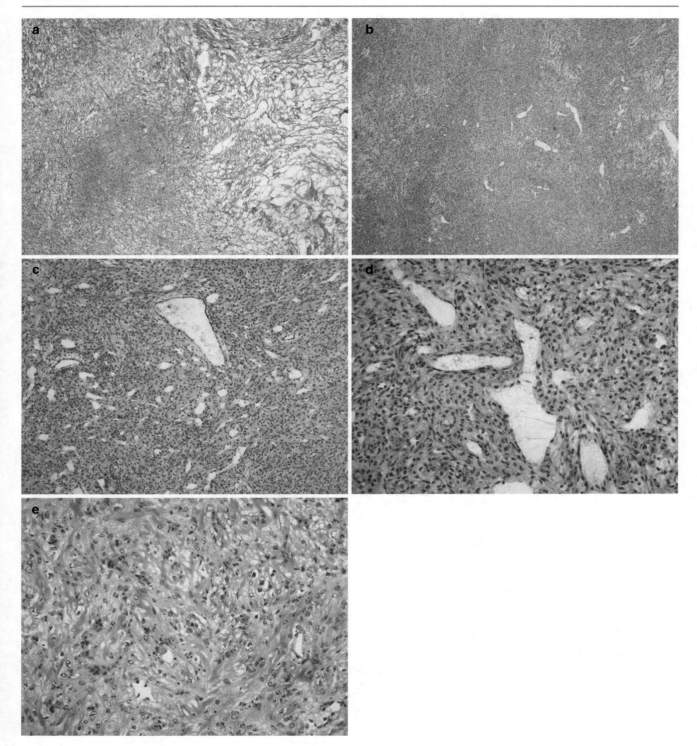

Fig. 10.22 Sclerosing stromal tumor has a characteristic pseudo-lobular pattern on low magnification with alternating hypo- and hyper-cellular areas (**a**). The vessels are thin-walled, branching with a "hemangiopericytoma-like" appearance (**b, c**). The tumor cells are oval or spindled and may show a disorderly storiform pattern. No significant nuclear atypia is seen (**d, e**)

References

1. Lurie S. Meigs' syndrome: the history of the eponym. Eur J Obstet Gynecol Reprod Biol. 2000;92:199–204.
2. Samanth KK, Black 3rd WC. Benign ovarian stromal tumors associated with free peritoneal fluid. Am J Obstet Gynecol. 1970;107:538–45.
3. Gorlin RJ. Nevoid basal-cell carcinoma syndrome. Medicine (Baltimore). 1987;66:98–113.
4. Mak CW, Tzeng WS, Chen CY. Computed tomography appearance of ovarian fibrothecomas with and without torsion. Acta Radiol. 2009;50:570–5.
5. Cho YJ, Lee HS, Kim JM, Joo KY, Kim ML. Clinical characteristics and surgical management options for ovarian fibroma/fibrothecoma: a study of 97 cases. Gynecol Obstet Invest. 2013;76:182–7.
6. Prat J, Scully RE. Cellular fibromas and fibrosarcomas of the ovary: a comparative clinicopathologic analysis of seventeen cases. Cancer. 1981;47:2663–70.
7. Irving JA, Alkushi A, Young RH, Clement PB. Cellular fibromas of the ovary: a study of 75 cases including 40 mitotically active tumors emphasizing their distinction from fibrosarcoma. Am J Surg Pathol. 2006;30:929–38.
8. Young RH, Scully RE. Ovarian stromal tumors with minor sex cord elements: a report of seven cases. Int J Gynecol Pathol. 1983;2:227–34.
9. Zhang J, Young RH, Arseneau J, Scully RE. Ovarian stromal tumors containing lutein or Leydig cells (luteinized thecomas and stromal Leydig cell tumors)–a clinicopathological analysis of fifty cases. Int J Gynecol Pathol. 1982;1:270–85.
10. Bhat RA, Lim YK, Chia YN, Yam KL. Sertoli-Leydig cell tumor of the ovary: analysis of a single institution database. J Obstet Gynaecol Res. 2013;39:305–10.
11. Staats PN, McCluggage WG, Clement PB, Young RH. Luteinized thecomas (thecomatosis) of the type typically associated with sclerosing peritonitis: a clinical, histopathologic, and immunohistochemical analysis of 27 cases. Am J Surg Pathol. 2008;32:1273–90.
12. Sun HD, Lin H, Jao MSm Wang KL, Liou WS, Hung YC, et al. A long-term follow-up study of 176 cases with adult-type ovarian granulosa cell tumors. Gynecol Oncol. 2012;124:244–9.
13. Stenwig JT, Hazekamp JT, Beecham JB. Granulosa cell tumors of the ovary. A clinicopathological study of 118 cases with long-term follow-up. Gynecol Oncol. 1979;7:136–52.
14. Norris HJ, Taylor HB. Prognosis of granulosa-theca tumors of the ovary. Cancer. 1968;21:255–63.
15. van Meurs HS, Bleeker MC, van der Velden J, Overbeek LI, Kenter GG, Buist MR. The incidence of endometrial hyperplasia and cancer in 1031 patients with a granulosa cell tumor of the ovary: long-term follow-up in a population-based cohort study. Int J Gynecol Cancer. 2013;23:1417–22.
16. Young RH, Oliva E, Scully RE. Luteinized adult granulosa cell tumors of the ovary: a report of four cases. Int J Gynecol Pathol. 1994;13:302–10.
17. Norris HJ, Taylor HB. Virilization associated with cystic granulosa tumors. Obstet Gynecol. 1969;34:629–35.
18. Young RH, Scully RE. Ovarian sex cord-stromal tumors with bizarre nuclei: a clinicopathologic analysis of 17 cases. Int J Gynecol Pathol. 1983;1:325–35.
19. Schumer ST, Cannistra SA. Granulosa cell tumor of the ovary. J Clin Oncol. 2003;21:1180–9.
20. Iavazzo C, Gkegkes ID, Vrachnis N. Fertility sparing management and pregnancy in patients with granulosa cell tumour of the ovaries. J Obstet Gynaecol. 2015;35:551–5.
21. Young RH, Dickersin GR, Scully RE. Juvenile granulosa cell tumor of the ovary. A clinicopathological analysis of 125 cases. Am J Surg Pathol. 1984;8:575–96.
22. Young RH, Scully RE. Ovarian Sertoli-Leydig cell tumors. A clinicopathological analysis of 207 cases. Am J Surg Pathol. 1985;9:543–69.
23. Sigismondi C, Gadducci A, Lorusso D, Candiani M, Breda E, Raspagliese F, et al. Ovarian Sertoli-Leydig cell tumors. A retrospective MITO study. Gynecol Oncol. 2012;125:673–6.
24. Gui T, Cao D, Shen K, Yang J, Zhang Y, Yu Q, et al. A clinicopathological analysis of 40 cases of ovarian Sertoli-Leydig cell tumors. Gynecol Oncol. 2012;127:384–9.
25. Tavassoli FA, Norris HJ. Sertoli tumors of the ovary. A clinicopathologic study of 28 cases with ultrastructural observations. Cancer. 1980;46:2281–97.
26. Oliva E, Alvarez T, Young RH. Sertoli cell tumors of the ovary: a clinicopathologic and immunohistochemical study of 54 cases. Am J Surg Pathol. 2005;29:143–56.
27. Roth LM, Sternberg WH. Ovarian stromal tumors containing Leydig cells. II. Pure Leydig cell tumor, non-hilar type. Cancer. 1973;32:952–60.
28. Paraskevas M, Scully RE. Hilus cell tumor of the ovary. A clinicopathological analysis of 12 Reinke crystal-positive and nine crystal-negative cases. Int J Gynecol Pathol. 1989;8:299–310.
29. Sternberg WH, Roth LM. Ovarian stromal tumors containing Leydig cells. I Stromal-Leydig cell tumor and non-neoplastic transformation of ovarian stroma to Leydig cells. Cancer. 1973;32:940–51.
30. Hayes MC, Scully RE. Ovarian steroid cell tumors (not otherwise specified). A clinicopathological analysis of 63 cases. Am J Surg Pathol. 1987;11:835–45.
31. Chalvardjian A, Scully RE. Sclerosing stromal tumors of the ovary. Cancer. 1973;31:664–70.
32. Qureshi A, Raza A, Kayani N. The morphologic and immunohistochemical spectrum of 16 cases of sclerosing stromal tumor of the ovary. Indian J Pathol Microbiol. 2010;53:658–60.
33. Yen E, Deen M, Marshall I. Youngest reported patient presenting with an androgen producing sclerosing stromal ovarian tumor. J Pediatr Adolesc Gynecol. 2014;27:e121–4.
34. Ismail SI, Adams SA. A large sclerosing stromal tumour of the ovary presenting with irregular uterine bleeding: first case report from the UK. J Obstet Gynaecol. 2010;30:322–3.
35. Vang R, Bague S, Tavassoli FA, Prat J. Signet-ring stromal tumor of the ovary: clinicopathologic analysis and comparison with Krukenberg tumor. Int J Gynecol Pathol. 2004;23:45–51.
36. Ramzy I. Signet-ring stromal tumor of ovary. Histochemical, light, and electron microscopic study. Cancer. 1976;38:166–72.
37. Dickersin GR, Young RH, Scully RE. Signet-ring stromal and related tumors of the ovary. Ultrastruct Pathol. 1995;19:401–19.
38. Irving JA, Young RH. Microcystic stromal tumor of the ovary: report of 16 cases of a hitherto uncharacterized distinctive ovarian neoplasm. Am J Surg Pathol. 2009;33:367–75.

Nonneoplastic Lesions of the Ovary and Miscellaneous Primary Ovarian Tumors

11

Introduction

Nonneoplastic—physiologic or reactive—conditions of the ovary may present as a mass lesion and mimic a malignant process clinically or radiologically and may result in a diagnostic dilemma on frozen section examination. Familiarity with the clinical context, the spectrum of frozen section histomorphology, and the potential technical artifacts can help avoiding overinterpretation of these benign lesions. Precise classification of benign findings, however, is rarely required for intraoperative management.

This chapter, in addition to presenting a brief overview of the most common nonneoplastic ovarian entities, also includes a few rare primary ovarian tumors, i.e., lymphomas and small cell carcinomas.

Nonneoplastic Lesions of the Ovary

Cortical Inclusion Cysts

- Very common, typically incidental findings beneath the ovarian surface.
- Measure <1 cm in size.
- Single layer of epithelial cell lining, may be tubal type/ciliated or flattened (Fig. 11.1).
- Mild cytological atypia may be seen.
- May be associated with calcifications.
- No papillary epithelial proliferation or tufting.
- Diagnostic pitfalls/key intraoperative consultation issues
  - Cortical inclusion cysts with prominent calcification and mild epithelial atypia may raise suspicion for borderline/atypical proliferative serous tumor; however, they lack epithelial proliferation, or tufting.

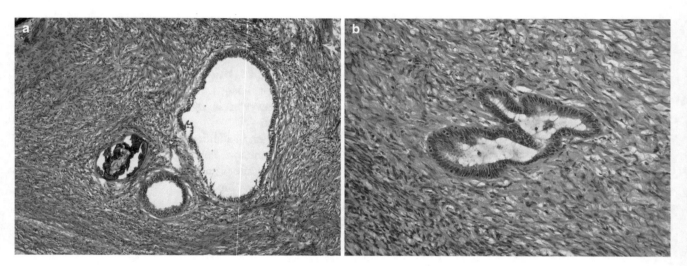

Fig. 11.1 Cortical inclusion cysts in the ovarian stroma with focal calcification (**a**). The lining epithelium is composed of a single layer of bland, flattened, or tubal-type cells (**b**)

Cystic Follicle/Follicle Cyst

- May occur at any age, although most common during the reproductive years.
- Lesions measuring less than 3 cm are typically designated as cystic follicle, while follicle cysts usually range between 3 and 8 cm in size.
- Cut surface shows a thin cyst wall, smooth inner surface, and clear or hemorrhagic fluid contents.
- Microscopically the cysts are lined by variable number of granulosa cell layers (Fig. 11.2).
  - Uniform, round to oval nuclei and small nucleoli.
  - Mitotic figures may be present.
  - Often luteinized with abundant eosinophilic cytoplasm.
  - Outer layer of luteinized theca cells is often seen.

- Differential diagnosis
  - Adult granulosa cell tumor (AGCT)
  - Juvenile granulosa cell tumor (JGCT)
- Diagnostic pitfalls/key intraoperative consultation issues
  - AGCT may be unilocular, cystic, mimicking a follicle cyst.
    - Luteinization is uncommon in cystic AGCT, while it is often seen in follicle cysts.
  - Cystic growth pattern and cytological features of JGCT show similarity to those of follicle cysts.
    - Follicle formation within the cystic granulosa cell lining is characteristic of JGCT [see Chap. 10] and not a feature of follicle cyst.

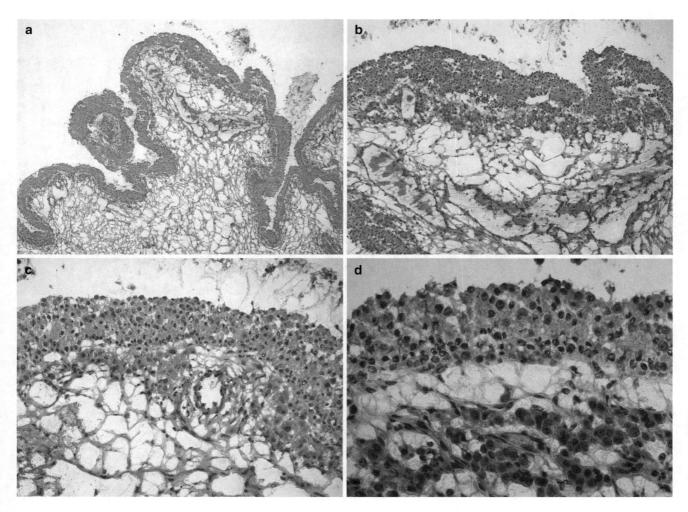

Fig. 11.2 Cystic follicle/follicle cyst. The cyst is lined by multiple layers of granulosa cells (**a**, **b**), characterized by uniform, round nuclei and often luteinized, eosinophilic cytoplasm (**b**, **c**). Luteinized theca cells are also present under the granulosa cell layer (**b–d**). Occasional mitotic figures may be seen among the granulosa cells (**d**)

Cystic Corpus Luteum/Corpus Luteum Cyst

- Enlarged, cystic corpus luteum is common during the reproductive years.
- Patients may present with abdominal pain, menstrual abnormalities, and rarely hemoperitoneum due to rupture [1].
- Yellow, cystic cut surface often with central hemorrhage.
- Thick, undulating lining composed of large luteinized granulosa cells (Fig. 11.3).
  - Uniform, round nuclei with small nucleoli
  - Abundant eosinophilic cytoplasm—may appear vacuolated on frozen sections
- Differential diagnosis
  - Luteinized follicle cyst
  - Steroid cell tumor
  - Leydig cell tumor

- Diagnostic pitfalls/key intraoperative consultation issues
  - Corpus luteum cyst is usually easily recognized on frozen sections.
  - Distinction between corpus luteum cyst and other benign entities—e.g., luteinized follicle cyst—is not critical for intraoperative management.
  - Steroid and Leydig cell tumors lack the characteristic undulating arrangement of cells.
    - Cystic change is not a feature of steroid or Leydig cell tumors.
    - Reinke crystals are absent in corpus luteum cyst.

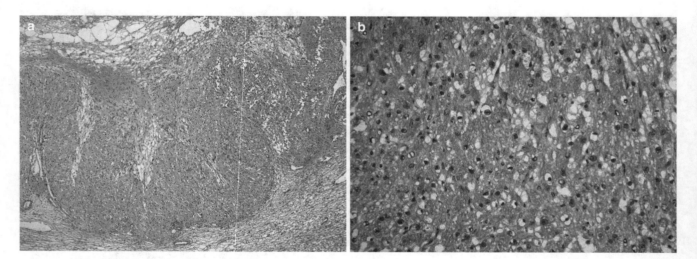

Fig. 11.3 Cystic corpus luteum/corpus luteum cyst. The cyst has thick, undulating layers of granulosa cells with relatively uniform, round nuclei and abundant eosinophilic cytoplasm (**a**). Cytoplasmic vacuolization may be seen on frozen sections (**b**)

Endometriosis/Endometriotic Cyst

- Endometriosis often involves the ovaries and may present with pelvic/abdominal mass and/or pain, irregular menstruation, dysmenorrhea, and infertility.
- Ovary may be significantly enlarged, often >10 cm in size.
- Ovarian surface adhesions and tubo-ovarian adhesions are often present.
- Cut surface may be solid, hemorrhagic, or cystic, filled with red-brown fluid ("chocolate cyst") (Fig. 11.4).
  - Cystic lesions may have intraluminal solid/polypoid protrusions—intraoperative frozen section sampling from these areas is important.
- Microscopic examination shows endometrial glandular epithelium and endometrial stroma often with abundant hemosiderin-laden macrophages (Fig. 11.5).
  - Characteristic vascular network of spiral arterioles in endometrial stroma helps distinguishing it from background ovarian stroma.
  - Epithelial lining may show metaplastic changes—tubal (ciliated), mucinous, hobnail, or eosinophilic (papillary syncytial) [2].
  - Cytological and/or architectural atypia may be seen—"atypical endometriosis" (Figs. 11.6 and 11.7; Fig. 11.7 clear cell carcinoma arising in atypical endometriosis).
  - Polypoid endometriosis resembles the growth pattern and architectural features of uterine endometrial polyps.
- Differential diagnosis
  - Hemorrhagic follicle cyst
  - Clear cell carcinoma arising in endometriosis
  - Endometrioid adenocarcinoma arising in endometriosis
- Diagnostic pitfalls/key intraoperative consultation issues
  - Atypical endometriosis—endometriosis with either cytological atypia or hyperplastic changes similar to eutopic (uterine endometrial) complex atypical hyperplasia—has been shown to have a benign clinical course and does not require extensive surgery [3].
  - Sampling for frozen section should focus on intraluminal polypoid masses and solid areas to rule out malignancy—most often clear cell and endometrioid carcinomas [see Chap. 8].
  - Distinction between endometriosis and other benign mimics is typically not crucial for intraoperative management.

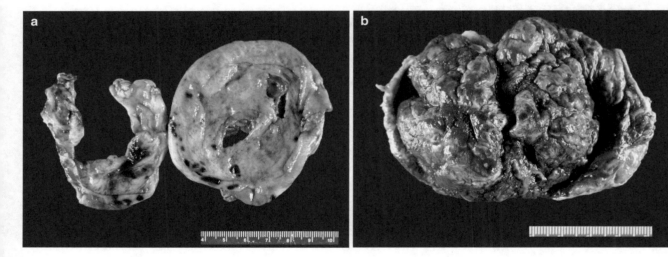

Fig. 11.4 Ovarian endometriosis. The lesion may appear grossly as a hemorrhagic cyst with a smooth, focally red-brown lining (**a**) or as a predominantly solid, hemorrhagic, tan-brown mass (**b**)

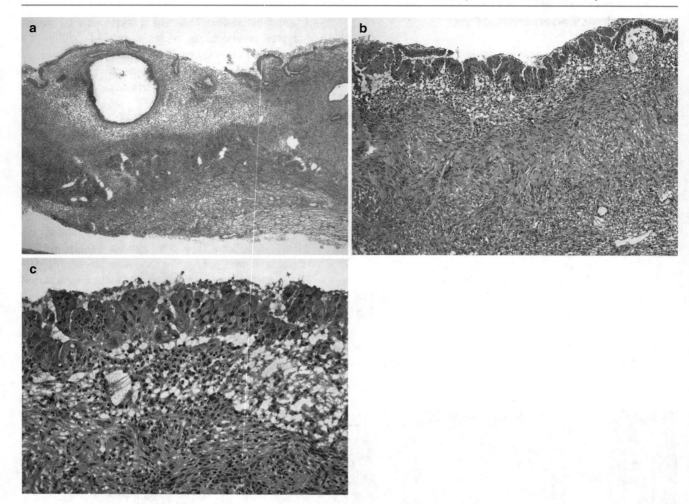

Fig. 11.5 Ovarian endometriosis. Histologically the lesion is characterized by variable proportions of endometrial stroma and endometrial glands/glandular epithelium (**a**). Note the distinctly different micro-scopic features of endometrial versus ovarian stroma (**b**). Mucinous metaplasia is common within the endometrial epithelium (**b**, **c**)

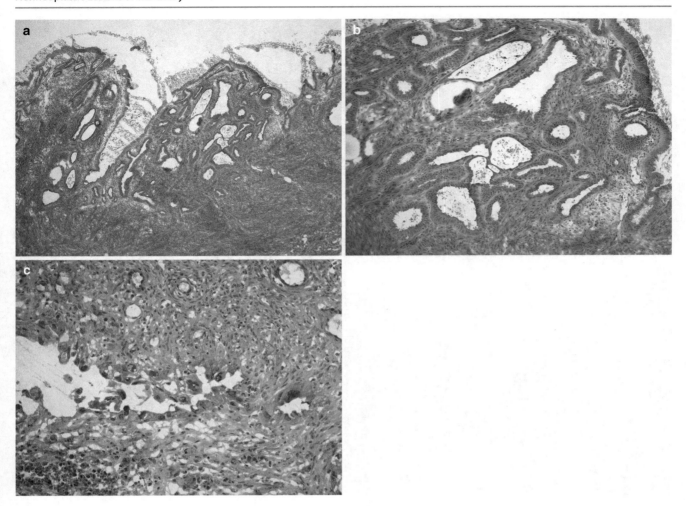

Fig. 11.6 Atypical endometriosis. Note the glandular crowding with complex architecture and atypia (**a**, **b**), similar to complex atypical hyperplasia of the eutopic endometrium, or marked cytological atypia of the endometrial glandular epithelium (**c**)

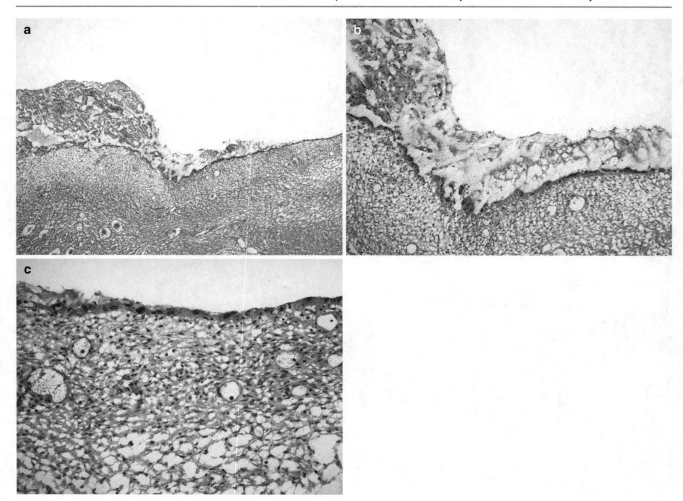

Fig. 11.7 Clear cell carcinoma of the ovary, arising in an endometriotic cyst. The endometrial epithelial lining shows marked cytological atypia (atypical endometriosis) (**a**, **b**, *right side of images*; **c**). Adjacent intraluminal tubulo-cystic proliferation represents a focus of clear cell carcinoma (**a**, **b**, *left side of images*)

Stromal Hyperthecosis

- May occur during the reproductive years and in postmenopausal patients.
- Patients may be asymptomatic or may present with endocrine manifestations (androgenic> estrogenic) [4].
- Ovaries are normal in size or slightly enlarged.
- Most often bilateral ovarian involvement.
- Solid, diffuse tan-yellow cut surface.
- Microscopically, stromal hyperthecosis is usually associated with ovarian stromal hyperplasia and shows luteinized cells—singly or in small nodules (less than 1 cm in size) (Fig. 11.8).
  - Luteinized cells have small, round, uniform nuclei and abundant eosinophilic (lipid-poor) or clear (lipid-rich) cytoplasm.
- Differential diagnosis
  - Stromal luteoma
  - Fibroma/thecoma
  - Metastatic signet-ring cell carcinoma (Krukenberg tumor)
- Diagnostic pitfalls/key intraoperative consultation issues
  - Distinction between stromal hyperthecosis and other benign entities—e.g., stromal luteoma, fibroma or thecoma—is not critical for intraoperative management.
  - Lipid-rich luteinized cells with clear cytoplasm may mimic signet-ring cells.
    - Nuclei of luteinized stromal cells are round and centrally located, unlike the eccentric, often crescent-shaped nuclei of Krukenberg tumor.
  - The ovarian stroma is often prominent/hyperplastic and may contain luteinized cells in Krukenberg tumors, giving the impression of stromal hyperplasia/hyperthecosis on low magnification. Cases with bilateral ovarian involvement by stromal hyperplasia should always be examined carefully on medium or high magnification to rule out presence of metastatic signet-ring cells.

Massive Edema

- Rare, benign condition occurring mostly in young patients (mean age: 20–22 years) [5, 6].

- Clinical presentation includes abdominal pain, menstrual abnormalities, and less commonly hormonal manifestations.
- Most often unilateral ovarian enlargement, up to 35 cm in size (mean size is around 10 cm) [5, 6].
- Tan, edematous, or gelatinous cut surface.
- Edematous, hypocellular ovarian stroma surrounding preexisting ovarian structures (e.g., follicles) and usually sparing the outer cortex.
- Differential diagnosis
  - Fibroma/thecoma with edema
  - Metastatic signet-ring cell carcinoma (Krukenberg tumor)

Ovarian Torsion

- May present at any age and occurs during pregnancy in up to 25 % of cases [7].
- Clinical symptoms include acute onset abdominal pain, nausea, vomiting, and fever.
- Most common predisposing lesions are ovarian cysts or benign cystic or solid neoplasms.
  - Less than 5 % of cases have an underlying ovarian malignancy [8].
  - May involve normal adnexa in pediatric patients.
- Hemorrhagic infarction microscopically may involve the entire ovary or may be focal.
- Thorough gross sampling is required to identify viable areas.
- Diagnosis of underlying ovarian pathology may be deferred to permanent sections if reasonable sampling on frozen section fails to show viable tissue.

Surface Papillary Stromal Proliferation

- Common incidental finding at any age
- Multiple small (<1 cm) papillary stromal projections on the ovarian surface lined by a single layer of surface epithelium
  - No pseudostratification or tufting
  - No significant nuclear atypia or mitotic activity
- Differential diagnosis
  - Serous borderline/atypical proliferative tumor

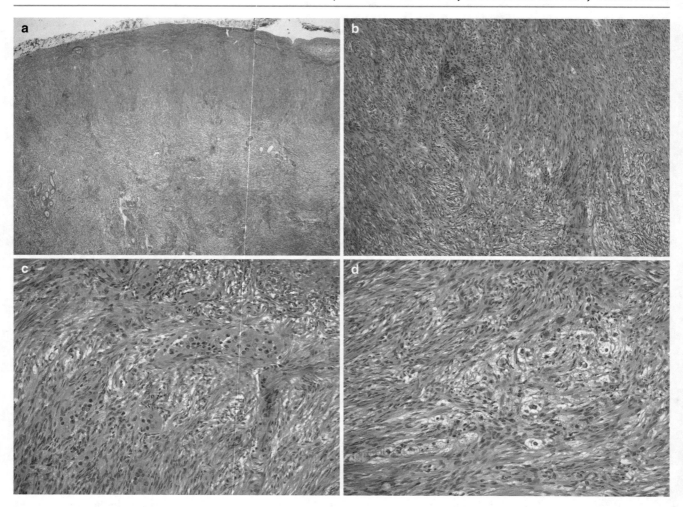

Fig. 11.8 Ovarian stromal hyperplasia/hyperthecosis. Note the diffuse proliferation of spindled ovarian stromal cells (**a**, **b**), admixed with small nests of round, uniform luteinized cells with abundant eosinophilic (**c**) or clear cytoplasm (**d**)

Tubo-ovarian Abscess

- Usually secondary to pelvic inflammatory disease.
  - Less commonly may be a result of direct spread from diverticulitis or appendicitis
- Clinical presentation includes abdominal pain/ mass, fever, nausea, and vaginal discharge or bleeding.
- Gross examination typically reveals enlargement of the adnexa with tubo-ovarian adhesions and heterogeneous cut surface often with apparent cystic yellow abscess cavity (Fig. 11.9).

- Surgery is more often performed for larger lesions (>10 cm in size), whereas smaller lesions may be treated conservatively [9].
- Most often polymicrobial—including *N. gonorrhoeae* and other aerobic and anaerobic species; less often caused by *Actinomyces* [9].
  - Mixed inflammatory infiltrate with neutrophils, histiocytes, lymphocytes, and plasma cells.
  - Actinomycotic ("sulfur") granules—round, basophilic aggregates of branching bacterial filaments in a radiating pattern—are diagnostic (Fig. 11.10).

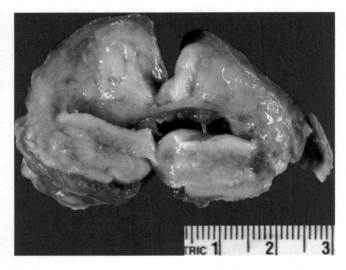

Fig. 11.9 Tubo-ovarian abscess shows a soft, tan-yellow cut surface and surface adhesions

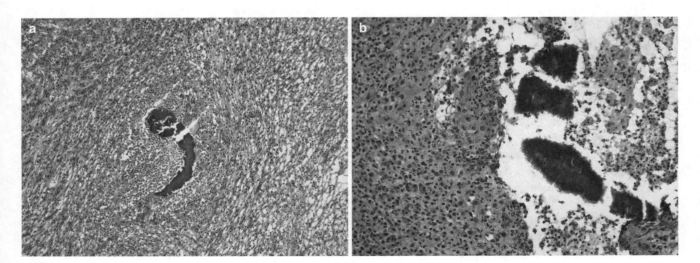

Fig. 11.10 Actinomycotic ("sulfur") granules in a tubo-ovarian abscess (**a**, **b**). Note the round, basophilic aggregates of branching bacterial filaments in a radiating pattern—surrounded by mixed (neutrophilic and lymphoplasmacytic) inflammatory infiltrate in the ovary

Miscellaneous Primary Ovarian Tumors

Lymphomas

- Primary ovarian lymphomas are rare.
  - Secondary involvement of the ovaries is more common [10].
- May occur at any age and present with abdominal mass/pain and often with general symptoms, i.e., fatigue, weight loss, and fever.
- Primary ovarian lymphomas are usually unilateral, except for Burkitt lymphoma [11].
- Size range is wide, ranging from microscopic to 20 cm [10].
- Cut surface is typically solid, nodular, tan-pink, fleshy, or rubbery (Fig. 11.11).
- Most common histological subtype is *diffuse large B-cell lymphoma (DLBL)*.
  - Microscopic appearance is similar to that of other sites:
    - Diffuse sheets of large cells with round to irregular nuclear contours (Fig. 11.12).
    - Small to moderate amount of cytoplasm, indistinct cytoplasmic borders.
    - Moderate to severe nuclear pleomorphism.
    - High mitotic activity.
    - Necrosis may be seen.
    - Histological feature unique to ovarian DLBL is stromal sclerosis, resulting in a storiform pattern or trabeculated arrangement of tumor cells.
- Differential diagnosis
  - Primary ovarian carcinomas
  - Metastatic carcinomas
  - Dysgerminoma
  - Adult granulosa cell tumor
- Diagnostic pitfalls/key intraoperative consultation issues
  - The differential diagnosis of undifferentiated round blue cell tumors should be wide at the time of frozen section to ensure appropriate triaging of tissue for ancillary studies.
    - If the morphology raises suspicion for a lymphoproliferative disorder, fresh tissue should be harvested for additional hematopathology workup.
  - There are no uniform guidelines regarding the extent of surgical debulking/staging; however, staging surgery is often performed, due to lack of definitive pre- or intraoperative diagnosis [12, 13].

- Conservative frozen section diagnostic approach should be considered in young patients wishing to preserve fertility—frozen section diagnosis of "Malignant neoplasm cannot rule out or favor lymphoma" can be communicated with deferral for permanent sections.

Small Cell Carcinoma, Hypercalcemic Type

- Rare, undifferentiated malignant tumor occurring in young patients (mean age is 24 years) [14, 15].
- Clinical presentation includes abdominal mass and paraneoplastic hypercalcemia in over half of the patients.
- Almost always unilateral, solid with a tan-white cut surface.
- Average tumor size is 15 cm [15].
- Diffuse growth pattern with follicle-like spaces.
  - Less often the tumor cells may form nests or cords.
- Small, round, hyperchromatic cells with high mitotic activity.
  - Large cell component with moderate to abundant cytoplasm is also seen in approximately half of the cases [15].
- Necrosis and hemorrhage are often seen.
- Differential diagnosis
  - Juvenile granulosa cell tumor
  - Clear cell carcinoma
  - Dysgerminoma
  - Lymphoma
  - Metastatic carcinoma
- Diagnostic pitfalls/key intraoperative consultation issues
  - Highly aggressive tumor, often with extraovarian spread at the time of presentation.
  - Fertility-sparing surgery with unilateral salpingo-oophorectomy and tumor debulking has been reported in rare cases [16–18].

Small Cell Carcinoma, Pulmonary Type

- Rare tumor, presenting in older patients (mean age around 60 years) [19].
- Patients usually present with an abdominal/pelvic mass.
- Large, solid tumor.
- Size may be over 20 cm.
- Often bilateral.

- Microscopic features resemble pulmonary small cell carcinoma.
  - Diffuse, or less often trabeculated, nested growth pattern.
  - Small- or medium-sized, hyperchromatic, round to oval nuclei.
  - Scant cytoplasm.
  - Brisk mitotic activity, abundant apoptotic bodies and necrosis.
  - Chromatin pattern and nuclear molding may be difficult to appreciate on frozen section slides.
- Not infrequently admixed with another histological subtype, i.e. endometrioid or mucinous carcinoma
- Rarely may arise in a mature teratoma [20, 21]

- Differential diagnosis
  - Other types of primary ovarian carcinoma, particularly high grade serous and endometrioid
  - Small cell carcinoma, hypercalcemic type
  - Metastatic small cell carcinoma
- Diagnostic pitfalls/key intraoperative consultation issues
  - Metastatic small cell carcinoma to the ovary should be ruled out, as it does not require comprehensive gynecologic staging surgery.
    - Clinical history and review of the patient's prior biopsies with morphological comparison is most helpful.

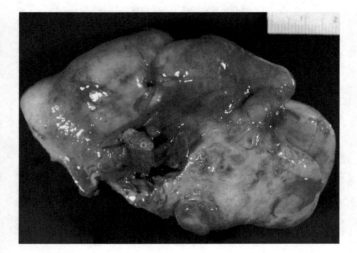

Fig. 11.11 Ovarian primary diffuse large B-cell lymphoma is grossly characterized by nodular, tan-pink, fleshy cut surface

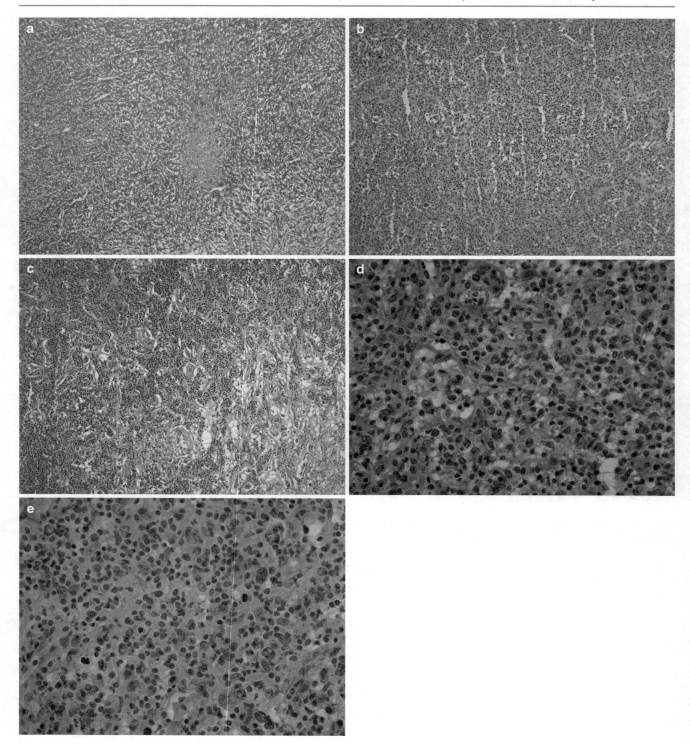

Fig. 11.12 Diffuse large B-cell lymphoma (DLBL). The tumor is composed of sheets (**a**, **b**) or cords (**c**) of large, markedly atypical lymphoid cells with high mitotic activity, irregular nuclear contours, and indistinct cell membranes (**d**, **e**). Stromal hyalinization is also a common feature of ovarian DLBL (**c**)

References

1. Hallatt JG, Steele Jr CH, Snyder M. Ruptured corpus luteum with hemoperitoneum: a study of 173 surgical cases. Am J Obstet Gynecol. 1984;149:5–9.

2. Fukunaga M, Ushigome S. Epithelial metaplastic changes in ovarian endometriosis. Mod Pathol. 1998;11:784–8.

3. Seidman JD. Prognostic importance of hyperplasia and atypia in endometriosis. Int J Gynecol Pathol. 1996;15:1–9.

4. Irving JA, McCluggage WG. Ovarian spindle cell lesions: a review with emphasis on recent developments and differential diagnosis. Adv Anat Pathol. 2007;14:305–19.

5. Young RH, Scully RE. Fibromatosis and massive edema of the ovary, possibly related entities: a report of 14 cases of fibromatosis and 11 cases of massive edema. Int J Gynecol Pathol. 1984;3: 153–78.

6. Roth LM, Deaton RL, Sternberg WH. Massive ovarian edema. A clinicopathologic study of five cases including ultrastructural observations and review of the literature. Am J Surg Pathol. 1979;3:11–21.

7. Sasaki KJ, Miller CE. Adnexal torsion: review of the literature. J Minim Invasive Gynecol. 2014;21:196–202.

8. Ganer Herman H, Shalev A, Ginath S, Kemer R, Keidar R, Bar J, Sagiv R. Clinical characteristics and the risk for malignancy in postmenopausal women with adnexal torsion. Maturitas. 2015;81: 57–61.

9. Lareau SM, Beigi RH. Pelvic inflammatory disease and tubo-ovarian abscess. Infect Dis Clin North Am. 2008;22:693–708.

10. Vang R, Medeiros LJ, Fuller GN, Sarris AH, Deavers M. Non-Hodgkin's lymphoma involving the gynecologic tract: a review of 88 cases. Adv Anat Pathol. 2001;8:200–17.

11. Lagoo AS, Robboy SJ. Lymphoma of the female genital tract: current status. Int J Gynecol Pathol. 2006;25:1–21.

12. Yadav BS, George P, Sharma SC, Gorsi U, McClennan E, Martino MA, et al. Primary non-Hodgkin lymphoma of the ovary. Semin Oncol. 2014;41:e19–30.

13. Ahmad AK, Hui P, Litkouhi B, Azodi M, Rutherford T, McCarthy S, et al. Institutional review of primary non-hodgkin lymphoma of the female genital tract: a 33-year experience. Int J Gynecol Cancer. 2014;24:1250–5.

14. Dickersin GR, Kline IW, Scully RE. Small cell carcinoma of the ovary with hypercalcemia: a report of eleven cases. Cancer. 1982;49:188–97.

15. Young RH, Oliva E, Scully RE. Small cell carcinoma of the ovary, hypercalcemic type. A clinicopathological analysis of 150 cases. Am J Surg Pathol. 1994;18:1102–16.

16. Walker NH, Sabanli M, Sykes PH, Russell P, Perez D. Successful reproductive outcome following treatment of advanced small cell carcinoma of the ovary. Gynecol Oncol Case Rep. 2012;2:115–7.

17. Powell JL, McAfee RD, McCoy RC, Shiro BS. Uterine and ovarian conservation in advanced small cell carcinoma of the ovary. Obstet Gynecol. 1998;91:846–8.

18. Distelmaier F, Calaminus G, Harms D, Sträter R, Kordes U, Fleischhack G, et al. Ovarian small cell carcinoma of the hypercalcemic type in children and adolescents: a prognostically unfavorable but curable disease. Cancer. 2006;107:2298–306.

19. Eichhorn JH, Young RH, Scully RE. Primary ovarian small cell carcinoma of pulmonary type. A clinicopathologic, immunohisto-logic, and flow cytometric analysis of 11 cases. Am J Surg Pathol. 1992;16:926–38.

20. Ikota H, Kaneko K, Takahashi S, Kawarai M, Tanaka Y, Yokoo H, Nakazoto Y. Malignant transformation of ovarian mature cystic teratoma with a predominant pulmonary type small cell carcinoma component. Pathol Int. 2012;62:276–80.

21. Lim SC, Choi SJ, Suh CH. A case of small cell carcinoma arising in a mature cystic teratoma of the ovary. Pathol Int. 1998;48: 834–9.

Metastatic Tumors of Ovary

12

Introduction

Metastatic tumors account for up to 15 % of ovarian malignancies in western countries [1, 2] and may present a significant diagnostic challenge during intraoperative frozen section consultation. The primary site is most commonly located in the gastrointestinal tract, with approximately 30 % of cases originating from the colon, followed by appendiceal, gastric, and pancreatobiliary primaries [3, 4]. Among non-gastrointestinal primaries, breast cancer is the most frequent source of ovarian metastases [3, 5], which may also be an incidental finding in prophylactic or therapeutic oophorectomy specimens. Metastatic endometrial and cervical carcinomas to the ovary occur at a lower frequency and generally have less severe implications on the intraoperative management at the time of frozen section compared to other metastatic sites. While comprehensive surgical staging is typically performed for primary ovarian malignancies, gynecologic staging surgery is unnecessary for extragenital primary tumors metastatic to the ovary. Intraoperative frozen section evaluation plays a critical role in this distinction and therefore guides the extent of surgery.

The most important first step in assessing the origin of tumor—primary versus metastatic—is thorough review of the patient's clinical history. However, the primary tumor may be occult and the metastasis may precede the diagnosis of primary tumor. In one study, 51 % of ovarian metastases of gastrointestinal origin were diagnosed prior to the discovery of the primary tumor [3]. The median age of patients with ovarian metastases is 53–55 years [4, 5], although patients with Krukenberg tumor typically present earlier (average age: 45 years) [6]. The clinical presentation may be similar to primary ovarian tumors—pelvic pain and mass effect, and rarely even hormonal (androgenic or estrogenic) manifestations, due to functioning stroma [6]. The macroscopic features may be helpful, as bilaterality, tumor size under 10 cm, ovarian surface involvement, and multinodular growth pattern are more common in metastatic tumors [7]; however, exceptions do occur. On microscopic examination, extensive lymphovascular invasion and ovarian hilus involvement are generally in favor of metastatic carcinoma. Comparison with the patient's known primary should be made if the prior specimen is available at the time of frozen section, although the histological features at the metastatic site may slightly be different from those of the primary tumor. For example, mucinous tumors metastatic to the ovary may demonstrate a "maturation phenomenon," mimicking a primary benign or borderline ovarian mucinous tumor [8]. Cystic growth pattern may be encountered in the ovarian metastasis, even when the primary tumor is predominantly solid [6].

The frozen section diagnosis—especially in difficult or equivocal cases—should not be made in isolation without intraoperative discussion with the surgeon. If only one ovary is received for frozen section, the surgeon should be inquired about the appearance of the other ovary and about the possibility of bilaterality, especially if dealing with a mucinous tumor. If a metastasis is suspected, intraoperative surgical evaluation of the pelvis and abdomen and sampling from any additional pelvic or intra-abdominal—intestinal, appendiceal, or gastric—lesions or enlarged intra-abdominal lymph nodes may be helpful. Intraoperative identification of pseudomyxoma peritonei by the surgeon or presence of extracellular mucinous material on the ovarian surfaces strongly favors appendiceal primary. Appendectomy is usually performed in this scenario even if the appendix appears grossly unremarkable.

Metastases to other gynecologic organs occur less commonly and may involve vagina, vulva, uterine cervix, endometrium, and fallopian tube—in decreasing order of frequency [5]. Metastatic tumors may mimic primaries at these sites and may be easily misinterpreted, especially due

© Springer International Publishing Switzerland 2015

P. Hui, N. Buza, *Atlas of Intraoperative Frozen Section Diagnosis in Gynecologic Pathology*,

DOI 10.1007/978-3-319-21807-6_12

to their rare occurrence. Unusual morphologic features—e.g., intestinal-type differentiation with goblet cells or extensive lymphovascular invasion—should raise suspicion for a possible metastatic origin.

This chapter summarizes the clinical, gross, and microscopic features and site-specific key intraoperative consultation issues of the most common metastatic tumors—intestinal, signet-ring cell, pancreatobiliary and appendiceal adenocarcinomas, and breast and gynecologic primaries—involving the ovary. Metastases from other primary sites—lung, urinary tract, melanoma, and sarcomas—occur rarely, and their clinical and histopathologic features depend largely on the primary tumor site.

Gastrointestinal Tract

Intestinal Adenocarcinoma

- Clinical and gross features
  - Most frequent tumor type among ovarian metastases.
  - May have functioning ovarian stroma.
  - Most common primary site is rectosigmoid (77 %), followed by cecum (9 %), ascending colon (9 %), and descending colon (5 %) [9].
  - Often bilateral, with a solid, or solid and cystic tan-yellow, or gray cut surface (Fig. 12.1).
  - Ovarian surface involvement and multinodular growth pattern are commonly seen.
  - Necrosis and hemorrhage are common.
- Microscopic features (Fig. 12.2)
  - Variably sized, often cystic, irregular glands.
  - Cribriform architecture may be seen.
  - "Dirty necrosis"—eosinophilic necrotic debris with karyorrhexis—within the gland lumens or surrounded by glandular epithelium in a garland pattern.
  - Moderate to severe nuclear atypia.
  - Rare mucin-containing goblet cells.
  - Infiltrative growth at least focally with desmoplastic stromal reaction.
- Differential diagnosis
  - Primary ovarian mucinous adenocarcinoma
  - Primary ovarian endometrioid adenocarcinoma
  - Sertoli-Leydig cell tumor with mucinous heterologous elements
- Diagnostic pitfalls/key intraoperative consultation issues
  - The ovarian metastasis may precede the diagnosis of colonic primary.

- Patients presenting with ovarian metastasis first tend to be younger compared with those who have a known colonic primary (mean age 48 versus 61 years, respectively) [10].
- Bilaterality, size <10 cm, ovarian surface involvement, multinodular growth pattern, and infiltrative growth with desmoplastic stromal reaction favor metastasis over ovarian primary (see Chap. 8, Table 8.1).
- Metastatic colorectal carcinomas may have a functioning ovarian stroma with androgen or estrogen production.
- Distinction between primary ovarian mucinous adenocarcinoma and metastatic colorectal carcinoma may not be possible at the time of frozen section especially in the absence of a known primary.
  - It is important to correctly identify mucinous differentiation and raise the possibility of a metastasis, as it gives the opportunity for thorough intraoperative surgical evaluation of the abdominal cavity—including intestines—and possibly additional sampling.
- Metastatic intestinal/colorectal carcinoma may also mimic primary endometrioid adenocarcinoma of the ovary.
  - Most helpful distinctive microscopic feature of endometrioid adenocarcinoma is squamous differentiation, which is absent in intestinal-type adenocarcinomas.
  - If only one ovary is sent for frozen section, the surgeon should be inquired about the appearance of the other ovary and the possibility of bilaterality.
- Association with mature teratoma favors ovarian primary.

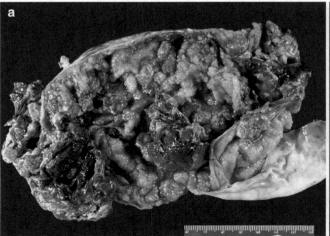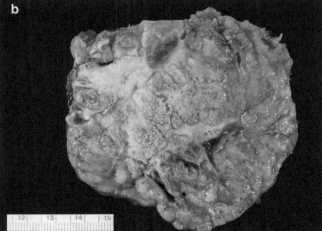

Fig. 12.1 Metastatic colorectal adenocarcinoma. Note the predominantly cystic (**a**) or solid, tan-pink, and multinodular cut surface (**b**)

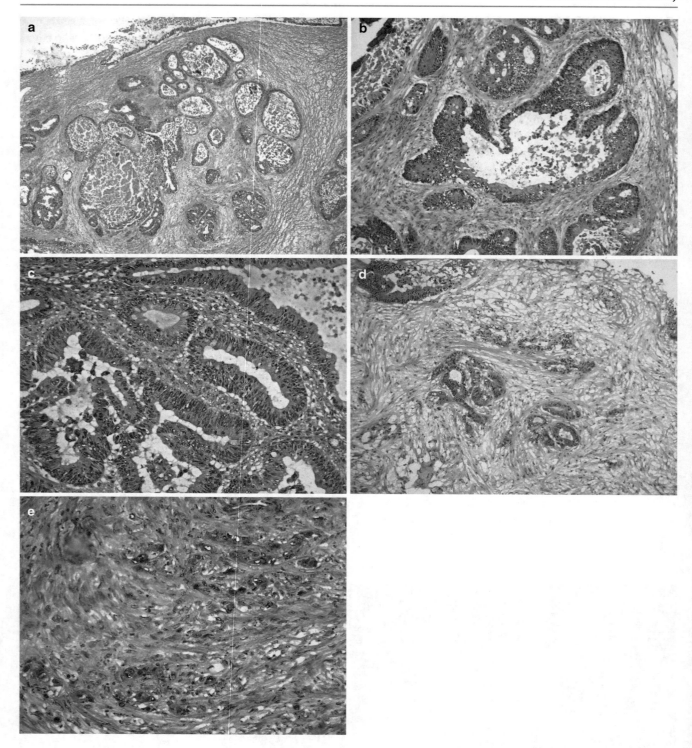

Fig. 12.2 Metastatic colorectal adenocarcinoma. Note the variably sized, irregular, and cystically dilated glands (**a**) with intraluminal necrotic debris (**b**) and moderate to severe nuclear atypia (**c**). Goblet cells are present but often are few in number (**c**). Stromal infiltration with desmoplastic reaction (**d**) and single cell infiltrative pattern (**e**) are helpful microscopic features

Metastatic Adenocarcinoma with Signet-Ring Cells/Krukenberg Tumor

- Clinical and gross features
  - The primary tumor is located in the stomach (often pylorus) in approximately 70 % of cases, less commonly in the colorectum, appendix, breast, and pancreatobiliary system [6, 11].
  - Often presents in young patients, the average age is 45 years [11].
  - May have functioning ovarian stroma resulting in endocrine manifestations.
  - Other symptoms may include abdominal swelling or pain.
  - Ascites has been reported in over 40 % of cases [11].
  - At least 80 % of tumors are bilateral [6].
  - Average tumor size is 10.4 cm, with most tumors falling between 5 and 20 cm [11].
  - Irregular ovarian surface, often involved by tumor.
  - Cut surface is most often solid, tan-yellow or white, and multinodular; may also be firm or soft and gelatinous—depending on the mucin content and proportion of fibrous stroma (Fig. 12.3).
  - Hemorrhage may be seen; necrosis is not common.
- Microscopic features (Fig. 12.4 stomach, Fig. 12.5 colon, Fig. 12.6 breast)
  - Low magnification may show a pseudo-lobular pattern with alternating hyper- and hypocellular—edematous—areas or diffusely cellular dense stroma.
  - Signet-ring cells infiltrate individually, or form small clusters, diffuse sheets or small tubular structures.
    - Eccentric nuclei with abundant basophilic, eosinophilic, or clear cytoplasm
    - Variable nuclear pleomorphism and mitotic activity, but most often only mild atypia and relatively low mitotic rate
  - Extracellular mucin pools may be present.
  - Stroma may be prominent and may contain luteinized cells.
- Differential diagnosis
  - Benign stromal tumors of ovary: fibroma, cellular fibroma, thecoma, sclerosing stromal tumor, and signet-ring stromal tumor
  - Stromal hyperplasia/hyperthecosis
  - Sertoli-Leydig cell tumor (versus tubular Krukenberg tumor)
  - Goblet cell (mucinous) carcinoid
- Diagnostic pitfalls/key intraoperative consultation issues
  - Signet-ring cells may be missed on low magnification in the background of a densely cellular stroma.
  - High magnification assessment is recommended before the diagnosis of fibroma/fibrothecoma is made, to rule out metastatic signet-ring cell carcinoma.
  - Krukenberg tumors are very often bilateral (~80 % of cases), whereas bilaterality is rare among benign ovarian stromal and sex cord—stromal tumors; only approximately 8 % of ovarian fibromas are bilateral.

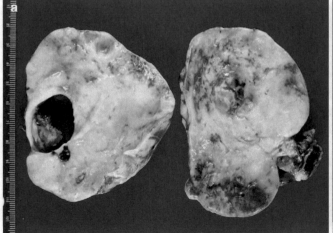
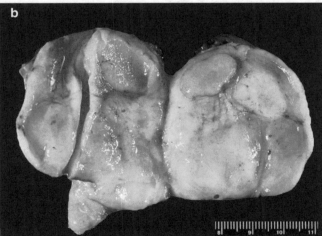

Fig. 12.3 Krukenberg tumor/metastatic signet-ring cell carcinoma (**a**, **b**). Note the characteristic solid, tan-yellow, multinodular, and often gelatinous (**b**) gross appearance

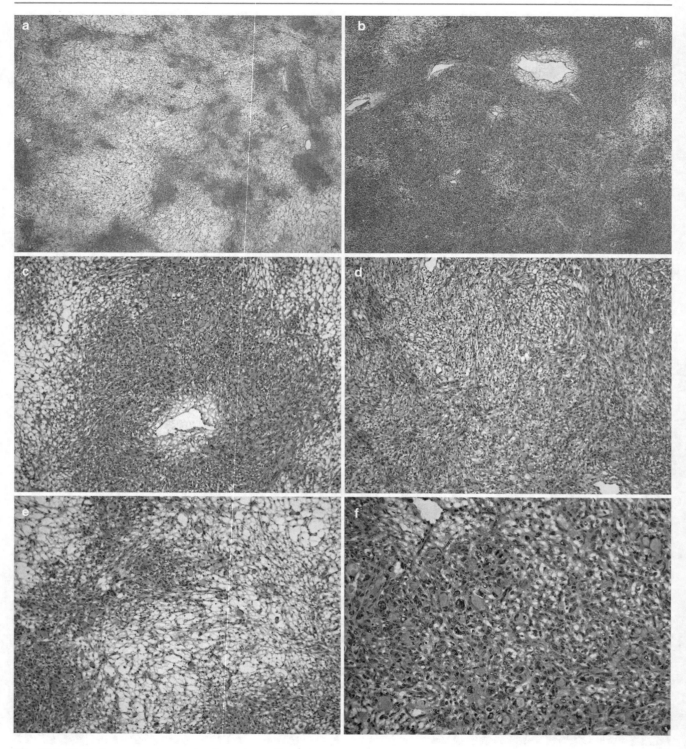

Fig. 12.4 Krukenberg tumor/metastatic signet-ring cell carcinoma from a gastric primary. Low magnification reveals a pseudo-lobular pattern with alternating hypo- and hypercellular areas (**a**). Densely cellular ovarian stroma may mimic an ovarian stromal tumor (**b**). Scattered individual tumor cells with relatively bland, small, eccentrically located nuclei and abundant pale basophilic or eosinophilic cytoplasm infiltrate the stroma (**c–e**). Less often marked nuclear atypia and brisk mitotic activity may be seen (**f**)

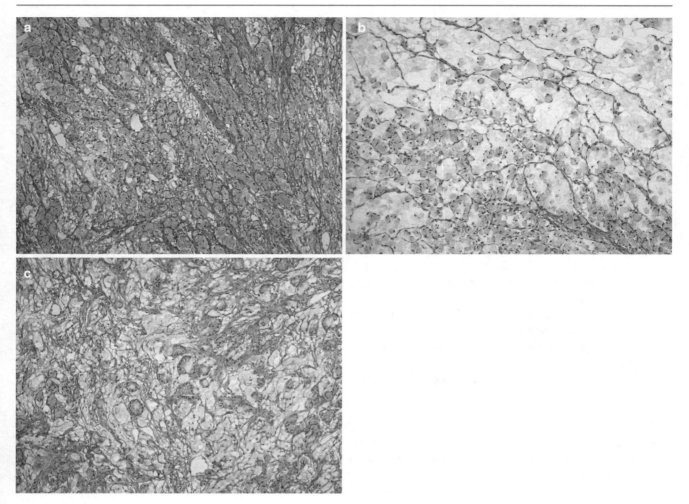

Fig. 12.5 Krukenberg tumor/metastatic signet-ring cell carcinoma from a colonic primary (**a–c**). Signet-ring cells are forming small clusters and tubules. Abundant extracellular mucin is also present

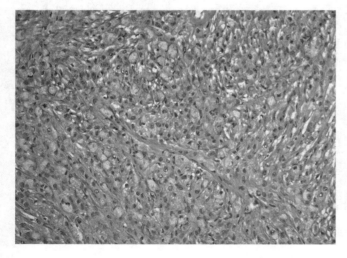

Fig. 12.6 Metastatic signet-ring cell carcinoma from a breast primary. Metastatic lobular carcinoma of the breast may have signet-ring cell morphology infiltrating the ovarian stroma in single cell files

Pancreatobiliary Adenocarcinomas

- Clinical and gross features
  - Relatively uncommon metastatic tumor in the ovary.
  - Mean patient age is 58–59 years [12, 13].
  - Most often bilateral (>80 % of cases).
  - Mean tumor size is around 10 cm [12, 13].
  - Cut surface may be solid or multiloculated cystic (Fig. 12.7a pancreas, Fig. 12.7b gallbladder).
  - Nodular growth pattern and surface involvement are common.
- Microscopic features (Figs 12.8 pancreas, Figs. 12.9 gallbladder)
  - Variably sized neoplastic glands, often forming cystic structures.
  - Areas mimicking a mucinous cystadenoma or mucinous borderline tumor are common ("maturation phenomenon").
    - Nuclear atypia may show a wide range from minimal to severe within the same tumor.
  - Intraluminal and extracellular stromal mucin may be abundant.
  - Infiltrative growth pattern with desmoplastic stroma.
    - Single tumor cell infiltration.
    - Signet-ring cells may be seen.
- Differential diagnosis
  - Primary ovarian mucinous tumors: mucinous cystadenoma, borderline (atypical proliferative) mucinous tumor, and mucinous carcinoma

- Diagnostic pitfalls/key intraoperative consultation issues
  - Metastatic pancreatobiliary adenocarcinomas may have a deceptively bland morphology and a cystic growth pattern, mimicking a benign or borderline (atypical proliferative) primary ovarian mucinous tumor.
  - Multiple blocks may need to be sampled for frozen section to identify areas with infiltrative growth and/or significant cytological atypia.
  - Morphologic comparison with the patient's known primary tumor—if slides are available—should be made.
  - Bilaterality favors metastasis over primary ovarian mucinous tumor.
  - Association with mature teratoma favors ovarian primary.

Appendiceal Tumors

- Most tumors with ovarian involvement are *low-grade mucinous neoplasms.*
- Less commonly primary, appendiceal intestinal-type adenocarcinomas, high-grade mucinous adenocarcinomas, signet-ring cell carcinomas, and mucinous (goblet cell) carcinoid tumors may also spread to the ovary.
- Metastatic intestinal-type and signet-ring cell adenocarcinomas are discussed earlier in this chapter.

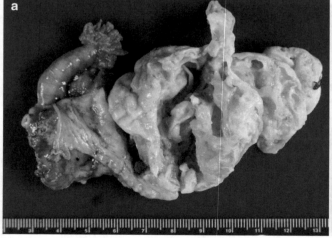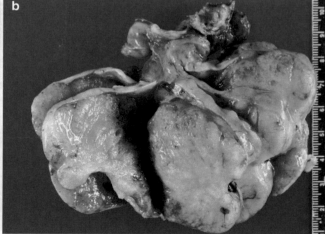

Fig. 12.7 Metastatic pancreatobiliary adenocarcinomas of the ovary. Note the multiloculated cystic (**a**) or predominantly solid, tan-yellow (**b**) cut surface

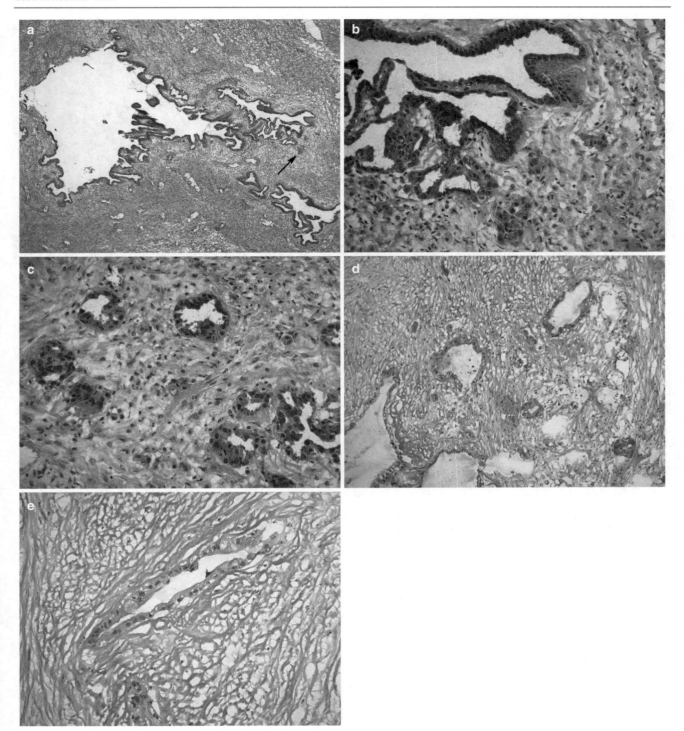

Fig. 12.8 Metastatic pancreatic adenocarcinoma. The tumor forms variably sized mucinous glands, which are often cystic and may mimic a primary ovarian—benign or borderline—mucinous tumor (**a**, **b**). Presence of stromal infiltration by small clusters or individual tumor cells is a helpful diagnostic clue (**a**, *arrow*; **b**, **c**). Desmoplastic stromal response and extracellular mucin pools may be seen (**d**). The nuclear atypia may be deceptively minimal (**e**)

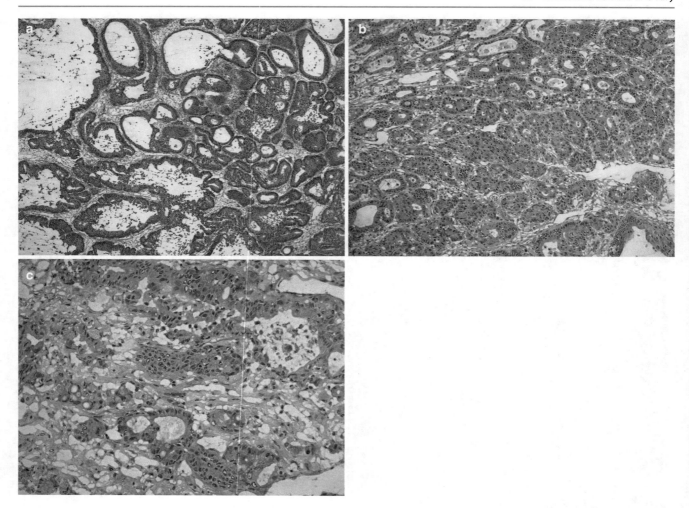

Fig. 12.9 Metastatic gallbladder carcinoma. Note the irregular, variably sized glands, with intraluminal necrosis (**a**) or mucinous material (**b**). Occasional signet-ring cells and extracellular mucin are also seen (**c**)

Low-Grade Appendiceal Mucinous Neoplasm (LAMN)

- Clinical and gross features
  - Mean patient age is around 50 years [14, 15].
  - Most patients present with symptoms related to ovarian metastases—pelvic mass/pain, increased abdominal girth, and the appendiceal mass is usually discovered synchronously.
  - Often associated with pseudomyxoma peritonei (see Chap. 13).
  - Frequent bilateral ovarian involvement and predominance of right-sided involvement among unilateral cases [14, 15].
  - Mean tumor size is 16 cm [14].
  - The cut surface is typically multiloculated, cystic with tan-gray mucoid appearance (Fig. 12.10a).
    - Ovarian surface involvement is common.
  - The appendix is grossly abnormal in most cases with a dilated tip filled with mucus (Fig. 12.10b).
    - Rupture and surface involvement may be grossly apparent.
- Microscopic features (Fig. 12.11)
  - Cystic glands lined by flat or undulating mucinous epithelium.
  - Abundant basophilic mucinous material is seen within the cystic gland lumens and spilling into/dissecting the ovarian stroma ("pseudomyxoma ovarii"), and is often also present on the ovarian surface.
  - Tall columnar tumor cells with bland, relatively uniform basally located nuclei.

- Abundant pale eosinophilic or basophilic cytoplasm.
- Goblet cells are present in variable proportions.
- No significant mitotic activity.
- Differential diagnosis
  - Primary ovarian mucinous borderline (atypical proliferative) tumor and mucinous cystadenoma
- Diagnostic pitfalls/key intraoperative consultation issues
  - Presence of pseudomyxoma peritonei, bilaterality, and ovarian surface involvement favor metastasis over ovarian primary.
  - Subepithelial clefts, scalloped glands, and pseudomyxoma ovarii have been found more commonly in metastatic LAMN than in primary ovarian mucinous borderline (atypical proliferative) tumors [16].
  - Association with a mature teratoma favors ovarian primary.
    - Teratoma-associated primary mucinous ovarian tumors may show morphologic features similar to LAMN and may present with pseudomyxoma peritonei.
  - The surgeon should be inquired about the intraoperative findings:
    - Pseudomyxoma peritonei
    - Gross appearance of the appendix
    - Gross appearance of the other ovary and the possibility of bilaterality (if only one ovary was sent for frozen section)
  - Appendectomy and frozen section evaluation of the appendix should be considered even in the absence of obvious gross abnormalities.

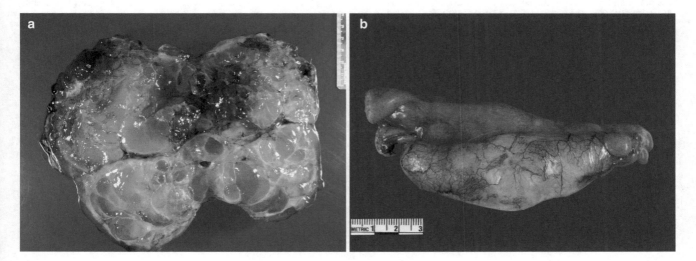

Fig. 12.10 Metastatic low-grade appendiceal mucinous neoplasm. The tumor typically appears as a multiloculated, cystic ovarian mass, filled with thick mucinous contents (**a**). The appendix is abnormally dilated due to the primary tumor (**b**)

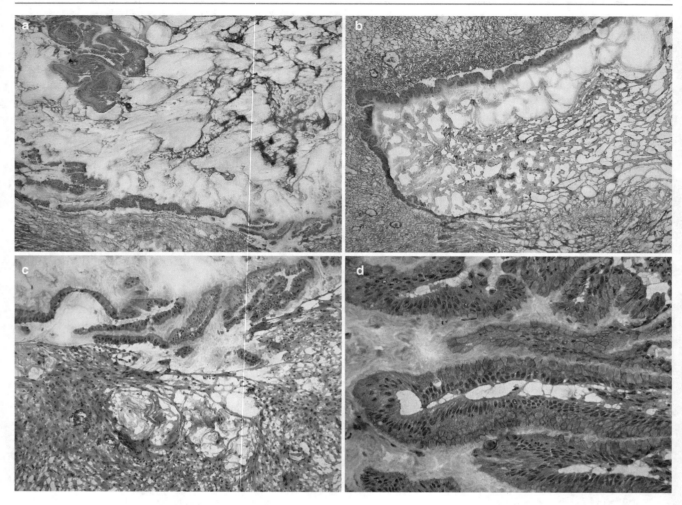

Fig. 12.11 Metastatic low-grade appendiceal mucinous neoplasm. The tumor microscopically appears as cystic structures filled with abundant basophilic mucinous material (**a, b**) and lined by flat or undulating mucinous epithelium (**a, b**). Mucin extravasation—pseudomyxoma ovarii is often seen (**c**). The tumor cells are relatively uniform with basally located nuclei and abundant mucinous cytoplasm (**d**). Goblet cells are usually numerous (**c, d**)

Breast

- Clinical and gross features
  - Most patients have known breast cancer.
  - Often found incidentally in prophylactic and therapeutic salpingo-oophorectomy specimens.
  - In rare cases, the ovarian metastasis may be symptomatic and precedes the diagnosis of breast primary [17].
  - Median time between breast cancer diagnosis and ovarian metastasis was 5 years in a recent study [18]
  - The metastatic tumors are often bilateral and small (<5 cm in size)
  - Cut surface is solid, tan-white, or yellow and may appear multinodular (Fig. 12.12.)
    - Small incidental metastatic tumors may have normal gross appearance.
- Microscopic features (Fig. 12.13)
  - Although the frequency of ovarian metastases is higher among invasive lobular carcinomas (ILC) than invasive ductal carcinomas (IDC) [19], most metastatic breast carcinomas in the ovary are of ductal histological type due to the much higher incidence of IDC.
  - Metastatic ductal carcinomas may have a solid, micropapillary, cribriform, or glandular pattern with variable degree of tubule formation.
    - The tumor cells most often show moderate to severe nuclear atypia and high nuclear to cytoplasmic ratio.
  - Metastatic lobular carcinomas typically show single cell spread haphazardly or arranged in linear cords.
    - May appear as diffuse sheets of tumor cells.
    - Eccentric small nuclei often with only mild to moderate atypia.

- Intracytoplasmic lumens with "targetoid" secretions may be seen.
- Less often signet-ring cell features are present (See Krukenberg tumor, Fig. 12.6).
- Differential diagnosis
  - Primary ovarian carcinomas—high-grade serous carcinoma and endometrioid adenocarcinoma
  - Adult granulosa cell tumor
  - Lymphoma
- Diagnostic pitfalls/key intraoperative consultation issues
  - In most cases, the breast cancer diagnosis precedes the ovarian metastasis, although the time interval between the primary and metastatic tumor may be quite long (up to 20 years) [18].
    - Clinical history of breast cancer may not be provided at the time of frozen section, especially if the clinical suspicion for a primary ovarian tumor is high.
    - The surgeon should be inquired about the clinical history and intraoperative findings—gross appearance of the other ovary and the possibility of bilaterality (if only one ovary was sent for frozen section).
  - Metastatic lobular carcinoma with diffuse growth pattern may mimic adult granulosa cell tumor or a lymphoproliferative process at low magnification.
    - Presence of larger cytoplasm and intracytoplasmic vacuoles on higher magnification can help to rule out the above entities.
  - Morphologic comparison with the patients known primary—if the slides are available—should be pursued.

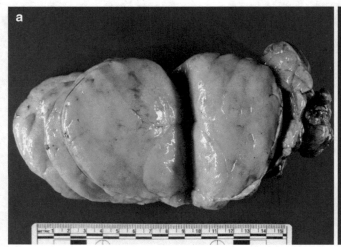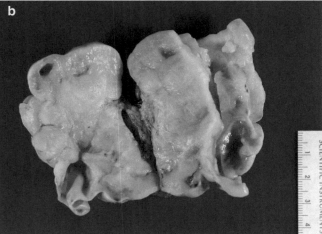

Fig. 12.12 Metastatic breast carcinoma macroscopically appears as a solid, tan-yellow or tan-white, multinodular mass (**a**, **b**)

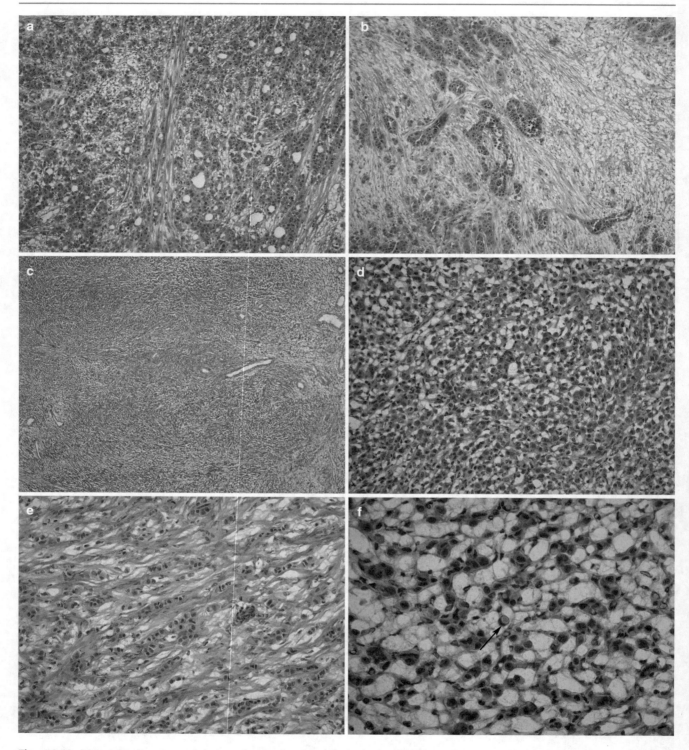

Fig. 12.13 Metastatic breast carcinoma, microscopic features. Metastatic ductal carcinoma has variable degree of tubule formation and moderate to severe nuclear atypia (**a**, **b**). Intraluminal necrotic debris is also seen (**b**). The tumor cells in metastatic lobular carcinoma may be diffusely "sprinkled" in the ovarian stroma (**c**, **d**) or may be arranged in single cell files (**e**). The nuclei are typically small with mild to moderate atypia (**d–f**). Intracytoplasmic targetoid secretions may be seen (**f**, *arrow*)

Gynecologic Organs

Cervical Adenocarcinoma, Usual Type

- Clinical and gross features
  - Ovarian metastases from cervical carcinomas are uncommon: approximately 5 % of cervical adenocarcinomas and less than 1 % of cervical squamous cell carcinomas spread to the ovary [20].
  - The primary endocervical tumor may be small or may lack unequivocal stromal invasion [21].
    - Ovarian mass may be the first clinical presentation of an unsuspected cervical adenocarcinoma.
  - The mean size of ovarian metastasis is 12.7 cm [21].
  - Unilateral in more than half of the cases.
  - Cut surface is often cystic and may contain viscous/mucoid material (Fig. 12.14).
- Microscopic features (Fig. 12.15)
  - Most often the tumor shows expansile growth; infiltrative stromal invasion is rare.
  - Confluent glandular, villoglandular, or cribriform architectural pattern.
    - Sharply angulated tips of the villoglandular structures are characteristic.
  - Columnar endocervical-type glandular cells with moderate amount of pale basophilic or eosinophilic cytoplasm.
  - Moderate nuclear atypia, nuclear hyperchromasia, and crowding, small nucleoli.
  - Frequent mitotic figures, located in the apical portion of cells—"jumping mitoses."
  - Abundant karyorrhectic debris at the basal portion of tumor cells.

- Differential diagnosis
  - Ovarian mucinous borderline (atypical proliferative) tumor
  - Ovarian endometrioid borderline (atypical proliferative) tumor
  - Primary ovarian mucinous carcinoma
  - Primary ovarian endometrioid adenocarcinoma
- Diagnostic pitfalls/key intraoperative consultation issues
  - The tumor growth pattern on low magnification may mimic ovarian mucinous and endometrioid borderline tumors.
  - The endocervical primary may be occult.
    - Gross and microscopic examination of the uterine cervix should be performed if the hysterectomy specimen was also received for frozen section.
  - Apical mitotic figures and basal apoptotic bodies are characteristic of usual type endocervical adenocarcinoma.

Endometrial Adenocarcinoma

- Endometrial and ovarian involvement by endometrioid or serous carcinoma may represent synchronous independent primaries or ovarian metastasis from the endometrial primary and vice versa.
  - Distinction between these possibilities is often impossible at the time of frozen section and is usually not critical for the intraoperative surgical management.
- Detailed histological features of endometrial adenocarcinomas are discussed in Chap. 4.

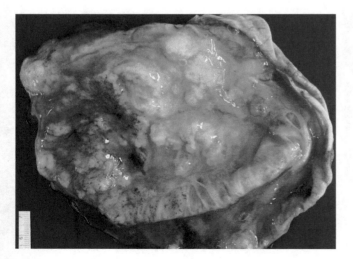

Fig. 12.14 Metastatic endocervical adenocarcinoma. The tumor shows a cystic cut surface with solid, irregular intraluminal growth and thick, viscous fluid contents

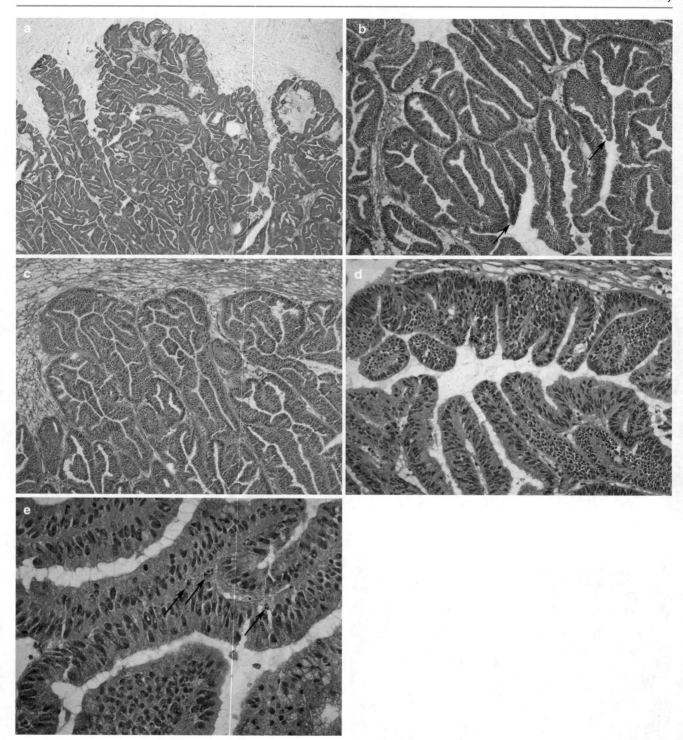

Fig. 12.15 Metastatic endocervical adenocarcinoma. The tumor demonstrates confluent glandular proliferation (**a**) with sharply angulated tips of the glandular/villoglandular structures (**b**, *arrows*). Expansile growth pattern without stromal reaction is most common (**c**). Moderate nuclear atypia, hyperchromasia, crowding, and numerous apically located mitotic figures are seen on high magnification (**d**, **e**). Frequent apoptotic bodies are also characteristic (**e**, *arrows*)

References

1. Ulbright TM, Roth LM, Stehman FB. Secondary ovarian neoplasia. A clinicopathologic study of 35 cases. Cancer. 1984;53:1164–74.
2. de Waal YR, Thomas CM, Oei AL, Sweep FC, Massuger LF. Secondary ovarian malignancies: frequency, origin, and characteristics. Int J Gynecol Cancer. 2009;19:1160–5.
3. Skirnisdottir I, Garmo H, Holmberg L. Non-genital tract metastases to the ovaries presented as ovarian tumors in Sweden 1990–2003: occurrence, origin and survival compared to ovarian cancer. Gynecol Oncol. 2007;105:166–71.
4. Moore RG, Chung M, Granai CO, Gajewski W, Steinhoff MM. Incidence of metastasis to the ovaries from nongenital tract primary tumors. Gynecol Oncol. 2004;93:87–91.
5. Mazur MT, Hsueh S, Gersell DJ. Metastases to the female genital tract. Analysis of 325 cases. Cancer. 1984;53:1978–84.
6. Young RH. From krukenberg to today: the ever present problems posed by metastatic tumors in the ovary: part I. Historical perspective, general principles, mucinous tumors including the krukenberg tumor. Adv Anat Pathol. 2006;13:205–27.
7. Yemelyanova AV, Vang R, Judson K, Wu LS, Ronnett BM. Distinction of primary and metastatic mucinous tumors involving the ovary: analysis of size and laterality data by primary site with reevaluation of an algorithm for tumor classification. Am J Surg Pathol. 2008;32:128–38.
8. Young RH, Scully RE. Differential diagnosis of ovarian tumors based primarily on their patterns and cell types. Semin Diagn Pathol. 2001;18:161–235.
9. Lash RH, Hart WR. Intestinal adenocarcinomas metastatic to the ovaries. A clinicopathologic evaluation of 22 cases. Am J Surg Pathol. 1987;11:114–21.
10. Judson K, McCormick C, Vang R, Yemelyanova AV, Wu LS, Bristow RE, Ronnett BM. Women with undiagnosed colorectal adenocarcinomas presenting with ovarian metastases: clinicopathologic features and comparison with women having known colorectal adenocarcinomas and ovarian involvement. Int J Gynecol Pathol. 2008;27:182–90.
11. Kiyokawa T, Young RH, Scully RE. Krukenberg tumors of the ovary: a clinicopathologic analysis of 120 cases with emphasis on their variable pathologic manifestations. Am J Surg Pathol. 2006; 30:277–99.
12. Meriden Z, Yemelyanova AV, Vang R, Ronnett BM. Ovarian metastases of pancreaticobiliary tract adenocarcinomas: analysis of 35 cases, with emphasis on the ability of metastases to simulate primary ovarian mucinous tumors. Am J Surg Pathol. 2011;35: 276–88.
13. Khunamornpong S, Lerwill MF, Siriaunkgul S, Suprasert P, Pojchamarnwiputh S, Chiangmai WN, Young RH. Carcinoma of extrahepatic bile ducts and gallbladder metastatic to the ovary: a report of 16 cases. Int J Gynecol Pathol. 2008;27:366–79.
14. Young RH, Gilks CB, Scully RE. Mucinous tumors of the appendix associated with mucinous tumors of the ovary and pseudomyxoma peritonei. A clinicopathological analysis of 22 cases supporting an origin in the appendix. Am J Surg Pathol. 1991;15:415–29.
15. Seidman JD, Elsayed AM, Sobin LH, Tavassoli FA. Association of mucinous tumors of the ovary and appendix. A clinicopathologic study of 25 cases. Am J Surg Pathol. 1993;17:22–34.
16. Stewart CJ, Ardakani NM, Doherty DA, Young RH. An evaluation of the morphologic features of low-grade mucinous neoplasms of the appendix metastatic in the ovary, and comparison with primary ovarian mucinous tumors. Int J Gynecol Pathol. 2014;33:1–10.
17. Young RH, Carey RW, Robboy SJ. Breast carcinoma masquerading as primary ovarian neoplasm. Cancer. 1981;48:210–2.
18. Bigorie V, Morice P, Duvillard P, Antoine M, Cortez A, Flejou JF, et al. Ovarian metastases from breast cancer: report of 29 cases. Cancer. 2010;116:799–804.
19. Arpino G, Bardou VJ, Clark GM, Elledge RM. Infiltrating lobular carcinoma of the breast: tumor characteristics and clinical outcome. Breast Cancer Res. 2004;6:R149–56.
20. Shimada M, Kigawa J, Nishimura R, Yamaguchi S, Kuzuya K, Nakanishi T, et al. Ovarian metastasis in carcinoma of the uterine cervix. Gynecol Oncol. 2006;101:234–7.
21. Ronnett BM, Yemelyanova AV, Vang R, Gilks CB, Miller D, Gravitt PE, Kurman RJ. Endocervical adenocarcinomas with ovarian metastases: analysis of 29 cases with emphasis on minimally invasive cervical tumors and the ability of the metastases to simulate primary ovarian neoplasms. Am J Surg Pathol. 2008;32: 1835–53.

Peritoneum

13

Introduction

Peritoneal biopsies are often performed and sent for frozen section evaluation during gynecologic surgeries. Intraoperative assessment of peritoneal surfaces is an integral part of surgical staging procedure for gynecologic malignancies. Peritoneal/omental nodules are usually more easily accessible at the beginning of the surgical procedure than other pelvic/gynecologic organs, and the frozen section diagnosis provides guidance for the type and extent of the surgery. While the peritoneum is often involved by various benign and malignant tumors originating from the gynecologic tract, tumors of other histogenetic origins and reactive conditions also occur and may pose a significant diagnostic challenge on frozen section.

Mullerian Epithelial Tumors

- Serous tumors—serous borderline (atypical proliferative) tumor, low-grade and high-grade serous carcinoma—may arise from the peritoneum as a primary site, and their histological features and diagnostic criteria are essentially identical to those of ovarian origin. (See Chap. 8—for detailed clinicopathologic features.)
- Primary ovarian serous tumors often show peritoneal involvement—implants of serous borderline (atypical proliferative) tumor or carcinoma.
    - The primary tumor site—ovarian versus peritoneal—often cannot be determined based on a small peritoneal biopsy alone.
    - There is no significant difference in intraoperative surgical management between primary ovarian and peritoneal serous tumors.
- Recognition of atypical/neoplastic nature of the process and serous (Mullerian) histological subtype are the most important for clinical management at the time of frozen section.
- Various nonneoplastic/reactive and neoplastic mimics exist and will be discussed in detail in this chapter.

P. Hui, N. Buza, *Atlas of Intraoperative Frozen Section Diagnosis in Gynecologic Pathology*, DOI 10.1007/978-3-319-21807-6_13

Mesothelial Tumors

Malignant Mesothelioma

- Clinical features
  - Majority of patients are male with history of occupational asbestos exposure [1].
  - Most common location is pleura, while peritoneal mesothelioma represents only 10–30 % of cases [1, 2].
  - Female patients with peritoneal mesothelioma less often have history of asbestos exposure and present at a mean age of 47.4 years (range 17–92 years) [3].
  - Most common clinical presentation of peritoneal mesothelioma includes pelvic mass/pain, ascites, and increased abdominal girth, although it may also be an incidental finding [3, 4].
- Gross pathology
  - Diffuse involvement of peritoneal surfaces by nodules, plaques, or papillary excrescences [3]
- Microscopic features (Fig. 13.1)
  - Epithelioid cells arranged in tubular, papillary, or solid architectural patterns—often multiple patterns within the same tumor.
    - Compressed tubular structures may resemble a reticular pattern.
  - Polygonal or round tumor cells with moderate amount of eosinophilic cytoplasm.
    - "Hobnail" and "cobblestone" appearance may be seen.
  - Mild to moderate atypia in most cases; rarely severe nuclear atypia.
  - Mitotic activity is usually low; less than 5/10 high-power field in most tumors [3].
  - Pale basophilic material may be seen in the lumen of tubules or within the cytoplasm.
  - Stromal infiltration is usually present; desmoplastic response may be seen.
  - Stroma may be hyalinized or less often myxoid.
  - Psammomatous calcifications may be present.
  - Rare histological variants—sarcomatoid, deciduoid, signet-ring cell, and multicystic—are also known to occur.
- Differential diagnosis
  - Mullerian serous tumors—high-grade and low-grade serous carcinoma, serous borderline (atypical proliferative) tumor
  - Metastatic carcinomas from other primaries
  - Well-differentiated papillary mesothelioma
  - Reactive mesothelial hyperplasia
- Diagnostic pitfalls/key intraoperative consultation issues
  - Malignant mesothelioma in women is much less common than Mullerian serous tumors.
  - The surgeon should be inquired about the intraoperative gross appearance of the lesion: a small, solitary nodule favors well-differentiated papillary mesothelioma.
    - The biopsy sent for frozen section is often small, and the histological features may be misleading without knowledge of the clinical context and gross appearance/extent of disease.
  - The mitotic activity is usually higher and the nuclear pleomorphism is more severe in high-grade serous carcinomas, compared with malignant mesothelioma.
  - Intraluminal and intracytoplasmic basophilic material may be seen in mesotheliomas, but it is not a feature of Mullerian serous tumors.
  - Desmoplastic and/or myxoid stromal reaction and intraluminal basophilic material may mimic metastatic adenocarcinoma, especially from gastrointestinal or pancreatobiliary primaries.
  - Definitive diagnosis of malignant mesothelioma on frozen section (i.e., on morphology alone, without ancillary studies) may be very challenging; however, based on the clinical and gross features and microscopic characteristics of tumor, the possibility of mesothelioma should be raised.

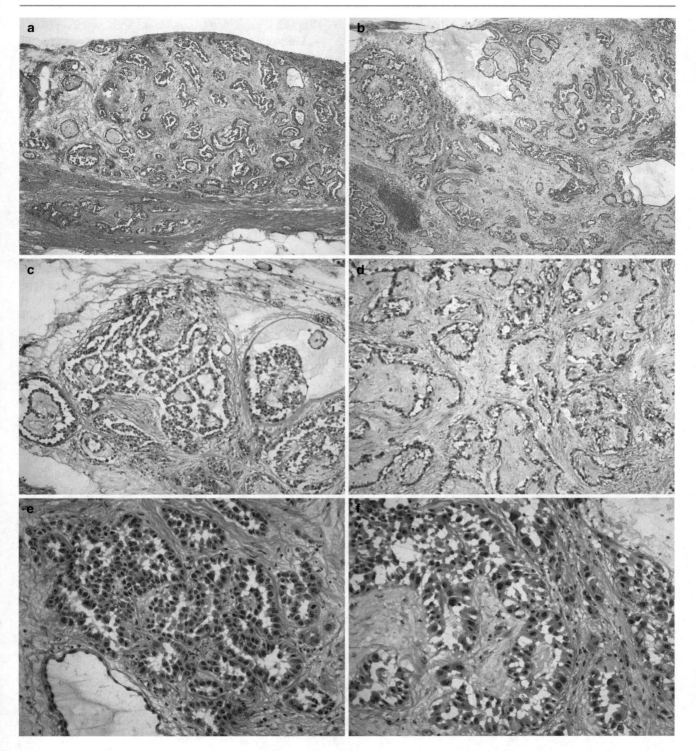

Fig. 13.1 Malignant mesothelioma. Note the plaque-like growth on the peritoneal surface (**a**) with papillary (**b, c**) and reticular (**d**) architecture. Pale basophilic intraluminal material (**b, c**) and myxoid stroma (**d**) may be seen. The cells show mild to moderate atypia and "hobnail" or "cobblestone" appearance (**e, f**)

Well-Differentiated Papillary Mesothelioma

- Clinical features
  - Most common in females, median age is 47 years [5, 6].
  - Most often an incidental finding during surgery.
- Gross pathology
  - Usually presents as a solitary or multiple small nodule(s), less than 2 cm in size [6]
- Microscopic features (Fig. 13.2)
  - Papillary or tubulo-papillary architecture.
  - Single layer of flat or cuboidal, bland mesothelial cells.
  - No significant atypia or mitotic activity.
  - Lack of stromal infiltration.
  - Psammoma bodies may be seen.
- Differential diagnosis
  - Malignant mesothelioma
  - Mullerian serous tumors—low-grade serous carcinoma and serous borderline (atypical proliferative) tumor

- Diagnostic pitfalls/key intraoperative consultation issues
  - Well-differentiated papillary mesothelioma typically shows a benign clinical course.
    - Rare cases may recur or have a more aggressive clinical behavior [6–8].
  - Intraoperative gross appearance of the lesion is very helpful: malignant mesothelioma is typically diffuse, nodular, or plaque-like, whereas well-differentiated papillary mesothelioma presents as a small, solitary nodule.
  - Significant nuclear atypia and apparent mitotic activity are in favor of malignant mesothelioma.
  - Stromal invasion is typically present in malignant mesothelioma but not in well-differentiated papillary mesothelioma.
  - Low-grade serous tumors—low-grade carcinoma and serous borderline (atypical proliferative) tumor—typically show more pronounced epithelial proliferation, multiple cell layers, and tufting, compared with well-differentiated papillary mesothelioma.

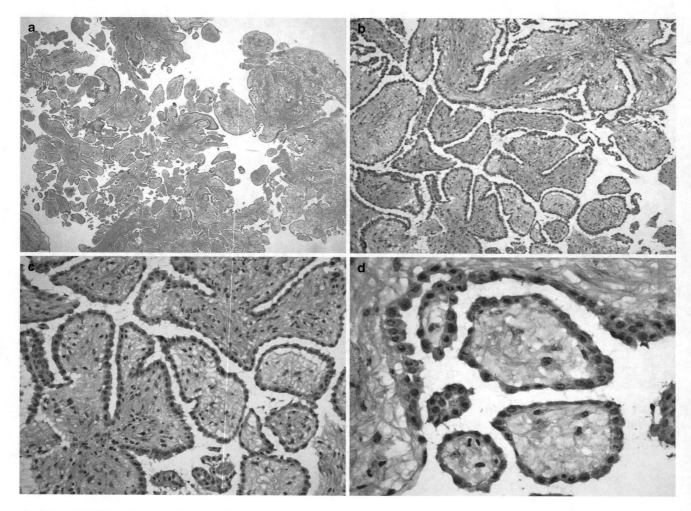

Fig. 13.2 Well-differentiated papillary mesothelioma. The tumor has papillary architecture on low magnification (**a**, **b**) without epithelial stratification or tufting. The papillae are lined by flat or cuboidal, bland mesothelial cells (**c**, **d**)

Mesenchymal Tumors

Leiomyomatosis Peritonealis Disseminata

- Rare, benign lesion
- Multiple small nodules on the peritoneal surfaces and omentum
- Composed of bland smooth muscle cells, histologically similar to uterine leiomyomas [see Chap. 5]
  - No significant nuclear atypia or mitotic activity
- Differential diagnosis: gastrointestinal stromal tumor, leiomyosarcoma; other benign and malignant spindle cell proliferations
  - See Chap. 5 for detailed histological features and differential diagnosis of smooth muscle tumors.

Gastrointestinal Stromal Tumor (GIST)

- Clinical features
  - Gastrointestinal stromal tumors may present—primarily or on recurrence—as an omental, mesenteric, or retroperitoneal mass [9–11].
  - Most common in middle-aged adults; median age of patients with omental presentation is around 60 years [9].
  - Patients may present with abdominal mass/pain or it may be an incidental finding during surgery.
- Gross pathology (Fig. 13.3)
  - Single or multiple masses, with a gray-tan or yellowish, predominantly solid cut surface.
  - May be attached to stomach or small intestine or there may not be evidence of gastrointestinal tract involvement.
  - Median tumor size is 14 cm [9].
  - Necrosis, hemorrhage, or cystic change may be seen.

- Microscopic features (Fig. 13.4)
  - The most common histological pattern is spindle cell, followed by epithelioid and mixed spindle and epithelioid patterns.
  - Significant nuclear pleomorphism is relatively uncommon, more often seen in epithelioid tumors.
  - Cellularity is variable.
  - Nuclear palisading and perinuclear vacuoles may be seen.
  - Mitotic activity is highly variable.
  - Myxoid change may be seen.
  - Necrosis and hemorrhage may be present.
  - Infiltration of peritumoral fat may occur.
- Differential diagnosis
  - Leiomyoma
  - Leiomyosarcoma
  - Metastatic carcinoma
  - Solitary fibrous tumor
  - Inflammatory myofibroblastic tumor
  - Fibromatosis
- Diagnostic pitfalls/key intraoperative consultation issues
  - Degree of atypia and mitotic activity are usually lower than those of malignant smooth muscle tumors.
  - Definitive diagnosis may be very challenging on frozen section and a descriptive diagnosis of "spindle cell lesion, final classification deferred for permanent sections" can be made, or a smooth muscle tumor or GIST may be favored, depending on the morphologic features and level of diagnostic certainty.
  - Epithelioid GIST may demonstrate significant nuclear pleomorphism, mimicking metastatic carcinoma.
    - Clinical history of prior epithelial malignancy should raise suspicion for metastatic carcinoma.
    - Identification of a spindle cell component may raise the possibility of GIST; sampling multiple blocks for frozen section may be helpful.

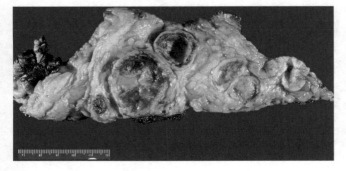

Fig. 13.3 Gastrointestinal stromal tumor (GIST) presenting as an omental mass, forming multiple solid and cystic nodules within the fibroadipose tissue

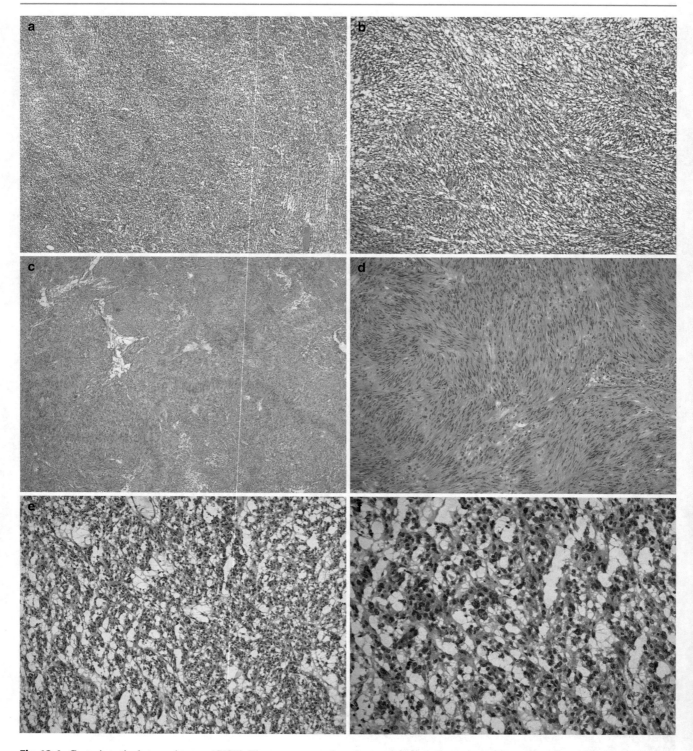

Fig. 13.4 Gastrointestinal stromal tumor (GIST). The tumor most often shows a spindle cell pattern (**a, b**), occasionally with nuclear palisading (**c, d**). Epithelioid GIST may have myxoid change and significant nuclear atypia (**e, f**), mimicking carcinoma

Tumors of Uncertain Histogenesis

Desmoplastic Small Round Cell Tumor (DSRCT)

- Clinical features
  - Rare malignant tumor typically occurring in adolescents or young adults [12, 13].
  - Male predominance [13].
  - Most patients present with abdominal mass/pain.
- Gross pathology (Fig. 13.5)
  - Multiple, variably-sized tumor nodules (mean size: 10 cm) [13].
  - Cut surface is solid, firm, multilobulated, and gray-white.
  - Necrosis, hemorrhage, and cystic change may be seen [14].
- Microscopic features (Fig. 13.6)
  - Sharply demarcated islands or sheets of small round blue cells in a desmoplastic stroma.
  - Uniform, round to ovoid, hyperchromatic nuclei and inconspicuous nucleoli.
  - Less commonly gland-like and rosette-like structures and peripheral palisading may be seen.
  - High mitotic activity.

- Scant, ill-defined cytoplasm.
- Single cell—or geographic necrosis
- Differential diagnosis
  - Other small round blue cell tumors, i.e., rhabdomyosarcoma, Ewing sarcoma, neuroblastoma, and lymphomas
  - Small cell carcinoma of ovary, hypercalcemic, and pulmonary types
- Diagnostic pitfalls/key intraoperative consultation issues
  - Location and distribution of tumor nodules is helpful in ruling out a primary ovarian tumor.
    - Intraoperative evaluation of ovaries by the surgeon is recommended.
    - Rare cases with ovarian involvement may mimic an ovarian primary [15].
  - Definitive diagnosis of DSRCT typically requires ancillary studies—immunohistochemistry, cytogenetics, or molecular methods; frozen section diagnosis of "small round blue cell tumor, final classification is deferred for permanent sections" is usually sufficient to guide intraoperative management.
    - Fresh tissue should be triaged for ancillary studies.

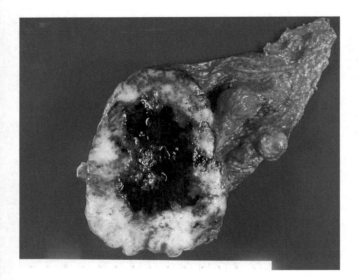

Fig. 13.5 Desmoplastic small round cell tumor. Note the solid, centrally cystic, and hemorrhagic tumor involving fibroadipose tissue

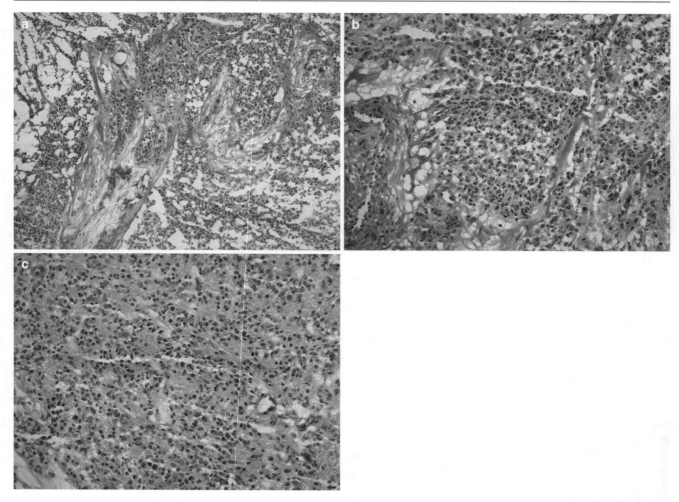

Fig. 13.6 Desmoplastic small round cell tumor. The tumor cells are forming islands in a desmoplastic stroma (**a**). Focal necrosis is often present (**a**, *left side of image*). Relatively uniform, round to oval nuclei and scant cytoplasm are characteristic (**b**, **c**). Rosette-like structures may be seen (**c**)

Metastatic Tumors

Pseudomyxoma Peritonei

- Peritoneal involvement by abundant brown-yellow mucinous material (Fig. 13.7).
- Most often the primary tumor is a low-grade appendiceal mucinous neoplasm (LAMN) [see Chap. 12].
    - Rare cases originate from a low-grade mucinous neoplasm associated with an ovarian teratoma.
    - Secondary involvement of ovaries by metastatic LAMN may be seen [see Chap. 12].
- Most patients are middle-aged and present with increased abdominal girth and/or pain.
- Microscopic examination shows extracellular mucin pools dissecting fibroadipose tissue, with variable amounts of mucinous epithelium—either as small fragments "floating" in mucin or forming cystic glands (Fig. 13.8).
    - Epithelial cells have mild to moderate nuclear atypia and abundant mucinous cytoplasm.
    - In some cases, the amount of neoplastic mucinous epithelium is very scant and may be difficult to identify on frozen sections.
        - Additional level sections or tissue blocks may help identifying the epithelial component.
        - Intraoperative implications of acellular mucin pools on the peritoneal surfaces or within the omentum are similar; surgical exploration of the abdominal cavity and pelvis is required to identify the primary site.
        - Rare cases of ruptured primary ovarian mucinous tumors may be associated with "mucinous ascites,"

which is typically a more localized process and lacks epithelial cells and stromal fibrosis.
- Stromal fibrosis and hyalinization are often seen and may also be accompanied by chronic inflammation and calcifications.
- If a peritoneal biopsy shows the above-described morphologic features of pseudomyxoma peritonei, a descriptive frozen section diagnosis can be made and the appendix should be surgically evaluated for a possible primary.

Metastatic Carcinomas

- Metastatic carcinomas involving the omentum most commonly originate from the gynecologic tract (ovaries), followed by gastrointestinal primaries.
- The surgical procedure for gastrointestinal versus gynecologic primaries are markedly different; therefore, an attempt should be made to separate them on frozen section based on identification of histological subtype.
    - Serous, clear cell and endometrioid histologies are characteristic of Mullerian origin (see Chap. 10 for detailed morphologic description).
    - Mucinous carcinomas may originate from both gastrointestinal and gynecologic organs; intraoperative surgical evaluation and clinical correlation are helpful.
    - Signet-ring cell carcinomas may also involve the omentum spreading from gastric, colorectal, appendiceal, or breast primaries.

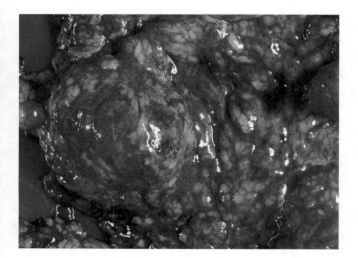

Fig. 13.7 Pseudomyxoma peritonei. Abundant glistening mucinous material is seen within the omental fibroadipose tissue

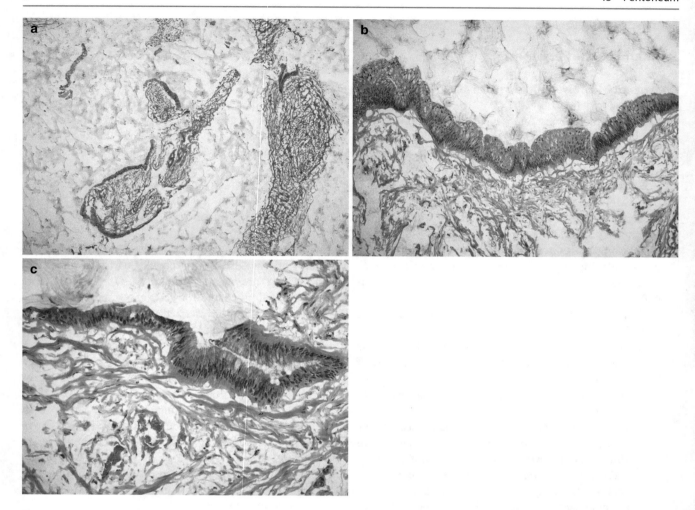

Fig. 13.8   Pseudomyxoma peritonei. Microscopic features include extracellular mucin pools with variable amounts of "floating" mucinous epithelium (**a**). The tumor cells show mild nuclear atypia and abundant mucinous cytoplasm (**b**, **c**)

Nonneoplastic/Reactive Conditions

Reactive Mesothelial Proliferation/Hyperplasia

- Reactive, nonneoplastic proliferation of mesothelial cells most commonly occurs in response to chronic inflammation, ovarian/pelvic mass lesions, and endometriosis.
- May be biopsied by the surgeon due to abnormal gross appearance associated with fibrosis, inflammation and/or endometriosis.
- Microscopic patterns include nested, trabeculated, papillary, or tubular proliferation of mesothelial cells (Figs. 13.9 and 13.10).
  - Mild to moderate nuclear atypia.
  - Mitotic figures may be seen.
  - Abundant eosinophilic or amphophilic cytoplasm; may contain cytoplasmic vacuoles resembling signet-ring cells.
  - Reactive mesothelial cells entrapped in fibrous tissue typically show linear arrangement, parallel to the surface.

- "Cobblestone" appearance is often seen and helps confirming mesothelial origin of cells.
- Differential diagnosis
  - Malignant mesothelioma
  - Well-differentiated papillary mesothelioma
  - Serous tumors—borderline (atypical proliferative) tumor or low-grade serous carcinoma
  - Metastatic carcinomas—especially signet-ring cell carcinoma
- Diagnostic pitfalls/key intraoperative consultation issues
  - In the presence of dense peritoneal adhesions, endometriosis, or significant inflammatory changes, the possibility of metastatic carcinoma (signet-ring cell or other type) should only be raised with caution, as overinterpretation of reactive mesothelial proliferation presents a significant diagnostic pitfall.
  - In patients with prior history of malignancy, morphological comparison with the prior specimen(s)—if available at the time of frozen section—should be made.

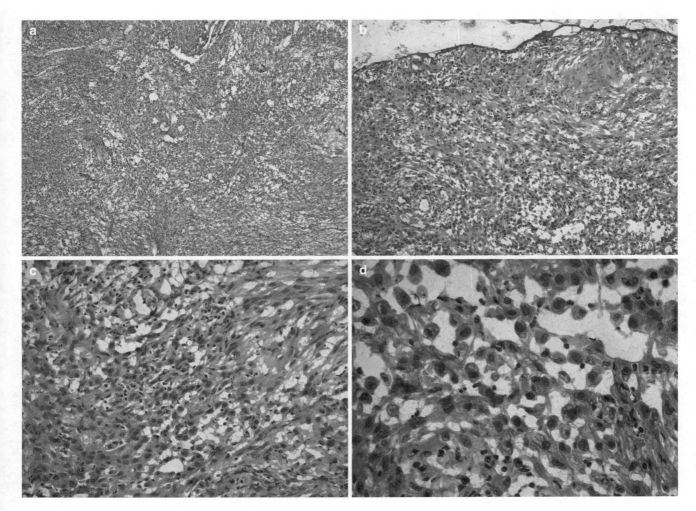

Fig. 13.9 Exuberant reactive mesothelial proliferation associated with endometriosis. The mesothelial cells form trabecular and tubular patterns (**a**, **b**) and show mild nuclear atypia and abundant eosinophilic cytoplasm (**c**). Note the presence of small, basophilic intracytoplasmic vacuoles (**d**)

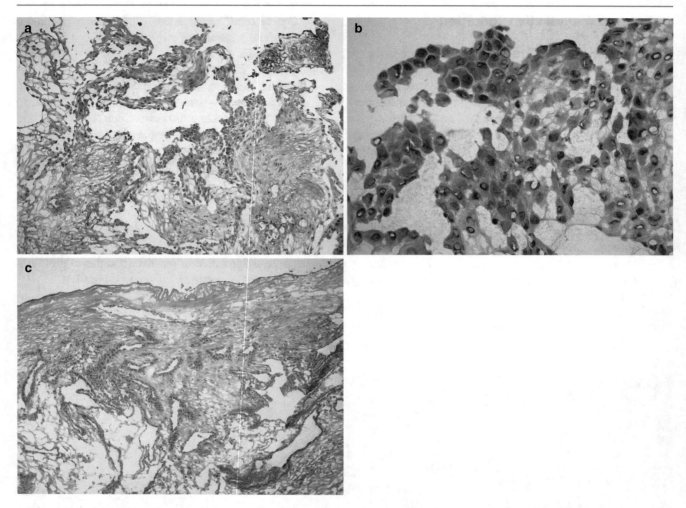

Fig. 13.10 Reactive surface papillary mesothelial proliferation. Note the papillary configuration of mesothelial cells (**a**) with mild nuclear atypia and "cobblestone" appearance (**b**). Tubular structures are also seen (**c**), mimicking a neoplastic glandular proliferation

Endometriosis

- Common finding, especially during the reproductive years.
- May appear as red, bluish, or brown nodules, patches, or puckered areas.
- May be associated with dense fibrosis and adhesions.
- Variable proportions of endometrial glandular epithelium and endometrial stroma microscopically (Fig. 13.11).

- Hemorrhage and hemosiderin-laden macrophages are common.
- Epithelium may show metaplastic changes or reactive atypia [see Chap. 11 for atypical endometriosis].
- The most important intraoperative diagnostic pitfall is overdiagnosis of endometriosis as an epithelial or mesenchymal (endometrial stromal) malignancy.

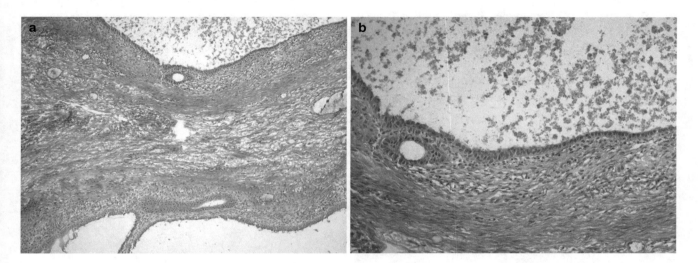

Fig. 13.11 Peritoneal endometriosis with typical endometrial stroma, glands, and intraluminal hemosiderin (**a**, **b**)

Endosalpingiosis

- Benign glands lined by tubal-type epithelium in peritoneal or omental fibrous tissue.
- May also be seen in retroperitoneal lymph nodes [see Chap. 8].
- Usually an incidental finding during the reproductive years and is often seen in patients with serous tumors (borderline/atypical proliferative or low-grade serous carcinoma).
- Single layer of tubal-type bland epithelial cells (Fig. 13.12).
    - No significant epithelial proliferation, papillary growth, or tufting
- No significant nuclear atypia or mitotic activity.
- Endometrial-type stroma is absent.

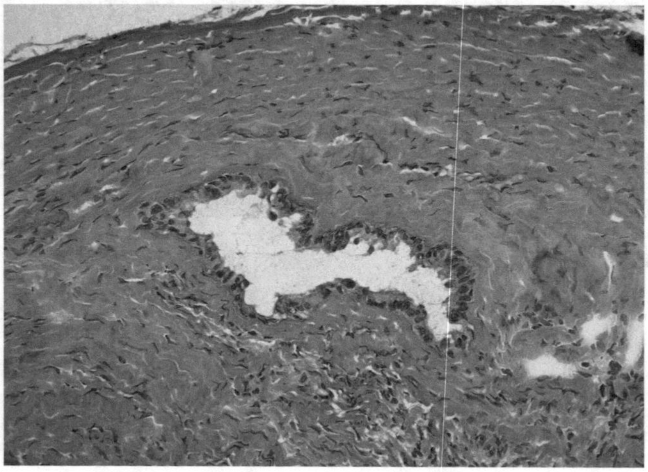

- Psammomatous calcifications are common.
- Differential diagnosis
    - Serous borderline/atypical proliferative tumor—primary peritoneal or implants from ovarian primary
- Diagnostic pitfalls/key intraoperative consultation issues
    - Detailed diagnostic criteria of ovarian serous borderline/atypical proliferative tumor and its implants are described in Chap. 8 and apply to peritoneal lesions as well.
    - Peritoneal lesions that lack significant epithelial proliferation and cytological atypia should not be over-interpreted, even in the context of an ovarian serous borderline/atypical proliferative tumor.
        - Morphological comparison with the ovarian tumor—if available on frozen section—is helpful.

Fig. 13.12 Endosalpingiosis in peritoneal dense fibrous tissue—a small glandular structure is lined by bland, tubal-type ciliated epithelium

Endocervicosis

- Benign endocervical-type glands involving peritoneum, lymph nodes, and most commonly the urinary bladder.
  - Bladder involvement usually presents as a mass lesion—up to 2.5 cm in size—on the posterior wall or bladder dome [16].
- Microscopic examination shows irregular, often cystic endocervical-type glands involving the peritoneum or bladder muscularis propria (Fig. 13.13).
  - Columnar endocervical mucinous epithelium
  - Basally located, small nuclei and abundant basophilic cytoplasm
  - No significant atypia or mitotic activity
  - Absence of goblet cells

- Differential diagnosis
  - Mucinous adenocarcinoma, primary or metastatic
- Diagnostic pitfalls/key intraoperative consultation issues
  - Significant nuclear atypia and infiltrative growth pattern with stromal desmoplastic response should raise suspicion for malignancy.
  - In patients with prior history of malignancy, morphological comparison with the prior specimen(s)—if available at the time of frozen section—should be pursued.
  - In difficult cases, intraoperative evaluation of other pelvic and/or abdominal structures by the surgeon may be helpful.
    - Biopsies of any additional suspicious lesions should be requested and examined on frozen section to rule out malignancy.

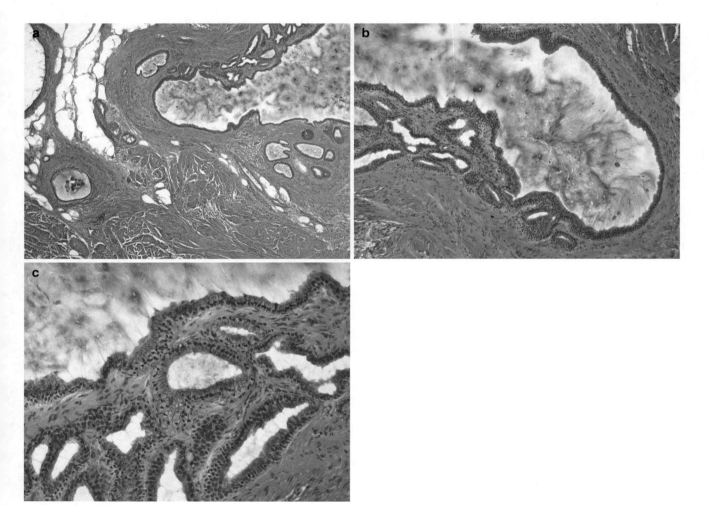

Fig. 13.13 Endocervicosis involving peritoneum and bladder wall. Irregular, cystic endocervical-type glands within smooth muscle bundles of muscularis propria of the urinary bladder (**a**). The glands are lined by endocervical-type mucinous cells with small, basally located nuclei and abundant basophilic cytoplasm (**b**, **c**). Goblet cells are absent

Peritoneal Inclusion Cyst

- Uni- or multilocular benign cystic mesothelial proliferation.
- May be associated with prior abdominal surgery, endometriosis, or pelvic inflammatory disease.
- Median size is 13 cm [17].

- Thin cyst wall typically lined by a single layer of flattened or cuboidal mesothelial cells (Fig. 13.14).
- No significant nuclear atypia or mitotic activity
- Differential diagnosis
  - Cystic lymphangioma
  - Adenomatoid tumor
  - Malignant mesothelioma

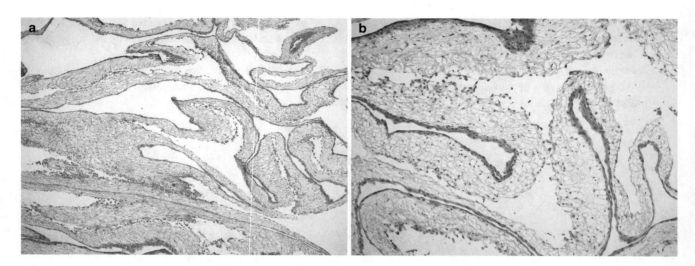

Fig. 13.14 Peritoneal inclusion cyst (**a**, **b**). The lesion is characterized by folded, thin fibrous cyst wall and a single layer of flattened or cuboidal, bland mesothelial cell lining

References

1. Britton M. The epidemiology of mesothelioma. Semin Oncol. 2002;29:18–25.

2. Asensio JA, Goldblatt P, Thomford NR. Primary malignant peritoneal mesothelioma. A report of seven cases and a review of the literature. Arch Surg. 1990;125:1477–81.

3. Baker PM, Clement PB, Young RH. Malignant peritoneal mesothelioma in women: a study of 75 cases with emphasis on their morphologic spectrum and differential diagnosis. Am J Clin Pathol. 2005;123:724–37.

4. Mohamed F, Sugarbaker PH. Peritoneal mesothelioma. Curr Treat Options Oncol. 2002;3:375–86.

5. Daya D, McCaughey WT. Well-differentiated papillary mesothelioma of the peritoneum. A clinicopathologic study of 22 cases. Cancer. 1990;65:292–6.

6. Malpica A, Sant'Ambrogio S, Deavers MT, Silva EG. Well-differentiated papillary mesothelioma of the female peritoneum: a clinicopathologic study of 26 cases. Am J Surg Pathol. 2012;36: 117–27.

7. Lee YK, Jun HJ, Nahm JH, Lim TS, Park JS, Ahn JB, et al. Therapeutic strategies for well-differentiated papillary mesothelioma of the peritoneum. Jpn J Clin Oncol. 2013;43:996–1003.

8. Butnor KJ, Sporn TA, Hammar SP, Roggli VL. Well-differentiated papillary mesothelioma. Am J Surg Pathol. 2001;25:1304–9.

9. Miettinen M, Sobin LH, Lasota J. Gastrointestinal stromal tumors presenting as omental masses–a clinicopathologic analysis of 95 cases. Am J Surg Pathol. 2009;33:1267–75.

10. Plumb AA, Kochhar R, Leahy M, Taylor MB. Patterns of recurrence of gastrointestinal stromal tumour (GIST) following complete resection: implications for follow-up. Clin Radiol. 2013;68:770–5.

11. Reith JD, Goldblum JR, Lyles RH, Weiss SW. Extragastrointestinal (soft tissue) stromal tumors: an analysis of 48 cases with emphasis on histologic predictors of outcome. Mod Pathol. 2000;13: 577–85.

12. Gerald WL, Miller HK, Battifora H, Miettinen M, Silva EG, Rosai J. Intra-abdominal desmoplastic small round-cell tumor. Report of 19 cases of a distinctive type of high-grade polyphenotypic malignancy affecting young individuals. Am J Surg Pathol. 1991;15: 499–513.

13. Lae ME, Roche PC, Jin L, Lloyd RV, Nascimento AG. Desmoplastic small round cell tumor: a clinicopathologic, immunohistochemical, and molecular study of 32 tumors. Am J Surg Pathol. 2002;26: 823–35.

14. Ordonez NG. Desmoplastic small round cell tumor: I: a histopathologic study of 39 cases with emphasis on unusual histological patterns. Am J Surg Pathol. 1998;22:1303–13.

15. Young RH, Eichhorn JH, Dickersin GR, Scully RE. Ovarian involvement by the intra-abdominal desmoplastic small round cell tumor with divergent differentiation: a report of three cases. Hum Pathol. 1992;23:454–64.

16. Young RH. Tumor-like lesions of the urinary bladder. Mod Pathol. 2009;22 Suppl 2:S37–52.

17. Ross MJ, Welch WR, Scully RE. Multilocular peritoneal inclusion cysts (so-called cystic mesotheliomas). Cancer. 1989;64:1336–46.

Index

© Springer International Publishing Switzerland 2015
P. Hui, N. Buza, *Atlas of Intraoperative Frozen Section Diagnosis in Gynecologic Pathology*,
DOI 10.1007/978-3-319-21807-6